Baillière's
# CLINICAL
# ANAESTHESIOLOGY
INTERNATIONAL PRACTICE AND RESEARCH

Baillière's

# CLINICAL ANAESTHESIOLOGY

INTERNATIONAL PRACTICE AND RESEARCH

Volume 1/Number 3
September 1987

# Burns and Plastic Surgery

KEITH C. JUDKINS MB ChB, FFARCS
*Guest Editor*

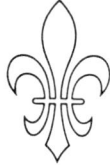

Baillière Tindall
**London Philadelphia Toronto Sydney Tokyo**

Baillière Tindall   24–28 Oval Road,
W.B. Saunders    London NW1 7DX

West Washington Square
Philadelphia, PA 19105, USA

1 Goldthorne Avenue
Toronto, Ontario M8Z 5T9, Canada

Harcourt Brace Jovanovich Group (Australia) Pty Ltd,
Post Office Box 300, North Ryde, NSW 2113, Australia

Exclusive Agent in Japan:
Maruzen Co. Ltd. (Journals Division)
3–10 Nihonbashi 2-chome, Chuo-ku, Tokyo 103, Japan

ISSN 0950-3501

ISBN 0-7020-1204-1 (single copy)

*Baillière's Clinical Anaesthesiology* is published four times each year by Baillière Tindall. Annual subscription prices are:

| TERRITORY | ANNUAL SUBSCRIPTION | SINGLE ISSUE |
| --- | --- | --- |
| 1. UK & Republic of Ireland | £35.00 post free | £15.50 post free |
| 2. USA & Canada | US$60.00 post free | US$25.00 post free |
| 3. All other countries | £45.00 post free | £18.50 post free |

The editor of this publication is David Dickens, Baillière Tindall, 24–28 Oval Road, London NW1 7DX.

*Baillière's Clinical Anaesthesiology* was published from 1983 to 1986 as *Clinics in Anaesthesiology*.

Typeset by Phoenix Photosetting, Chatham.
Printed and bound in Great Britain by Mackays of Chatham Ltd.

# Contributors to this issue

**C. J. BARHAM** MB BS, FFARCS, MRCS, LRCP, Consultant Anaesthetist, The Queen Victoria Hospital, Holtye Road, East Grinstead, West Sussex RH19 3DZ, UK.

**DAVID F. COCHRANE** MB BCh, FFARCS, Frenchay Hospital, Bristol BS16 1LE, UK.

**DEREK J. DYE** MB ChB, FFARCS, Consultant Anaesthetist, Welsh Regional Unit for Burns, Plastic and Maxillofacial Surgery, St. Lawrence Hospital, Chepstow, Gwent NP6 5YX, UK.

**WILLIAM R. HAIN** MB BS, FFARCS, Consultant Anaesthetist, Nottingham Hospitals Clinical Teacher, University of Nottingham, Department of Anaesthesia 'C' Floor, University Hospital, Nottingham NG7 2UH, UK.

**CONSTANCE C. M. HOWIE** MB ChB, DA, FFARCS, Consultant Anaesthetist, Bangour General Hospital, Broxburn, West Lothian, Scotland, UK.

**KEITH C. JUDKINS** MB ChB, FFARCS, Consultant Anaesthetist, Queen Victoria Hospital, Holtye Road, East Grinstead, West Sussex RH19 3DZ, UK.

**CHUNGSOOK KIM** MS, PhD, Instructor in Anesthesiology, Harvard Medical School; Research Associate in Pharmacology (Anesthesia), Massachusetts General Hospital and Shriners Burns Institute, Boston, MA 02114, USA.

**J. C. LAWRENCE** PhD, C.Biol, FIBiol, Research Director, MRC Burns Research Group, Birmingham Accident Hospital, Bath Row, Birmingham B15 1NA; Bacteriologist-in-Charge, West Midland Regional Burns Unit, Birmingham B15 1NA, UK.

**PETER J. LAWRENCE** MB BS, FFARACS, Senior Specialist in Charge, Intensive Care Unit, Repatriation General Hospital, Concord, NSW 2139, Australia.

**D. J. F. MACDONALD** MB ChB, FFARCS, DA, DTM&H, Division of Anaesthesia, Royal Infirmary, Glasgow G31 3ER; Glasgow and West of Scotland Regional Centre for Plastic Surgery, Canniesburn Hospital, Bearsden, Glasgow G61 1QL, UK.

**J. A. JEEVENDRA MARTYN** MD, FFARCS, Associate Professor of Anesthesiology, Harvard Medical School; Associate Director of Anesthesia, Massachusetts General Hospital and Shriners Burns Institute, Boston, MA 02114, USA.

**H. P. PATEL** FFARCS, MD, Consultant Anaesthetist, Queen Victoria Hospital, Holtye Road, East Grinstead, West Sussex RH19 3DZ, UK.

**JOHN A. D. SETTLE** OBE, M.Phil, MRCS, LRCP, DA, Consultant in Clinical Physiology, Medical Director, Yorkshire Regional Burns Centre, Pinderfield General Hospital, Wakefield, West Yorkshire WF1 4DG, UK; Honorary Clinical Lecturer, Department of Surgery, University of Leeds.

**ANNE B. SUTHERLAND** MD, FRCSE, Consultant Plastic Surgeon, Regional Plastic Surgery Unit, Bangour General Hospital, Broxburn, West Lothian, Scotland; Royal Hospital for Sick Children, Edinburgh Clinical Teaching Staff, Department of Surgery, Edinburgh University, UK.

**FRANK J. M. WALTERS** MA, MB BChir, FFARCS, Consultant Anaesthetist, Frenchay Hospital, Bristol BS16 1LE, UK.

**MICHAEL ELLIOTT WARD** MB BS (London), MRCS, FFARCS (Eng), Consultant Anaesthetist, Nuffield Department of Anaesthetics, John Radcliffe Hospital, Oxford OX3 9DU; Clinical Lecturer, University of Oxford Medical School, John Radcliffe Hospital, Oxford OX3 9DU, UK.

# Table of contents

## FORTHCOMING ISSUES

December 1987
**Update on Opiates**
K. BUDD

## RECENT ISSUES

March 1987
**Thoracic Anaesthesia**
J. W. W. GOTHARD

June 1987
**Anaesthesia for Neurosurgery**
D. A. JEWKES

# Foreword

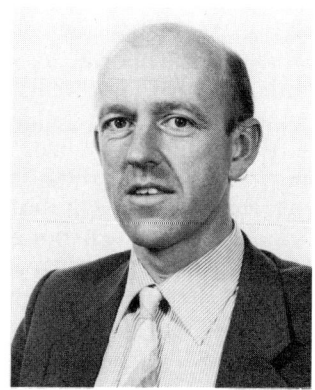

This edition of Baillière's Clinical Anaesthesiology is devoted to an area of medical practice that has traditionally been the province of the plastic surgeon, certainly in the UK and perhaps also elsewhere; in the past, anaesthesiologists have been called in when anaesthesia was required and for little else.

In recent years, this has changed. Although the plastic surgeon rightly remains in control, the anaesthesiologist has developed a crucial role in burns and plastic surgery. Two things have influenced this evolutionary process: one is the realization that more aggressive and technological advances in intensive care and in pain relief, fields in which anaesthesiologists have developed a special interest, have a real contribution to make to burns care; the other is the ability of the anaesthesiologist to tailor the surgical environment to enhance the quality of work which the surgeon can carry out. The beginning of this latter cooperation included the advent of hypotensive anaesthesia in the 1950s, a subject which continues to generate controversy.

The primary aim of this volume is to bring together a series of papers by working clinicians. The first paper in each section is, for want of a better word, 'philosophical' in content; that is, while the advice given is intensely practical, the authors have addressed the factors, such as communication, cooperation and involvement in a team, which ensure that the anaesthesiologist's contribution is used to maximum advantage for the good of the patient. The initiative for the team approach may come from the surgeon or from the anaesthesiologist but, once established, it often falls naturally to the anaesthesiologist to maintain a rapport between disparate groups of staff.

The first section is devoted to first principles in the care of the burned patient. The variety of factors which have to be taken into account is evident, and provides the fascination which those of us involved regularly in burns find so stimulating. It is useful to be able to collate this information in one book for the benefit of the interested anaesthesiologist. The authors are all intimately involved in the work about which they write and represent a range of medical disciplines, emphasizing again the cooperative nature of burns care.

Two possible chapters are 'missing': burns in children and the problem of catabolism. Children account for about one-third of burn admissions. The differences in their care have been clarified where necessary by the individual authors, so a separate chapter was considered unnecessary. Catabolism is a major problem in burns and is alluded to especially in the sections on nutrition, pharmacology and sepsis. Its practical implications are therefore covered. The pathophysiological background to the catabolic response is very complex; after much thought, it was concluded that a presentation that would do justice to the subject was not possible in the available space. The interested reader is therefore referred to Davies (1982) for a very thorough review of the background to this important problem.

The second section assumes that the reader knows how to give a good basic anaesthetic. A group of challenges was identified which face the anaesthesiologist in plastic surgery and the authors were again chosen for their extensive practical experience in those areas. There is more than one way to skin a rabbit and none of the writers would claim that the approaches they describe are the final word on the subject. However, I have no doubt in my mind that the reader will find their contributions interesting and highly informative, as I have done during the editing process.

I will not waste space describing the piece of serendipity that involved me as editor in the first place. Many have much more experience and are much better known in burns and plastics anaesthesia than myself. Suffice it to say that, apart from my personal enthusiasm for the team approach, I have tried to avoid emphasizing any one aspect to the detriment of others. Some of the writers are internationally known in their areas of expertise, both as first-rate clinicians and as contributors to the literature. Others may be less well known, but in their clinical work have made thorough practical application of principles and techniques well described by others; their ability to review a subject clearly and practically has therefore been an important consideration in choosing them to write.

There are anaesthesiologists who consider anaesthesia in plastic surgery to be dull and uninteresting. That this is not the case will be evident to all who read this volume and if more interest and investigation in the field is stimulated as a result, it will have served its purpose.

KEITH C. JUDKINS

## REFERENCE

Davies JWL (1982) *Physiological Responses to Burning Injury*, 649 pp. London: Academic Press.

# Burns (including Clinical Physiology and Intensive Care)

# 1

# The role of the anaesthetist in burns care

## W. R. HAIN

A symposium in 1971 (Davies, 1972) led to further meetings of anaesthetists in the UK concerned with the management of the burned patient, and subsequently to the formation of an association devoted to its study.* It demonstrated that the anaesthetist possesses and can develop skills of particular value to the burns unit. Emphasis was placed on the attenuation of pain and distress accompanying dressing changes and to the especial vulnerability of children, who form the larger proportion of burned patients (Figure 1).

Interest in burns problems is increasing and it appears that within the UK an expectation of the inclusion of an anaesthetist within the burns unit team is leading to appointments at consultant level with advertised or implied interest in this field. For many an anaesthetist, however, a sessional commitment will currently be mainly or exclusively to the operating list. He will often have received only scant notice of his patient's imminent surgery and not have been involved in prior therapy. He will be expected to anaesthetize safely, attend to fluid replacement, prescribe a modicum of postoperative analgesic drugs, and abandon his responsibilities once recovery from anaesthesia is recognizable.

By contrast, this chapter seeks to explore the concept of the anaesthetist as an integral member of a team caring for the burned patient. To achieve assimilation it may be necessary to demonstrate both an interest in and an aptitude for participation in the various aspects of care that are traditionally the responsibility of practitioners in other specialities. Strictly adhered to, a sessional commitment will be incompatible with continuity of care.

## RESUSCITATION

Established staff in accident and emergency departments generally, and particularly those in reception facilities within a dedicated burns unit, will be familiar with the priorities of management to be afforded the severely burned. It will nevertheless be appropriate if within a particular unit written guidelines are established as a protocol for newer staff members. The

* Plastic Surgical and Burns Anaesthetists (PSABA): Hon. Secretary: Dr FJ Walters, Frenchay Hospital, Bristol, England, BS16 1LE.

anaesthetist will be aware of its provisions (he might be the author) and, if he can regard himself as 'on-call' for the admission of severe burns cases, has skills of value in their assessment and resuscitation. These include the establishment of intravenous access, the assessment and maintenance of respiratory performance and the provision of appropriate analgesia or anaesthesia.

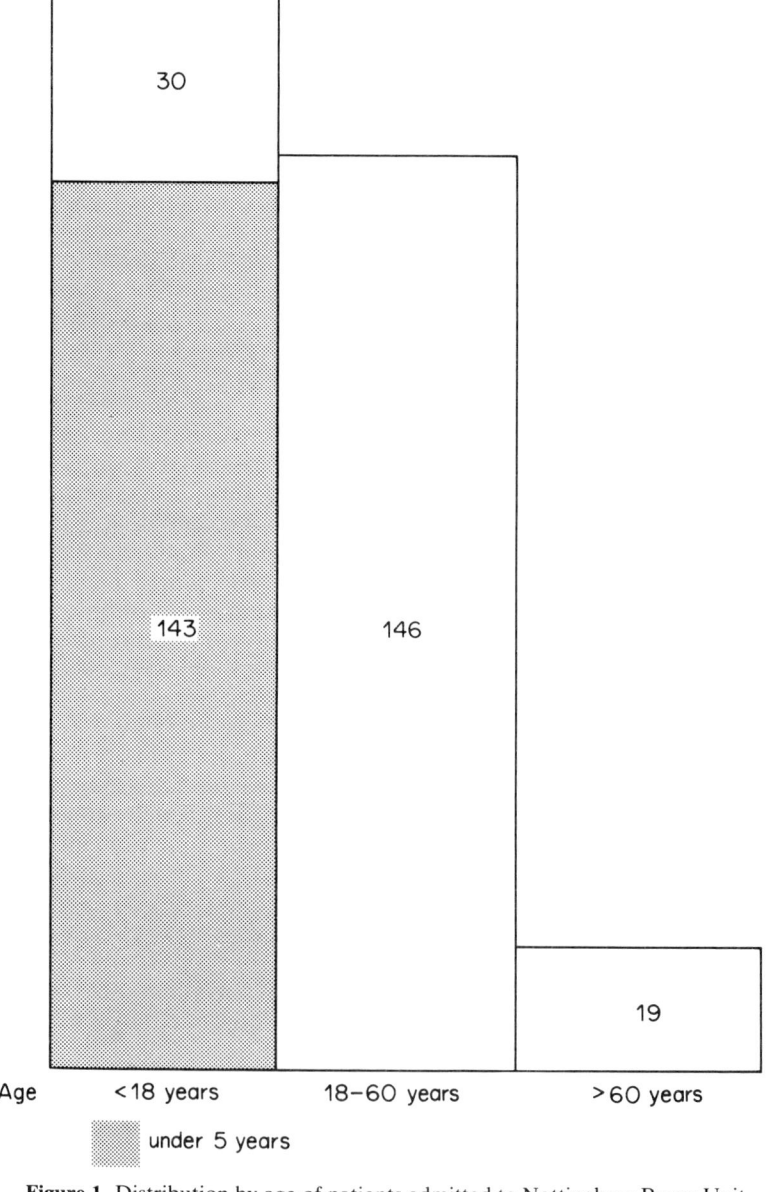

Figure 1. Distribution by age of patients admitted to Nottingham Burns Unit.

### Intravenous access

Early reliable infusion of fluids is vital, and conservation of veins whenever possible is important to subsequent management. The anaesthetist is particularly practised in gaining appropriate access to both peripheral and central veins, and, when necessary, to arteries. His task will be the easier the earlier in management he is involved, before attempts by the less experienced have lessened the chances of early success.

### Respiratory management

The anaesthetist is accustomed to making rapid clinical assessment of respiratory function, interpreting any appropriate investigation, and dealing generally with the emergency situation.

Endotracheal intubation, inspection of the airway, and possibly bronchoscopy using either local (Clark et al, 1983) or general anaesthesia are indicated when respiratory distress is present as a complication of the burn injury. These are all techniques very familiar to trained anaesthetists. The indications for them and details of management are discussed in Chapter 3.

### Anaesthesia and analgesia

The psychological impact of the burn injury is very considerable, particularly upon children (Breslin, 1975). It behoves the concerned anaesthetist to use his knowledge and skills so as to minimize the adverse effects both of the injury and of its management, in part by meticulous attention to the prevention of pain.

The narcotic analgesic agents continue to represent the first line of defence against pain. Anaesthetists can now choose from a wide array of techniques for their administration, including continuous infusion by intramuscular, subcutaneous or intravenous routes; epidural and intrathecal placement; not forgetting oral and rectal ingestion. For adults, patient-activated systems with sophisticated safeguards are available. Children need the surveillance and initiative of well-taught nurses.

The intravenous route will usually be preferable and is one with which the anaesthetist is thoroughly familiar. It should not be accepted that the distressed burned patient need suffer the onslaught of resuscitation without adequate analgesic therapy. Occasionally, indeed, the best conditions for the rapid institution of all necessary resuscitative measures in the restless, unco-operative child will be the induction of general anaesthesia, which advantageously also produces oblivion for the patient.

Pain prevention beyond the acute resuscitative phase is briefly discussed later. A detailed review of these topics appears in Chapter 5.

## INTENSIVE CARE

Within an introductory chapter of this nature it would be impossible to review the full panoply of care that an anaesthetist might be called upon to offer the critically ill, burned patient. Currently in Britain it would be highly unlikely that any consultant anaesthetist could be appointed who had not during his training received in-depth teaching and experience in intensive care management. However, any future development of intensive care as a separate speciality may diminish the intensive care content of anaesthetic training.

All major burns require the minute-by-minute attention from skilled personnel implied by the term 'intensive care' for at least 48 hours. Whether such care is offered within a burns unit or in a satellite intensive care unit (ICU) catering mainly for a variety of other critically ill patients will be a matter for local decision. The availability of nursing staff, particularly those with the requisite skills, may well determine that the most severely burned patients be managed in an established ICU. This is particularly likely to be the case where lung damage or other, possibly multiple, injuries compound the problems of burns management.

At all times the seriously ill patient will benefit from regular assessment by the team anaesthetist who, with his surgical colleagues, will be particularly concerned with adequacy of pain relief, electrolyte and fluid balance, nutritional status, renal and pulmonary function and mental security.

While his experience and interest is crucial to the welfare of such patients retained within the burns unit itself, especially where sophisticated techno-logical support is required, the burns team anaesthetist has also a pivotal role once his patient is housed in another's facility. He must act as liaison officer and as adviser on all aspects of care as they affect, or are affected by, the burn injury.

The altered activity of drugs in burned patients (see Chapter 6), the hazards and management of convulsions occurring during resuscitation, usually in a child, and the intense catabolic response dictating a vigorous approach to maintenance of nutrition (see Chapter 7) are among several areas of particular concern with which the burns team anaesthetist will be familiar and hence on which he will be able to give advice likely to assist his colleagues from the same or other specialities.

The presence of a burned patient within a general ICU is rightly con-sidered a significant infection hazard. It will be demanded that as soon as the need for full intensive care management is over, the patient should be discharged to the burns unit for further management. The anaesthetist must be able to agree when that time is reached and assure himself that the facilities there are indeed appropriate to optimum subsequent management. Future designs of intensive care units should make appropriate provision for this factor if burned patients are among those likely to be admitted.

The availability, accessibility and sterilization of all equipment which may be needed in an acute emergency will all be further concerns for the anaesthetist, who should institute regular checking procedures. He will also need to assure himself that those who may have to use the equipment know the whereabouts, function, operation and limitations of it.

Funds for purchasing new equipment will usually come from three sources: a budget agreed with hospital or university, non-budgeted sums made available for small purchases at short notice, and gifts from charitable sources. The anaesthetist will, for both replacement and new equipment, find it helpful to maintain an up-to-date 'shopping list' ranked in order of priority within different cost groupings. The list should include the name and ordering address of the manufacturer, a recent written quotation (VAT included) and a prepared case of need. Items donated through charity moneys need not incur VAT. It would be unwise to decline any additional resource in this area requiring so much 'high technology' assistance.

## ANAESTHESIA

The anaesthetist will need to know that the operating facility matches the particular requirements of burns surgery. Of prime importance are maintenance of a warm operating environment, particularly in prolonged surgery, and when needed the prompt receipt by patients of properly cross-matched blood products.

The mechanism for ordering blood and blood products must be clearly defined with the blood bank and with all staff involved with their provision. Few failures of organization can be so potentially dangerous as the late discovery that blood believed ordered at the right time in the appropriate manner was in fact mislabelled, or ordered for the wrong date, or for some other reason is not available when required. Newcomers to the team may require instruction in local arrangements: repeated unwarranted demands for emergency crossmatching will endanger that close co-operation of blood bank with burns team which is essential if optimum care is to be afforded the burned patient.

The anaesthetic management of patients requiring grafting procedures is discussed in Chapter 4. The importance of providing generous venous access while seeking to conserve veins for future use cannot be overstressed. Induction of anaesthesia by inhalation or, in unco-operative children, by intramuscular injection (Hain, 1986), usually facilitates uncomplicated venous cannulation.

The security of all cannulae is a particular responsibility of the anaesthetist. The appropriate use of sutures, strapping and extension tubes, with manual checking of all connections which are then further reinforced with adhesive tape, should be undertaken before surgery begins. Traction and torsion on lines, particularly at times of repositioning the patient or applying dressings, should be regarded as avoidable perils. Access to lines intra-operatively should not depend on burrowing beneath the surgical drapes.

## Recovery

It remains unfortunately true that many patients spend this critical period of their perioperative management in relatively unsupervised conditions. Following major burns surgery it is the duty of the anaesthetist to ensure that the level of care offered to his patient in the recovery area matches any existing or potential challenge to patient welfare.

It should be axiomatic that the estimated blood volume loss be replaced

before the patient leaves the operating table, and any tendency to hypothermia reversed. Appropriate orders concerning postoperative pain prevention, further drug and fluid therapy, monitoring, patient posture,
resumption of fluid intake etc., should all be clearly written down. The
anaesthetic record sheet should be complete and legible and accompany the
patient to the ward. The anaesthetist should discourage surgeons from
retaining records in the operating suite for later attention: the ward staff may
need information urgently.


## ANALGESIA

Techniques of analgesia are discussed in detail in Chapter 5. They aim to
provide comfort both to the undisturbed patient and to the patient who must
undergo procedures such as late graft application and dressing change. The
two cases may need quite different approaches. For the patient to derive
maximum benefit, considerable time, care and attention must be given by a
committed anaesthetist.

Various regional techniques using local anaesthetic agents have also a
place in the prevention of pain. Their use in burns is, however, often
constrained by the geography of the burned areas, by the infection risk and
by any inability of the patient to co-operate with their performance.

General anaesthesia using techniques favourable to early resumption of
food intake will often prove preferable to excessive sedative and/or narcotic
medication with the accompanying risk of prolonged drowsiness, respiratory depression and reluctant appetite.

Much work remains to be done to establish which approach in any given
situation will be preferable. Advantages need to be balanced against
inherent disadvantages. Anaesthetists are the best qualified to make the
appropriate judgements.


## LIAISON

Anaesthetists have much experience and usually interest in co-ordinating
other professionals in the provision of care for their patients. Cultivation of
the blood bank is implied above. Other groups with whom contact should be
continuous and effective include the surgical team, the nursing staff and the
hospital administration.

The individual anaesthetist is furthermore directly responsible for the
welfare of his patients at all times while they are receiving or reacting to
therapy directed by him. Disagreements between the anaesthetist and other
members of the burns unit team may occasionally arise, yet conflict within a
medical team cannot be advantageous to patient care. Consensus must be
sought.

Management protocols to be followed within the unit should be
developed with the participation of the anaesthetist, and amended if these
fail to resolve particular difficulties without rancour. Attempts by the

anaesthetist to alter the proposed course of intensive care or surgical management must be undertaken with tact and irrefutable argument. Once he is an accepted equal in a team, the anaesthetist should find his advice readily sought and accepted. The newcomer may first have to establish his credentials. Brusque attempts to abandon wholesale an existing regime, no matter how effective the proposed alternative has been found in other units, are likely to provoke resentment and the suspicion, often justified, that the would-be innovator has blinkered vision and limited experience.

The co-operation, even enthusiasm, of senior nursing staff is essential if any improvement is to be made in the management of pain. Studies invariably conclude that the recognition of pain and the response are too often unsatisfactory. Unfortunately, many of the more satisfactory techniques for relieving pain depend upon added tasks and responsibilities devolving upon nurses, and the relevant skills and knowledge may not have been included in their training.

Recommendations to be followed in Britain when nurses are asked to undertake tasks for which their training has not prepared them are contained in a memorandum (Royal College of Nursing, 1978) published jointly by the British Medical Association and the Royal College of Nursing.*

The anaesthetist who wishes to institute modalities of care requiring the co-operation, supervision and active participation of members of the nursing staff must himself accept responsibility for inculcating enthusiasm and for teaching the relevant techniques and background information required. In Britain at least, he will need to ensure that senior nursing staff and employing authorities are in agreement that the nurses may be so involved. Example, encouragement and support are required from the anaesthetist who wishes to offer his patients the widest possible range of appropriate techniques.

The talents of the hospital administrator are customarily derided or ignored by the medical profession, yet his interest and assistance can greatly

---

* Relevant extracts from this document include:
a) 'There should be full consideration of all relevant circumstances including the competence of the nurse who should have had appropriate training and supervised experience in the techniques in question. The nurse should satisfy herself/himself that she/he is competent to take the new duty or responsibility.'
b) 'In order to reach agreement on the procedure to be undertaken by the nursing staff in a particular health authority . . . joint committees of medical staff should be set up on a local basis. These committees should include *inter alios* the head of the nursing service and a senior representative of the medical staff.'
c) 'When agreement is reached which involves a nurse in any work outside her/his current scope of nursing practice, this should be communicated to and approved by the employer.'
d) 'Health authorities are expected to undertake the defence of a nurse in any proceedings commenced against her/him . . . This does not absolve the nurse from personal liability for her/his own actions.'
e) 'Every nurse should be a member of the appropriate professional organisation which provides for individual legal representation. Membership of the RCN provides such representation through its indemnity insurance scheme which covers the nurse for any incident arising out of her/his professional duties.'
The recommendations apply to individual nurses. It cannot be assumed that a nurse new to the unit will be willing to undertake first training and subsequently responsibility in techniques with which he/she was previously unfamiliar.

ease the path of the clinician. Improved patient care is the aim of both disciplines.

The anaesthetist is uniquely fitted to clarify priorities in treating severely injured patients and to co-ordinate other specialities in their care. He can therefore profitably discuss with the relevant administrative officer ambitions for the development of the burns unit, and problems concerning organization, mechanical maintenance, equipment provision, the printing of protocols, liaison with voluntary organizations, secretarial provision, etc. Contact should not be restricted to exasperated complaint when, for example, the theatre heating system fails—again! Appropriate action in an emergency is more probable when the usual situation is known and understood.

## TEACHING

The anaesthetist who accepts responsibility for burned patients outside the cosy confines of the operating theatre has a clear duty to teach nurses in the recognition and management of pain in its various degrees, using perhaps the therapeutic modalities described in Chapter 5. He will also be able to contribute teaching in other aspects of burn care, including resuscitation, fluid therapy, and preoperative and postoperative management as required.

The anaesthetist will naturally be involved also with training junior staff. In-depth teaching is best achieved by a semi-structured 'immersion' course rather than by intermittent irregular contact between pupil and teacher. It will therefore be preferable when possible for junior staff to be assigned to the burns unit anaesthetist for a period of days, weeks or months, according to circumstance, in a training module through which appropriate grades of staff rotate. The establishment of a suitable module, the structure and content of the didactic teaching involved and the regard which his activities attract from colleagues will depend critically on the anaesthetist's enthusiasm as well as his position.

## RESEARCH

Research is a broad term which may be taken to include case reports, surveys and reviews as well as clinical, animal and laboratory investigations. These publishable activities are all needed so that individual practitioners can share in the advances and observations made by others. Undoubtedly, continued activity by clinicians is needed to reduce mortality and morbidity associated with burns injury.

Computer-compatible records will facilitate storage, retrieval and analysis. Carefully completed, they will enable both prospective and retrospective analyses to be undertaken confidently. Given modern monitoring practice much information may be gained by 'pencil and paper' observation concerning current practices. The clinical assessment of newer approaches may be formalized by appropriate forethought into an assessment of scientific validity of value to others. Trials must, of course, be planned with care such that the patient at all times receives the best known practicable treatment, offering only potential benefit and no discernible risk of harm in the interests of 'science'.

Many of the important advances made already have been made by alert clinicians rather than by professional research workers. More are eagerly awaited.


## SUMMARY

The anaesthetist has the potential to be involved usefully at all stages in the care of the burned patient, not just in the operating theatre. His particular skills equip him well for participation in resuscitation, pain relief and intensive care, as well as in training and administration. The chapters (2–8) that follow in this section summarize well the considerations relevant to this demanding but fascinating role.


## REFERENCES

Breslin PW (1975) The psychological reactions of children to burn traumata—a review. *Illinois Medical Journal* **148:** 519–524 (Part I), 595–602 (Part II).

Clark CJ, Reid WH, Telfer ABM & Campbell D (1983) Respiratory injury in the burned patient. *Anaesthesia* **38:** 35–39.

Davies RM (ed.) (1972) Anaesthesia in burns: the place of the anaesthetist in the overall care of the burnt patient. *Postgraduate Medical Journal* **48:** 121–161.

Hain WR (1986) Induction of anaesthesia in children. *Anaesthesia* **41:** 1272–1273.

Royal College of Nursing (revised 1978) The Duties and Position of the Nurse. RCN, 1, Henrietta St, London, WC1, UK.

# 2

## Resuscitation and fluid balance

JOHN A. D. SETTLE

### THE RATIONALE OF FLUID THERAPY

The abnormality of bodily function that dominates the first 48 h following an extensive burn is a gross derangement of those homeostatic mechanisms that control the movement of water and solutes between the intravascular, extracellular and intracellular compartments. This derangement is demonstrated by a progressive shift of fluid from the circulation into the interstitium, resulting in clinically obvious oedema in the region of the burn and, in some circumstances, in tissues remote from the burn. Furthermore, changes in cell membrane function may permit the intracellular movement of sodium and water, thereby adding to the functional sodium deficit that characterizes the electrolyte disturbance of severe burns injury.

The burn oedema is, in effect, an extension of the plasma volume and, in the absence of effective treatment, increases at the expense of that plasma volume. The patient, bleeding plasma into his own tissues, becomes increasingly hypovolaemic. At first, cardiac output is maintained to some extent by progressive tachycardia and blood pressure is supported by peripheral and splanchnic vasoconstriction. However, if the plasma loss is large enough these compensatory mechanisms will eventually fail, to be quickly followed by marked hypotension, stagnant hypoxia and death.

These fundamental haemodynamic changes associated with extensive burns were described in some detail more than 50 years ago (Underhill et al, 1923). Subsequently, the magnitude of the fluid shift was investigated (Blalock, 1931; Harkins, 1935) and these studies led on to the publication of budgets, forecasts and formulae whereby the fluid requirement of the burn patient could be predicted (Cope and Moore, 1947; Evans et al, 1952). In view of the intensive research, both experimental and clinical, that has been undertaken during the past 40 years into these phenomena and their treatment, it is perhaps surprising that so many widely different regimes of fluid therapy are in common use today. All the well-known formulae and fluid regimes have been validated in clinical practice, although the type of fluid recommended may be crystalloid, colloid, isotonic or hypertonic and the volume and salt loads given in the first 24 h may vary by a factor of two. In part, the explanation may be that the physiological reserve of the average burned patient allows this latitude in early postburn fluid resuscitation (Pruitt, 1981). However, consideration of several regimes that appear to be fundamentally different (Settle, 1982) suggests: (a) that there is more than one path to the goal of effective resuscitation; and (b) that some important differences are imposed by other aspects of burn care, e.g. the management of the burn wound.

## Effective resuscitation

It has often been assumed that the goal of effective resuscitation is the restoration of all vital bodily functions to as near normal as possible. However, because of the magnitude of the abnormality and the failure so far to devise any satisfactory method of preventing the fluid leak from the circulation, it may not be possible to correct all the pathophysiological abnormalities that result from this fluid shift. A less ambitious goal is that proposed by Pruitt (1981) as an acceptable consensus: 'The maintenance of vital organ function at the least immediate or delayed physiologic cost'. The volume of fluid required to produce this effect, although in general terms directly related to the severity of the injury, must always be adjusted, on a short time scale, to provide the actual requirements of the individual under-going treatment.

## Colloid versus crystalloid

In considering which path to follow in order to maintain vital organ function, it has to be recognized that different types of fluid therapy will confer different physiological advantages and exact different costs. For example, the use of Lactated Ringer's solution is associated with marked haemo-concentration, whereas a normal haematocrit can be maintained in a colloid regime (Hall and Sørensen, 1978). The implication that a colloid fluid is more effective in maintaining blood volume is supported by the observation that cardiac output is restored more quickly by a colloid fluid (Dorethy et al, 1977), and that a colloid fluid permits satisfactory resuscitation with a smaller volume of fluid (Goodwin et al, 1980) and with significantly less oedema in non-burned areas (Mason, 1980). However, the smaller volume of colloid fluid does not result in less lung water (Goodwin et al, 1980), haemodilution per se does not lead to pulmonary oedema in patients with intact capillaries, and the most important factor in preventing pulmonary oedema is the prevention of increase in capillary hydrostatic pressure (Peters and Hargens, 1981). Furthermore, it is claimed that a crystalloid regime can be supervised by less experienced staff (Hall and Sørensen, 1978) and it is obviously much cheaper than a colloid regime. The question then is not whether one regime is intrinsically better than the other, but rather which physiological costs are of most importance to burn patients in general and to an individual patient in particular.

## Hypertonic fluids

When the use of hypertonic fluids is considered, a further series of advan-tages and disadvantages can be listed. Hypertonic fluids deliver the necessary salt load in a smaller volume, minimize the burn oedema and, by producing hypertonicity of the extracellular fluid, prevent cellular over-hydration and minimize oedema in non-burned areas (Monafo et al, 1973). However, just because a hypertonic extracellular fluid would seem to be advantageous does not support the contention that the infused fluid must be hypertonic or, conversely, that a fluid regime with a net sodium concentration of less than 140 mmol/l will always result in hyponatraemia. To argue in this way is to ignore an aspect of water balance that is of the utmost relevance to the burned patient, i.e. extrarenal water loss by evaporation from the burn wound. If a patient with an extensive burn is exposed in a warm, dry environment, and a fluid with 140 mmol/l of Na is used for resuscitation, vast quantities of sodium-free water will also have to be given if serious hyper-natraemia is to be avoided (Eklund, 1970). Conversely, should evaporative water loss from the burn wound be prevented by, for example, covering the wound with wet soaks, a fluid regime with a net sodium concentration well above 140 mmol/l would be appropriate. Hence, the optimum sodium con-centration of the total fluid input is not really a free choice for the clinician, but is actually imposed by the method chosen for the treatment of the burn wound.

### Common ground of fluid therapy

From these and other considerations of validated fluid therapy (Settle, 1982) some common ground for safe and effective resuscitation can be identified. Salt and water are the essential requirements. The optimum sodium load is of the order of 0.5 mmol per kg body weight per % burn and the total volume of fluid (excluding the replacement of excessive evaporative loss) is likely to be between 2 and 4 ml/kg/%. The actual volume required can be reduced by including a suitable colloid, by using a hypertonic salt solution or by some combination of the two. The fluid regime should aim to produce a moderate extracellular hypertonicity. Sodium-free water may also have to be given in large quantities if extrarenal losses are great, but the quantity of sodium-free water administered should only be sufficient to prevent marked hyper-natraemia.

## PRACTICAL RESUSCITATION

### Initial assessment

The cause of the injury and the time that it occurred should be ascertained and recorded. Even quite experienced staff can mistake the depth of a burn and at this stage it is sufficient to distinguish between erythema and actual skin damage. There is, however, a need to make a quick estimate of the extent of the injury because this will indicate the urgency of intravenous fluid therapy. The estimate can be made mentally by using the rule of nine, which indicates, in an easily remembered form, the percentage of total body surface area accounted for by various parts of the body: 9% each for arms and head; 18% each for legs, front of trunk and back of trunk (Figure 1). For parts of the body that have only small areas of burn it is useful to remember that the palmar surface of the patient's hand constitutes about 1% of the body surface area.

Simple erythema is excluded from the estimate and, if the total burn is more than 15–20% in an adult, or 10–15% in a child, intravenous infusion is indicated. With extensive burns (+30%) it is both essential and urgent.

### Setting up the intravenous drip

Unless both arms are burned to the extent of deep charring, it will be possible to find a large vein in one or other forearm or antecubital fossa. If the vein can be seen, venipuncture is satisfactory; otherwise a cut-down

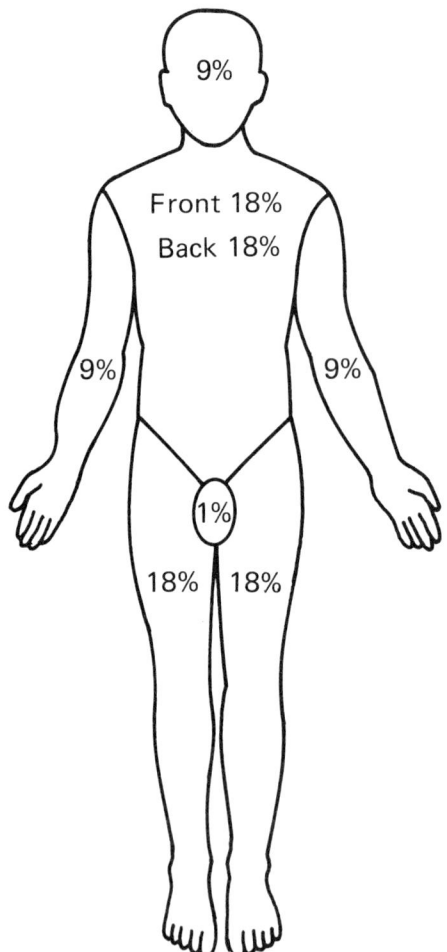

**Figure 1.** The 'rule of nine' in estimating percentage body surface area.

should be performed. In either case, the largest possible cannula should be inserted and secured firmly. A long narrow catheter is a bad choice. Flow rate is inversely proportional to the length of a tube and directly proportional to the third power of the diameter—double the bore gives eight times the flow rate. If it is necessary to cut through full thickness burn to get at the vein, so much the better. No analgesia will be needed, the wound will not need careful repair and a vein will have been used that in subsequent weeks will be inaccessible anyway. The long saphenous vein at the ankle is a bad choice for an intravenous route at this stage. Almost invariably it will go into spasm, giving endless trouble at a time when a reliable drip is essential. Furthermore, in the weeks to come, an ankle vein under intact skin will be a priceless asset for the many infusions that will be required.

### Blood samples

If a blood sample can be obtained from the cannula before the drip set is connected it will save time and the need for a venipuncture a few minutes later, but attempts to get this sample must not be allowed to prejudice the setting up of the drip. Ten millilitres minimum of blood will be required: 4 ml in a lithium heparin tube for haematocrit, urea and electrolytes; at least 4 ml in a plain tube together with 2 ml in a sequestrene tube for group and crossmatch.

### Choice of infusion fluid

Except that the fluid should contain 130–160 mmol Na/l, the exact composition is less important than the need to start the infusion. In the UK it is customary to use human plasma protein fraction solutions but other fluids are widely used in other parts of the world. When the burns are very extensive (+60%) or very deep (e.g. electrical current burns) or there has been delay of an hour or more in starting intravenous therapy, low molecular weight colloid fluids such as Rheomacrodex, Lomodex, Haemaccel or Gelofusine may be particularly useful in the first hour or two of fluid therapy. This is because of their marked though transient 'plasma expander' effect and because their rapid excretion via the kidney promotes a solute diuresis that may be beneficial if degraded haem pigments are present in the glomerular filtrate. They are *not* suitable for continued use in a regime designed for plasma, since their short half-life in the circulation and continued solute diuretic effect would require a regime specifically designed to take account of these properties.

### Catheterization of the bladder

Because knowledge of the flow rate and composition of the urine provides vital information concerning both the effectiveness of resuscitation and the functional status of the kidneys themselves, an indwelling catheter should be inserted if burns involve 25% or more of the body surface area. The bladder is emptied, the urine volume measured and a specimen kept, a drainage bag is connected to the catheter and the hourly urine volume measured thereafter.

## Reassessment of the patient

When the above priorities in treatment have been attended to, the need to support the airway considered (Chapter 3), and any necessary analgesia provided (Chapter 5), the patient's condition should be reassessed. Use of the rule of nine often results in an over-estimate of the extent of the burn and, at this stage, a more accurate assessment should be made using a Lund and Browder Chart (Figure 2). An attempt should now be made to distinguish

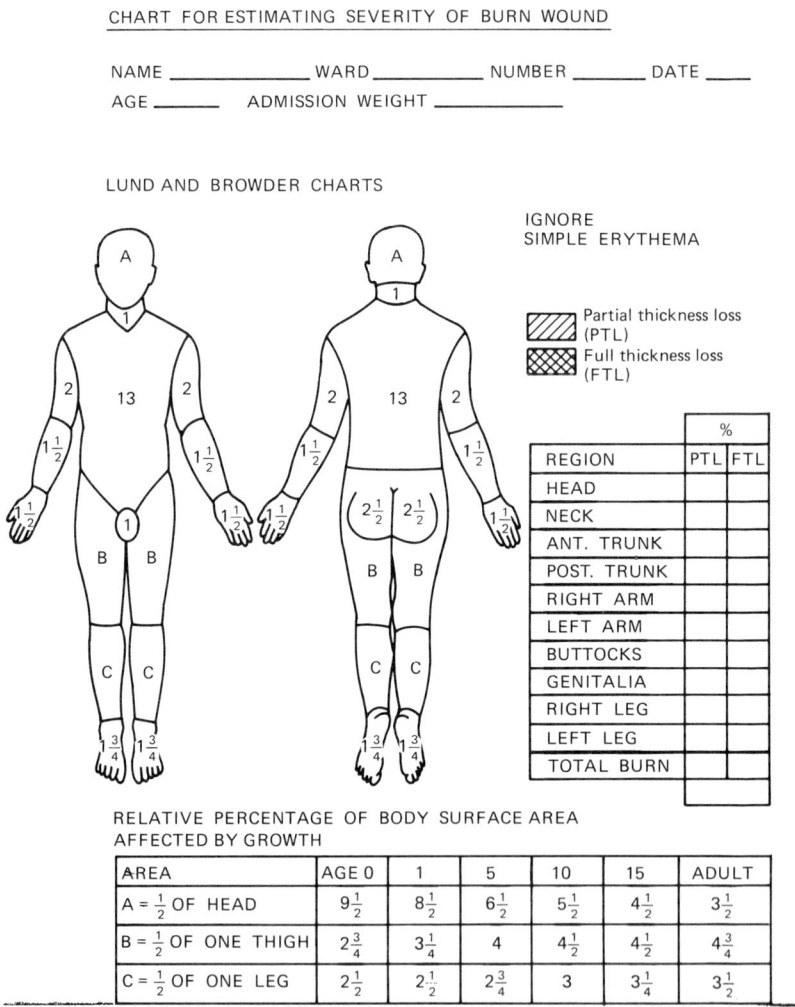

CHART FOR ESTIMATING SEVERITY OF BURN WOUND

NAME _____ WARD _____ NUMBER _____ DATE ____
AGE _____   ADMISSION WEIGHT _____

LUND AND BROWDER CHARTS

IGNORE SIMPLE ERYTHEMA

Partial thickness loss (PTL)
Full thickness loss (FTL)

| REGION | PTL | FTL |
|---|---|---|
| HEAD | | |
| NECK | | |
| ANT. TRUNK | | |
| POST. TRUNK | | |
| RIGHT ARM | | |
| LEFT ARM | | |
| BUTTOCKS | | |
| GENITALIA | | |
| RIGHT LEG | | |
| LEFT LEG | | |
| TOTAL BURN | | |

RELATIVE PERCENTAGE OF BODY SURFACE AREA AFFECTED BY GROWTH

| AREA | AGE 0 | 1 | 5 | 10 | 15 | ADULT |
|---|---|---|---|---|---|---|
| A = $\frac{1}{2}$ OF HEAD | $9\frac{1}{2}$ | $8\frac{1}{2}$ | $6\frac{1}{2}$ | $5\frac{1}{2}$ | $4\frac{1}{2}$ | $3\frac{1}{2}$ |
| B = $\frac{1}{2}$ OF ONE THIGH | $2\frac{3}{4}$ | $3\frac{1}{4}$ | 4 | $4\frac{1}{2}$ | $4\frac{1}{2}$ | $4\frac{3}{4}$ |
| C = $\frac{1}{2}$ OF ONE LEG | $2\frac{1}{2}$ | $2\frac{1}{2}$ | $2\frac{3}{4}$ | 3 | $3\frac{1}{4}$ | $3\frac{1}{2}$ |

**Figure 2.** Lund and Browder chart for accurate assessment of percentage body surface areas.

between partial thickness and full thickness skin loss and the burned area drawn on the chart can be suitably shaded to show this distinction. When this more accurate estimate of burn size has been made, the requirement for fluid therapy should be reassessed and a suitable plan devised.

### Resuscitation with oral fluids

When the burn involves less than 10% of the body surface area (BSA) in children or less than 15% BSA in adults, there is usually no difficulty in balancing the fluid loss by increasing the oral fluid intake. There is, however, still a requirement for salt and it is highly dangerous to attempt resuscitation in these patients simply by increasing the 'normal' fluid intake of water, tea, fruit-flavoured drinks etc. Such a policy will almost certainly result in the production of severe hyponatraemia. Because water diuresis is rarely possible during the first 12 or even 24 h following injury, even a moderate excess of sodium-free water intake may lead to water intoxication with possibly fatal consequences.

A suitable oral fluid for infants is Dextrolyte and, for young children, sachets of Dioralyte can be used to make up a satisfactory solution. Both these products are likely to be available in any hospital with a paediatric ward, since they are commonly used to replace the water and electrolyte loss caused by diarrhoea.

For older children and adults, Moyer's solution is a well-known and satisfactory oral replacement fluid which contains 4 g NaCl and 1.5 g $NaHCO_3$ per litre. Approximately this composition can be obtained by mixing one litre of 'normal' (0.9%) saline with one litre of tap water and then adding 100 ml of isotonic (1.26%) sodium bicarbonate solution. The resulting mixture is still rather salty and can be made more palatable by the addition of flavourings such as orange squash. The quantity of fluid required will obviously vary depending upon the size and nature of the burn and the size of the patient, but two or three times the normal hourly water intake, given *instead of* the normally sodium-free water intake, will usually be the maximum requirement.

For mass casualty situations, and in parts of the world where intravenous fluids are very expensive or in short supply, oral fluids may have to suffice for burns of up to 30% BSA and there are many reports of successful treatment of this kind. Moyer's solution should be used with a maximum volume equal to 10% of the patient's weight and given in hourly doses over a 24–36 h period.

### Resuscitation with intravenous fluid

In England and Wales until about 1979 and in Scotland until about 1984, reconstituted freeze-dried plasma was the fluid in general use for burns but it has now been superseded by human plasma protein fraction solutions (HPPF). There are some small differences between solutions provided by different suppliers but all contain about 4.5% human albumin and about 150 mmol Na/litre.

The formula most widely used in the UK to predict the likely fluid requirement and indicate an appropriate rate of infusion is that devised by Muir and Barclay (1987) in the late 1950s. This formula, derived from observations on patients treated with freeze-dried plasma, predicts the same total fluid requirement as that of Evans et al (1952) but, by considering sequential fluid budgets for much shorter periods than any previous formula, it throws into sharp focus the need for frequent clinical reassessment. The first 36 h following the injury are divided into six successive periods of 4, 4, 4, 6, 6 and 12 h. The estimate of the volume of plasma (in ml) that should be infused by the end of the *4th hour after burning* is derived from the equation:

$$\frac{\text{Total percentage area of burn} \times \text{weight in kg}}{2}$$

i.e. 0.5 ml/kg %

At the end of this first 4 h period an assessment is made of the state of the patient, and if the amount is judged to have been correct the same volume is given in the next period. If, however, the patient is judged to be over-transfused or undertransfused, the ration for the next period is decreased or increased accordingly. This same reassessment is carried out at the end of each period. The block graph shown in Figure 3 represents the fluid that would be given (if started immediately after injury) should no alterations be necessary. In practice, of course, a histogram of actual fluid given, though having this general shape, would be much less regular in outline.

Retrospective analysis of the actual volumes of freeze-dried plasma (and where appropriate some whole blood) given during the first 24 h postburn in a consecutive series of patients with burns of 30% and over, treated in the Yorkshire Regional Burns Centre between 1966 and 1979, gave the following results. The mean colloid load during the first 24 h postburn in 46 children was 2.87 ml/kg % and in 69 adults, 2.40 ml/kg % with an overall

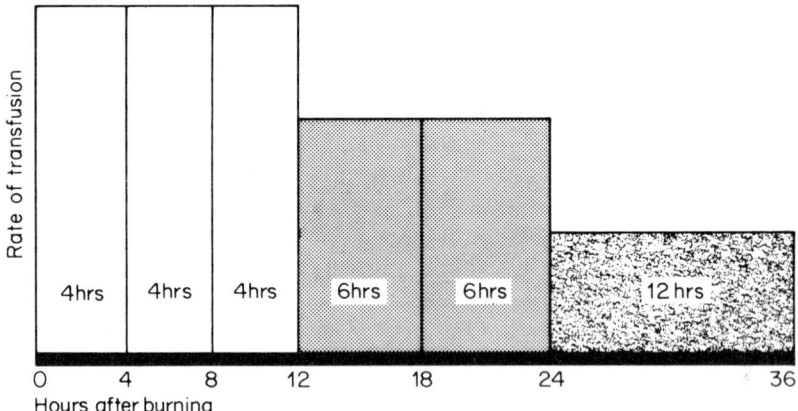

**Figure 3.** Histogram of Muir and Barclay transfusion scheme. The blocks represent equal volumes of transfusion fluid and show how the rate of transfusion is altered by varying the time during which the equal 'rations' are given.

mean of 2.58. This is virtually the same as the 2.50 ml/kg % predicted by the Muir and Barclay formula which was also derived from a mixed group of adults and children. During the period 1979–83, when HPPF had replaced freeze-dried plasma, the comparable figures are 3.52 ml/kg % in 19 children and 3.12 ml/kg % in 21 adults. This gives an overall mean of 3.31, which represents an increase of approximately 25% compared with freeze-dried plasma.

This finding, that effective resuscitation usually requires more HPPF than freeze-dried plasma, was evident soon after the introduction of HPPF, and some burn clinicians soon began to make a routine increase in the Muir and Barclay formula prediction by up to 30%. However, bearing in mind that any calculated prediction is simply a guide and not a precise prescription and that even moderate overtransfusion can have serious consequences, particularly if there are complications such as renal impairment or pulmonary damage, I believe that a more prudent approach is preferable. The plasma budget for the period up to 4 h postburn should be based on an expected requirement of between 0.5 and 0.65 ml/kg body weight/% burn (these limits being the Muir and Barclay formula prediction and that amount plus 25%). For example, a 75 kg patient with a 55% burn is likely to need between 2000 and 2600 ml of plasma in the first 4 h postburn. If the drip had not been started until 1 h postburn, it would be reasonable to give 1200 ml during the 2nd h, and 600 ml during each of the 3rd and 4th hours. A careful appraisal of the effectiveness of this regime would be made at 4 h postburn and a fluid budget decided for the next 4 h period.

**Calculated plasma deficit**

The actual volume of plasma missing from the circulation can be estimated if the haematocrit (HTC) is measured. Obviously, a number of assumptions and approximations have to be made: it has to be remembered that loss of red blood cells will result in an underestimate of the plasma deficit, it is assumed that the HTC was normal before the accident, it is assumed that the measured HTC is a reliable index of the red cell : plasma ratio in the total blood volume, and it is assumed that the HTC result can be known within 15 min of the sample being taken; otherwise the information becomes too out-of-date to be of much value. Because of the variables involved, the change in apparent plasma deficit calculated from sequential HTC measurements is usually of more value than a single determination. Ideally, the HTC should be measured in a side-room adjacent to the treatment area and the use of a Hawksley micro-haematocrit centrifuge makes it possible to know the HTC result within a few minutes of the specimen being taken. If this facility is available, HTC readings can be performed on capillary blood samples.

The calculation of plasma deficit is performed by using the formula:

$$\text{Deficit} = \text{Blood volume} - \left[\text{Blood volume} \times \frac{\text{Normal HTC}}{\text{Observed HTC}}\right]$$

(All volumes in ml)

### Deciding the plasma requirement for the second period

If the i.v. drip and urine collection were started at about 1 h postburn, a considerable amount of data should be available by 4 h postburn. In the case of the example given above (75 kg, 55% burn) this might be:

| | |
|---|---|
| 1 h postburn | Drip set up, bladder emptied. Obvious peripheral vaso-constriction, HTC = 49% (calculated plasma deficit 500 ml). |
| 2 h postburn | 1200 ml plasma given during past hour.<br>Urine output 30 ml (conc. 850 mOsm/l).<br>Shell temperature 33 °C. Core temperature 38 °C.<br>RChlorpromazine 25 mg i.v. and 600 ml plasma during next hour. |
| 3 h postburn | 600 ml plasma given during past hour.<br>Urine output 40 ml (conc. 750 mOsm/l).<br>Shell temperature 34.5 °C and core temperature 37 °C.<br>R600 ml plasma during next hour. |
| 4 h postburn | 600 ml plasma given during past hour.<br>Urine output 35 ml (conc. 800 mOsm/l).<br>Shell temperature 34 °C and core temperature 37 °C.<br>HTC 47 (calculated plasma deficit 220 ml). |

The implications of these findings are that the patient is being a little undertransfused. His urine is highly concentrated and barely adequate in volume. His peripheral perfusion is a little less than optimal and the HTC suggests a plasma deficit of about 200 ml. It would be appropriate to give an additional bolus of plasma to correct the deficit and also increase the plasma ration for the next 4 hours by a similar amount. A suitable scheme would be: 850 ml plasma in the next hour and 650 ml in each of the subsequent 3 hours.

### Red cell requirement

Muir (1961) has shown that a general relationship exists between the extent of whole thickness skin burn and the amount of red cell destruction. He recommended that when deep burns involve more than 10% of the BSA, the whole blood requirement is 1% of the patient's normal blood volume for each 1% deep burn. In an adult this would amount to one unit of blood or packed cells for each 10% of deep burn over and above the first 10%. In general, it is best to give the blood during the second 24 h, i.e. the 6th Muir and Barclay period; the transfusion of packed cells will cause a marked rise in HTC and interpretation of HTC changes during the subsequent hours can be quite difficult.

### Metabolic water requirement

The amount of sodium-free water required by the burn patient is directly related to evaporative and other extrarenal losses. If the burn wound is 'exposed' in a hot dry environment the water losses can be as great as 2 litres per 10% burn per 24 h. Obviously, in these circumstances, a comparably large water intake will be required. However, if the wounds are dressed conventionally with cream or tulle covered by a thick layer of absorbent material, the evaporative water loss is greatly reduced and the requirement of sodium-free water is usually in the range 1.5 to 2.0 ml/kg body weight/h with a minimum of 30 ml/h for infants. The water can be given by mouth if it is well tolerated, but otherwise intravenously as 5% dextrose solution.

It is important to remember that the quantity of sodium-free water given should only be sufficient to prevent significant hypernatraemia. If hyponatraemia is allowed to develop, intracellular overhydration will occur that can lead on to serious and even fatal complications. This is probably the mechanism, in many instances, of the so-called 'burn encephalopathy' syndrome associated with burns and scalds in children. The syndrome includes cerebral irritability, hyperpyrexia, vomiting, twitching, convulsions and coma and has had a fatal outcome in some cases. A common finding in many such cases has been a plasma Na level of less than 130 mmol/l at the time of onset of symptoms and a history of a significant sodium-free water load being given during the preceding hours. It seems that the resultant cerebral oedema produces (among other things) hypothalmic malfunction so that heat continues to be produced even to the extent of shivering occurring while peripheral vasoconstriction continues to minimize heat loss. Thus the core temperature rises while the shell temperature remains subnormal.

Prevention of this complication requires thoughtful control of fluid and electrolyte balance. Marked hypernatraemia due to an inadequate intake of sodium-free water should not be allowed to develop, but if it does it should be slowly and carefully corrected. Rapid correction will result in an osmotic drive between extracellular and intracellular compartments, thus producing a sudden influx of water to the cells. If the syndrome does develop and convulsions occur, they should be controlled by conventional drugs such as barbiturates. If hyperpyrexia occurs it will not respond to any attempts to cool the patient by use of fans, ice, cold water etc. Indeed, such measures will make matters worse. Successful treatment requires the production of peripheral vasodilation in order that heat can be lost, and drugs such as chlorpromazine or phenoxybenzamine may be required. Note that a low shell temperature in the burn patient will usually be the result of reduced peripheral perfusion due to persistent hypovolaemia, and it is essential to make sure that plasma replacement has been adequate before diagnosing that inequalities between shell and core temperatures are the result of hypothalmic malfunction.

**Monitoring the fluid therapy**

Frequent clinical reassessment is the lynchpin of effective resuscitation and should include consideration of the patient's general demeanour, skin colour (pallor, cyanosis etc.), filling of peripheral veins and capillary return. Clinical measurement should include heart rate, respiratory rate, arterial blood pressure, core (deep rectal) and shell (skin on big toe if unburned) temperatures and hourly urine volume. This information with laboratory investigations such as haematocrit and urine concentration (osmolarity) should enable the clinician to assess the adequacy of the tissue perfusion and thus the effectiveness of fluid therapy. If renal function remains unimpaired, the urine produced by the burn patient (certainly during most of the first 24 h postburn) will be persistently more concentrated than a glomerular filtrate and can be expected to have an osmolarity in the range 600–1000 mOsm/l. With adequate renal perfusion, the burn patient can be expected to produce this concentrated urine at the rate of about 0.5 ml/kg body weight/h. If there is a marked deviation from this value for two consecutive hours, serious consideration should be given to altering the plasma infusion rate.

Invasive measurement techniques should be avoided whenever possible because of the high incidence of bacteraemia associated with them and the serious risk of sepsis in the extensively burned patient. However, if there has been marked delay in starting resuscitation or if serious renal impairment or cardiac failure occurs, measurement of central venous pressure (and occasionally pulmonary wedge pressure) may be invaluable.

## Checking on the patient's progress

The doctor must decide for himself how frequently he will make a formal reassessment of the patient's condition. Usually he should take stock at the end of each of the periods of the Mount Vernon plan. During the first two periods, i.e. up to 8 h from burning, he should be aware of each hour's urine volume and whether the infusion rate per h is that which he intended. If all seems to be going well at this time, he should leave clear instructions of the circumstances which will necessitate him being called, e.g. if oral fluids are not being tolerated; if urine volume is less than $x$ ml/h for 2 h or more than $y$ ml/h for 2 h; if there is difficulty with the drip; if respiratory difficulties occur, etc. By setting these alarms the doctor will continue to provide a proper standard of care while proceeding with other duties or perhaps even having a few hours of well-earned sleep.

The use of volumetric infusion pumps has greatly facilitated the accurate administration of i.v. fluids to burn patients. With these devices it is possible to 'dial-up' the required hourly infusion rate and thus free the nursing staff from the tedious chore of frequently having to check the rate of infusion. However, if a suitable pump is not available, frequent visual checks (including counting the rate of the drops) *must* be carried out. It is clearly a futile exercise to attempt to alter subsequent hourly rations of fluid if there is no reliable knowledge of what has been given previously and no confidence that what is being prescribed will be given as requested. Giving sets containing calibrated burettes are a reasonable alternative to a volumetric pump, although they require a good deal of attention if they are to be put to good use, but vague instructions indicating $x$ bottles in $y$ hours are quite inappropriate for the treatment of burns shock. Indeed, there is no satisfactory alternative to the prescription, administration and recording of fluids on a strict ml/h basis, and the charts used should facilitate this approach.

Patients with extensive burns will require intravenous fluids for at least 36 h and commonly for 48 h or more; plasma and/or blood may still be required after the 'sixth period' (24–36 h postburn) but after 48 h other i.v.

fluids should be required only if oral intake is inadequate or complications have occurred.

## RENAL FUNCTION

### Urine output

Of all the viscera, the kidney is the one most likely to be damaged by uncontrolled hypovolaemic shock. Fortunately, however, careful examination of the urine being secreted can provide a useful guide to the haemodynamic circumstances under which the urine is being elaborated and the functional status of the kidney at the time of production.

In the early stages after any injury, the kidney is subjected to intense activity by the sympathetic nervous system, by circulating catecholamines, by angiotensin and by the antidiuretic hormone of the posterior pituitary (Le Quesne, 1954). Because of variability in these stimuli, changes in urine flow can be difficult to interpret. Some authorities, observing an apparent unpredictability and wide variation in hourly urine volumes, have concluded that urine volume is a totally unreliable index of the effectiveness of resuscitation (Barton and Laing, 1970), while others have used hourly urine volume as a main guide to infusion therapy (Baxter, 1971). However, in order to make any sense of urine output, the hourly urine volume and its concentration must be considered *together*; consequently, both should be measured.

It is reasonable to assume that following the occurrence of a burn large enough to require intravenous fluid therapy, antidiuretic hormone (ADH) will be present in the circulation for most of the first 24 h. During this time water diuresis will not be possible and the urine will remain significantly more concentrated than the glomerular filtrate (i.e. urine osmolarity will be two or three times greater than the normal plasma osmolarity of around 300 mOsm/l). This persistent antidiuresis does not mean that the hourly urine volume will inevitably be very small, because antidiuresis and oliguria are not synonymous; the former describes the concentration, the latter describes the volume. Indeed, it is in precisely the circumstances of maximal ADH activity that a direct linear relationship exists between total solute excretion and urine volume. Hence, an increase in filtered solute load, whether resulting from an increased glomerular filtration rate or from the presence of a disposable solute such as glucose, mannitol or low molecular weight dextran, will promote an increased urine volume, but with *an inverse fall in its concentration*. (It is *possible* for water diuresis to occur even within the first 8 h following a major burn (Settle, 1974) but it is usually a transient response to a dangerously large water load that has depressed plasma osmolarity below 275 mOsm/l; a hazardous situation that should be avoided by limiting the sodium-free water intake of the patient.)

In the absence of a large amount of disposable solute (glucose, mannitol etc.) in the glomerular filtrate and the avoidance of a massive sodium-free water intake, the final urine will be significantly concentrated

(600–900 mOsm/l) compared with the glomerular filtrate *unless serious impairment of renal function occurs*. If the doctor is certain that a concentrated urine is being produced, urine flow is a useful index of effective resuscitation. In these circumstances, a satisfactory flow rate is 0.5 to 1.0 ml/h/kg body weight, e.g. an hourly volume of 35–70 ml for an adult patient (Settle, 1974). An hourly volume below 0.5 ml/h/kg, with a concentration above 800 mOsm/l, is a reliable indication that infusion therapy is inadequate, while volumes well over 1.0 ml/h/kg, with a concentration of 350–450 mOsm/l, strongly indicate overtransfusion.

### Measurement of urine volume

A closed urinary drainage system should be connected to the indwelling catheter. The design should permit the accurate measurement of each hour's urine output and allow a small sample of that output to be removed without risk of bacterial contamination of the drainage system.

### Measurement of urine concentration

The time-honoured way of estimating urine concentration is by measuring specific gravity, i.e. the ratio of the density of the urine to that of pure water at 4 °C. Thus, specific gravity is an index of the weight of solute present in the urine. However, the biologically significant aspect of a urine's concentration is its osmotic potential or osmolarity, which is a consequence of the number of particles of solute in solution and not the weight of these particles. Because of this, it is possible for urines of identical osmolarity to have widely different specific gravities as a consequence of solutes such as glucose or protein being present in differing amounts. The truth of this may be seen from the fact that 0.9% saline (280 mOsml/l) has a specific gravity of 1.006, while 5% glucose solution (280 mOsm/l) has a specific gravity of 1.019. (Even greater discrepancies occur if refractive index is used as an indicator of urine concentration; e.g. an instance where urine with an osmolality of 350 mOsm/l gave specific gravity readings as high as 1.030 when 'measured' in a urine refractometer.)

If at all possible, urine concentration should be determined by measurement of urine osmolarity. Using a depression of freezing point method, this measurement can be performed on a sample as small as 0.2 ml and takes only 2 min. It has been a routine in the Yorkshire Regional Burns Centre since 1969, and in recent years has been performed by the nursing staff as each hourly urine is collected. Measurement of urine urea concentration and determination of urine/blood urea ratio provide an estimate of renal concentrating power that is useful in the diagnosis of renal failure, but any pathology laboratory that is capable of measuring urea concentration of hourly urine samples would almost certainly offer osmolarity measurement as a better alternative.

### Interpreting the urine output

It is most useful to plot the values for urine flow rate and osmolarity as graphs, one above the other, just as pulse rate and temperature are conventionally charted. When volume and concentration can be seen at a glance, the inverse relationship between them is obvious and the trends from hour to hour can easily be seen. Trends are much more important than single hourly values. For instance, a sharp fall in urine volume after several hours of adequate volumes of concentrated urine, particularly if the concentration of the small urine volume is similar to those of previous hours, is almost certainly a drainage problem rather than an indication of inadequate resuscitation or impairment of renal function. On the other hand, a gradual reduction of volume to barely adequate levels, with a reciprocal progressive rise in concentration, is clear evidence that fluid infusion should be increased.

## Impaired renal function

It is evident that renal failure is a potential complication in any patient with a large burn. Unless resuscitation with appropriate intravenous fluids is started early and continued effectively, the inevitable fall in cardiac output can be sufficient to reduce the effective renal perfusion to the point where classical acute tubular necrosis occurs. In the vast majority of burn patients, effective intravenous fluid therapy will prevent this very serious complication. However, if effective treatment is delayed, renal failure can occur even in patients with relatively small burns. For example, a 60 year old previously healthy male was admitted to the Yorkshire Regional Burns Centre 12 h after he had sustained a deep flame burn to his right buttock, thigh and leg amounting to 10% of his body surface area. He had not sought any medical assistance until 10 h postburn, and within a few hours of admission to the Burns Centre it was evident that oliguric renal failure was established. So catabolic was this patient that his blood urea level rose at a rate of over 15 mmol/24 h until checked by peritoneal dialysis. Subsequently, repeated haemodialysis was required to control his uraemia. At three weeks, spontaneous recovery of renal function commenced and, after the burn wounds had been closed by skin grafting, he was discharged home with perfectly satisfactory renal function 13 weeks after the injury.

Occasionally, patients with extensive burns develop early renal failure in spite of apparently adequate fluid therapy. For example, a 10 year old boy with 55% mainly very deep burns was admitted to the Yorkshire Regional Burns Centre during the 3rd hour postburn, effective intravenous fluid therapy having been commenced during the previous hour. In spite of rapid correction of moderate haemoconcentration, his urine output remained inadequate (mean value 0.5 ml/h/kg but with osmolarity fixed at about 350 mOsm/l). Peritoneal dialysis was commenced at 54 h postburn (blood urea 34 mmol/l; $K$ 6.2 mmol/l) and was continued for 10 days. Three major skin grafting sessions were required and he was discharged home 18 weeks after the injury (Settle, 1974).

The gravity of renal failure as a complication of burns can hardly be overstated. Because the survival of the patient during the first 36 h following extensive burns is dependent upon the infusion of vast quantities of fluid, it is inevitable that by the 2nd and 3rd days postburn there will be a large positive fluid balance in the form of burn oedema. Resolution of this burn oedema occurs as a consequence of a reverse shift from interstitial to intravascular compartments followed by diuresis. If this diuresis is not possible, which it certainly is not if renal failure supervenes, the burn oedema will be redistributed to the lungs and severe pulmonary oedema will occur. The extensively burned patient whose kidneys fail during or soon after effective fluid resuscitation is likely to drown in his own extracellular fluid long before hyperkalaemia reaches a fatal level—hence the need for early diagnosis and urgent and effective treatment of renal failure following extensive burns.

## Diagnosis of renal impairment

It has been reported that all patients with burns of more than 20% show some evidence of mixed glomerular and tubular damage during the first few days postburn (Yu et al, 1983). This damage shows itself in the form of proteinuria comprising high molecular weight proteins such as albumin (66 300 daltons), low molecular weight (LMW) proteins such as β-2-microglobulin (11 800 daltons) and tubular enzymes such as $N$-acetyl-β-D-glucosaminidase (NAG). The severity of total proteinuria is directly related to the severity of the burn but this phase of mixed glomerular and tubular proteinuria usually resolves once the patient is stabilized by effective resuscitation. There then follows a period of tubular proteinuria characterized by increased excretion of LMW proteins and a rising level of NAG. The final return to normal proximal tubular cell function in an uncomplicated patient may take several weeks. The initial proteinuria may be accompanied by other indications of acute renal insufficiency such as a falling glomerular filtration rate and failure to concentrate the urine, but if these are absent, renal damage is insufficient to affect normal excretory function of the kidney and its role in maintaining body water and electrolyte balance. However, these studies, together with routine urine osmometry during the past 17 years, have demonstrated a spectrum of renal impairment ranging from a transient and relatively insignificant proteinuria through to acute oliguric renal failure with total loss of urine concentrating power characteristic of acute tubular necrosis.

Acute oliguric renal failure occurring early in the shock phase should be diagnosed within hours of its onset. The characteristic findings are: (a) very low hourly urine volumes, e.g. 10 ml/h or less in an adult; (b) loss of urine concentration/dilution power with a 'fixed' urine osmolarity of about 350 mOsm/l; (c) urine/blood urea ratio of 5 or less; (d) high Na and low K levels in urine; (e) low urine creatinine levels; (f) rising blood creatinine level with very low creatinine clearance (10 ml/min or less); and (g) uraemia—azotaemia, hyperkalaemia, hyponatraemia and metabolic acidosis.

At the other end of the spectrum there is minor tubular damage in which the maximum urine concentration may be limited to 500 mOsm/l and urine/blood urea ratio lies in the range 15–20:1. This abnormality will be detected only if it is looked for actively or if urine osmolarity (or urea concentrating power) measurement is a frequent and routine investigation. If the patient is kept in good fluid and electrolyte balance this minor impairment of renal function will be of little significance. However, if the patient becomes hypernatraemic and hyperosmolar as a consequence of losing sodium-free water that is not being replaced (most likely if the burn wound is being treated by exposure and the vast evaporative water losses have not been appreciated), the inability of the kidney to correct body osmolar balance by excreting a highly concentrated urine may be a critical factor in the development of progressive hyperosmolarity.

Between these two extremes lies non-oliguric (or high output) renal failure. As Cason pointed out in 1966, when he reported a 5% incidence of renal failure in a series of 962 burn patients who had required active resuscitation, about half the cases of postburn renal failure are of a non-oliguric type. Ten years previously, Sevitt (1974) had described the post-mortem appearance of the kidney in such cases and concluded that the underlying pathology was a necrosis of the distal convoluted tubule, the condition being called 'lower nephron nephrosis'. Commonly, the complication is not recognized in the early stages, since urine flow may seem to be adequate and the unexpected finding of a high blood urea level at the end of the shock phase or even several days later may be the first indication that a serious complication has occurred. This unpleasant surprise can be avoided if the quality of the urine is examined in addition to measuring its quantity. Typically, the urine concentration in non-oliguric failure will lie in the 350–400 mOsm/l range, and the urine/blood urea ratio will be less than 10 and may be less than 5 (cf. normal of over 50). Often there will be casts in the urine and, in a high proportion of cases, a history of 'haemoglobinuria' during the early stages of the shock phase.

It may be thought that routine measurement of blood would also provide early warning of impending or actual renal failure. In our experience it is less useful than urine osmolarity measurement because many burn patients with good renal function can have a temporary rise in blood urea to levels between 10 and 15 mmol/l simply because of the hypercatabolism that accompanies the burn injury. Furthermore, we have seen blood urea levels of over 30 mmol/l in patients whose renal impairment was relatively minor and who certainly did not require dialysis.

## Management of renal impairment

The early recognition of loss of renal concentrating power is essential for two separate reasons. Firstly, it allows the clinician the option of attempting to restore renal function and, if this fails, to proceed with forms of treatment designed to prevent uraemia. Secondly, it signals the end of urine flow measurement as any sort of index of effective resuscitation. If the burn is extensive and the renal impairment judged to be serious, it is advisable to institute CVP measurement. This will provide a reliable means of judging the fluid therapy requirement in circumstances where the response to overtransfusion will be pulmonary oedema rather than diuresis.

There are occasions when persistent and inappropriate vasoconstriction may be responsible for 'physiological' impairment of renal function. This complication can be avoided if small doses of chlorpromazine are used during the shock phase, for in addition to its sedative and anti-emetic properties, it also has some alpha receptor blocking activity. A much more powerful drug in this respect is phenoxybenzamine but it should only be used with great care since its administration may be followed by a catastrophic fall in blood pressure. The doctor should be satisfied by CVP measurement that blood volume replacement has been adequate before phenoxybenzamine is given (0.5 mg/kg body weight, given in 250 ml of 0.9% saline over 30 min). CVP monitoring must be continued while the drug is being given and it is highly likely that additional fluid will need to be given to fill the vessels released from vasoconstriction.

When the renal impairment is of the non-oliguric type, the possibility of producing a diuresis should be considered. If the urine Na is less than 10 mmol/l, the tubule may respond to frusemide (1 mg/kg body weight given i.v.). Otherwise, a solute diuretic such as mannitol can be tried (1 g/kg body weight given as a 20% solution over 15–30 min). When mannitol works satisfactorily, the response is an obvious diuresis that continues, though gradually declining, over the next 12 h. If it does not work, it *must not* be repeated as this may lead to sudden pulmonary oedema. If a urine flow of several litres per day can be maintained by the use of a diuretic, urinary excretion of urea, potassium, etc. may be sufficient to prevent uraemia. However, very careful attention will need to be paid to the patient's water and electrolyte balance, and blood chemistry measurements should be performed at least twice per day.

If a satisfactory diuresis cannot be induced, it is best to proceed to dialysis at an early stage. Because the patient will very probably be hypercatabolic, conservative methods of management are seldom useful. Unless the clinician in charge of the burn patient is experienced in the techniques of dialysis it will be best to obtain the advice and assistance of a renal physician. However, peritoneal dialysis is a relatively straightforward technique that can reasonably be undertaken by any clinician who is competent to look after patients with severe burns.

### Technique of peritoneal dialysis

This can be performed through burned skin although intact skin is obviously preferred. Dialysis fluid, administration sets, catheters, and collection bags are commercially available, and carry clear instructions. Briefly, the technique is as follows:

1. Empty the bladder.
2. Choose the site of insertion (midline, one-third down from the umbilicus to the pubis, is best).
3. Infiltrate the site with local anaesthetic, and incise the skin with a scalpel.
4. Push the trochar, with obturator in place, into the peritoneal cavity.
5. Remove the obturator, and push the trochar in further.
6. Insert the cannula so that it lies in the left paracolic gutter, and test for patency before securing with a purse-string suture.

The principle of peritoneal dialysis is to run dialysate into the abdominal cavity, allow it to equilibrate with the blood in the mesenteric vessels, syphon it out and then run in some more. For an adult, 2 litres of dialysate would be used and each complete cycle would take about 1 h. The whole procedure may need to be continued for up to two weeks and great care must be taken to avoid peritonitis due to bacterial contamination of the fluids or the equipment. Useful instructions and advice come with the commercial dialysate which is available in two main forms. One has a glucose content of 1.36% and is moderately hypertonic, while the other, with 6.36% glucose, is strongly hypertonic and is used when the removal of a large positive water balance is required.

**Haemodialysis**

In the Yorkshire Regional Burns Centre we have had experience of several patients in whom the combination of acute oliguric renal failure and hyper-catabolism due to extensive burns resulted in blood urea levels rising at the rate of 15–20 mmol/l per day. With this rate of urea production it is unlikely that peritoneal dialysis will be able even to stop the blood urea level from rising, and haemodialysis will be required. In a recent case, haemodialysis using equipment with the maximal clearance rate available had to be repeated twice per day in order to control the blood urea level. This requirement was unprecedented in the experience of the renal physician concerned.

If gross overhydration is the main problem, the possibility of using a technique of ultrafiltration rather than dialysis should be considered.

**Haemoglobinuria**

Thermally degraded haem pigments from haemoglobin and myoglobin have a sinister reputation for producing renal damage, although the normal kidney can pass large quantities of normal haemoglobin without any damage occurring. Whether the urinary pigments sometimes seen in patients with deep or extensive burns are actually responsible for renal damage, or whether some other 'toxic' substance is responsible, is not yet clear. However, a diuresis that will clear haem pigments will also clear any other 'toxic' substance present, and most burn clinicians will give mannitol (1 g/kg body weight given i.v. as a 20% solution over 15–30 min). The caution given above about repeating mannitol should be observed. Most burn clinicians believe, like Dudley et al (1957), that they have, at some time, aborted renal failure by using mannitol, but objective proof is difficult to find.

**The prognosis of renal failure**

Twenty years ago, postburn renal failure was considered to be virtually always a fatal event (Cameron and Miller-Jones, 1967) and only a handful of survivors had been reported in the world literature. The position today is rather different. Early diagnosis and effective treatment can be expected to give the patient a good chance of surviving this complication. Thereafter, until he is healed, the patient's chance of surviving is probably not much worse than if the renal failure had not occurred.

## SUMMARY

Salt and water are the essential requirements for effective resuscitation of a patient with extensive burns. The optimum sodium load is of the order of 0.5 mmol/kg body weight/% burn, and the total volume of fluid (excluding the replacement of any large evaporative losses) is likely to be between 2 and 4 ml/kg body weight/% burn. Sodium-free water, given to replace any extrarenal losses, should be limited to an amount sufficient to prevent marked hypernatraemia.

The priorities in practical management are the establishment of a reliable intravenous line and the planned administration of a suitable salt-containing fluid, with the aim of maintaining vital organ function at the least immediate or delayed physiological cost. The effectiveness of the fluid therapy in correcting existing deficits and in keeping pace with continuing losses should be reviewed at frequent intervals, bearing in mind that the rate of loss decreases with time. Usually, at least one half of the total fluid requirement will have been given in the first 12 h, and periodic adjustments to the rate of infusion should be made in response to information gained by monitoring the patient's condition.

Urine produced during the first 24 h following extensive burns is usually concentrated, i.e. osmolarity between 500 and 1000 mOsm/l and water diuresis, i.e. osmolarity less than 300 mOsm/l, is rare. An hourly output of between 0.5 and 1.0 ml/kg body weight (using 12.5 kg as a minimum weight for infants) of concentrated urine is a useful index of satisfactory resuscitation; less than 0.5 ml/kg/h indicates undertransfusion, while an output well over 1.0 ml/kg/h suggests overtransfusion.

The hallmark of renal failure is severe tubular impairment that results in loss of concentrating power. If there is severe glomerular impairment as well, oliguria will be evident; otherwise the urine volume may be normal. Hence the importance of measuring urine concentration (osmolarity) or calculating the urine/blood urea ratio, which in normal health is usually 50 or more but in acute renal failure is less than 5. The triad of oliguria, loss of urine concentration and haem pigments in the urine is particularly ominous. A forced solute diuresis should be attempted (intravenous mannitol, 1 g/kg body weight as a 15 or 20% solution) whenever obvious 'haemoglobinuria' occurs, but should *not* be repeated if a marked diuresis does not ensue. When examination of the urine output indicates serious renal impairment, the advice of a renal specialist should be obtained without delay. The enormous positive fluid balance typically present at 48 h postburn will, in the absence of effective renal function, threaten the patient's life by pulmonary oedema long before he is at risk of dying from uraemia.

# REFERENCES

Barton GMG & Laing JE (1970) Control of intravenous therapy by blood volume estimations. In Matter P, Barclay TL & Konickova Z (eds) *Transactions of the 3rd International Congress on Research in Burns*, 20–25 September, Prague. Berne: Hans Huber.

Baxter CR (1971) Crystalloid resuscitation of burn shock. In Polk HC & Stone HH (eds) *Contemporary Burn Management*, pp 7–32. Boston: Little, Brown & Co.

Blalock A (1931) Experimental shock: importance of local loss of fluid in production of low blood pressure after burns. *Archives of Surgery* 22: 610–616.

Cameron JS & Miller-Jones CMH (1967) Renal function and renal failure in badly burned children. *British Journal of Surgery* 54: 132–141.

Cason JS (1966) Treatment of renal failure. In Wallace AB & Wilkinson AW (eds) *Research in Burns*. Edinburgh: Livingstone.

Cope O & Moore FD (1947) The redistribution of body water and fluid therapy of the burned patient. *Annals of Surgery* 126: 1010–1045.

Dorethy JF, Welch GW, Treat RC, Mason AD & Pruitt BA (1977) Sequential haemodynamic alterations in severe thermal injury in the military population. Colloid-crystalloid versus crystalloid fluid resuscitation. In *U.S. Army Institute of Surgical Research Annual Research Progress Report* pp 120–138.

Dudley HAF, Batchelor ADR & Sutherland AB (1957) The management of haemoglobinuria in extensive burns. *British Journal of Plastic Surgery* 9: 275–285.

Eklund J (1970) Renal regulation of body osmolal balance in burns. A clinical and experimental study with special reference to hyperosmolality. *Acta Chirurgica Scandinavica* supplement 410.

Evans EI, Purnell OJ, Robinett RW, Batchelor A & Martin M (1952) Fluid and electrolyte requirements in severe burns. *Annals of Surgery* 135: 804–817.

Goodwin CW, Lam V & Martin D (1980) Measurement of pulmonary tissue volume in thermally injured soldiers. The effect of crystalloid and colloid resuscitation on lung water following thermal injury. In *U.S. Army Institute of Surgical Research Annual Research Report* pp 255–262.

Hall KV & Sørensen B (1978) The treatment of burn shock: results of a 5 year randomized, controlled clinical trial of Dextran 70 vs Ringer lactate solution. *Burns* 5: 107–112.

Harkins HN (1935) Experimental burns. The rate of fluid shift and its relation to the onset of shock in severe burns. *Archives of Surgery* 31: 71–85.

Le Quesne LP (1954) Postoperative water retention with report of a case of water intoxication. *Lancet* i: 172–174.

Mason AD (1980) The mathematics of resuscitation. 1980 Presidential Address. American Burn Association. *Journal of Trauma* 20: 1015–1020.

Monafo WW, Chuntrasakul C & Ayvazian VH (1973) Hypertonic sodium solutions in the treatment of burn shock. *American Journal of Surgery* 126: 778–783.

Muir IFK (1961) Red cell destruction in burns. *British Journal of Plastic Surgery* 4: 273–302.

Muir IFK, Barclay TL & Settle JAD (1987) *Burns and Their Treatment*, 3rd edn. London: Butterworth.

Peters RM & Hargens AR (1981) Protein vs electrolytes and all of the Starling forces. *Archives of Surgery* 116: 1293–1298.

Pruitt BA (1981) Fluid resuscitation of extensively burned patients. *Journal of Trauma* 21(supplement 8): 690–692.

Settle JAD (1974) Urine output following severe burns. *Burns* 1: 23–42.

Settle JAD (1982) Fluid therapy in burns. *Journal of the Royal Society of Medicine* 75(supplement 1): 6–11.

Sevitt S (1974) Acute renal failure. In Sevitt S (ed.) *Reactions to Injury and Burns and their Clinical Importance*, pp 86–108. London: Heinemann.

Underhill FP, Carrington GL, Kapsinow R & Pack GT (1923) Blood concentration changes in extensive superficial burns and their significance for systemic treatment. *Archives of Internal Medicine* 32: 31–49.

Yu H, Cooper EH, Settle JAD & Meadows T (1983) Urinary protein profiles after burn injury. *Burns* 9: 339–349.

# 3

# Respiratory problems in burns

PETER J. LAWRENCE

The mortality associated with thermal injury has improved dramatically over the last three decades. Important factors in this progress have been the development of more appropriate fluid resuscitation, topical and systemic antibacterial therapy, burns centre care, earlier burn wound excision and nutritional support (Alexander, 1986). Another factor has been a better understanding and awareness of respiratory complications of inhalation injury and of cutaneous burn injury. It remains a frustration to those involved in the care of burn victims, however, that respiratory complications remain the most common cause of death in burn victims admitted to hospital.

Lung function is not greatly altered by cutaneous burns alone, but respiratory function may be compromised by direct thermal injury or by inhaled products of combustion. The term 'inhalation injury' includes both of these aetiologies of clinical conditions which usually, but not invariably, become apparent in the first 24–48 h of the injury.

Inhalation injury occurs in one-third of all burns admissions. The incidence shows a correlation with the extent of cutaneous burn injury (Thompson et al, 1986). The presence of an inhalation injury greatly increases the mortality for any given total body surface area (TBSA) burn and conversely the mortality of inhalation injury increases with increasing TBSA burn. When associated burns exceed 40% TBSA, the mortality may exceed 70% (Thompson et al, 1986). When early mechanical ventilation is required following combined inhalation and cutaneous injury the mortality may exceed 70% (Tranbaugh et al, 1983). The overall mortality of inhalation injury exceeds 50% in many series (Herndon et al, 1985).

Upper airway obstruction is the most common early respiratory problem. The ability to select safely those patients requiring airway intervention and respiratory support demands a clear understanding of the pathophysiology of inhalation injury, the effects of fluid resuscitation and the usefulness and limitations of a variety of clinical signs and investigations.

After the first 48 h, respiratory problems are predominantly those associated with sepsis, either pulmonary or extrapulmonary, especially of the burn wound. Treatment of these is but one part of the management of the septic, hypercatabolic, immunosuppressed patient often with dysfunction of other vital organs.

## THE FIRE ATMOSPHERE

Victims found dead at the fire scene die from carbon monoxide poisoning and asphyxia due to precipitous falls in ambient oxygen concentration during conflagration. Respiratory tract pathology is commonly absent (Zikria et al, 1972).

A major cause of respiratory injury in immediate survivors of fires is the inhalation of toxic products of combustion of various fuels (Table 1).

**Table 1.** Some toxic products of combustion.

| Fuel | Toxic products |
|------|----------------|
| Polyvinyl chloride<br>  Electrical insulation,<br>  furniture, acrylics, wall<br>  coverings, clothing | Hydrogen chloride<br>Phosgene<br>Chlorine |
| Nylon, wool, silk,<br>polyurethane | Hydrogen cyanide<br>Phosgene<br>Carbon monoxide |
| Petroleum products | Acrolein<br>Acetic acid<br>Formic acid<br>Oxides of sulphur<br>Carbon monoxide |
| Wood, cotton, paper | Acrolein and other aldehydes<br>Formic acid<br>Acetic acid<br>Carbon monoxide |
| Nitrocellulose film | Oxides of nitrogen, formic acid |

The composition of the fire atmosphere depends on the type of fuel, the temperature achieved and the degree of pyrolysis versus oxidation (Purser and Buckley, 1983). Oxidation of wood, cotton and other non-synthetic fuels results in the production of highly irritant and potentially lethal aldehydes. The concentrations of carbon monoxide and hydrogen cyanide (HCN), both common in the fire atmosphere, also vary with fuel type and are higher with pyrolysis at higher temperatures (Purser and Buckley, 1983). Polyvinyl chloride may release 40% of its weight as HCl, and other fuels may also release gases which dissolve in respiratory tract fluid to form strong acids.

The carbonaceous component of the fire atmosphere is not directly harmful but may act as a vehicle for heat and adsorbed toxic products of combustion. A variety of heavy metal salts have been found in soot removed from the lower respiratory tract at autopsy (Birky and Clarke, 1981). The most abundant has been antimony, which when inhaled as the hydride in a concentration of 40 ppm causes death from pulmonary oedema in an animal model. Other metals found include cadmium, lead, copper and zinc. Chu (1982) also found high levels of urinary arsenic in fire victims. The significance of these metals, which come predominantly from synthetic polymers and paints, is unknown.

## PATHOPHYSIOLOGY OF INHALATION INJURY

### Thermal injury

Animal studies have shown the lung parenchyma and subglottic airway to be relatively protected from direct thermal injury (Moritz et al, 1945). Super-heated dry gases entering the nose and mouth have a low heat content and are rapidly cooled by the mucosa before reaching the lower trachea. A degree of thermal injury to at least the upper tracheal mucosa does occur in rare circumstances in immediate survivors of fire. Glottic closure is protective but this mechanism is lost in the unconscious victim. An exception to the sparing of the lower respiratory tract from thermal injury occurs in steam inhalation, when tracheobronchial and alveolar damage may be severe because of the high heat content of water vapour.

The injury ranges from hyperaemia and oedema to frank mucosal ulceration and sloughing. Upper airway obstruction is the most common early major manifestation of inhalation injury and is due to oedema of the false cords but may also involve the true vocal cords. Diffuse supraglottic swelling occurs, and when obstructive symptoms and signs have developed, oedema of the arytenoids, aryepiglottic folds and epiglottis is usually present. Sputum pooling may be the final precipitant of total obstruction.

### Chemical injury

#### Upper airway

Thermal injury is probably the dominant cause of injury to the upper airway, including the nose and mouth, although chemical injury may also occur.

#### Lower airway

Infraglottic injury is essentially a chemical tracheobronchitis which in its mildest forms causes hyperaemia and oedema. There may be a more than 10-fold increase in tracheobronchial blood flow, contributing to oedema (Herndon et al, 1985). Severe injury produces necrosis and sloughing of mucosal shreds which may obstruct small airways. Larger airways may be obstructed by casts containing sloughed mucosa, secretions and neutrophils. Airflow obstruction with wheezing may occur due to true bronchospasm, mucosal oedema or airway plugging. Bronchorrhoea may occur, usually after 24 h or more, and these copious secretions often rapidly become purulent, denoting bacterial tracheobronchitis.

#### Lung parenchyma

Injury to lung parenchyma occurs as a result of alveolar cytotoxicity from inhaled products of combustion, and is associated with surfactant damage, alveolar macrophage depression and microatelectasis. Impaired oxygenation following inhalation injury occurs most commonly as a result of altered ventilation–perfusion ratios (Robinson et al, 1981) but some increase in shunt may also occur (Davies et al, 1983). Early severe pulmonary oedema due to major permeability changes, which is usually fatal, is fortunately uncommon.

## Effects of cutaneous burn and fluid resuscitation

Until recently it was believed that extensive cutaneous burns result in a diffuse capillary leak syndrome involving unburned soft tissue and the lungs. Harms et al (1982) studied a sheep model and demonstrated that no increase in lung permeability occurs. This has been confirmed in other animal models and is supported by the absence of any increase in extravascular lung water during massive crystalloid resuscitation of humans (Tranbaugh et al, 1980). The mistaken fear of producing pulmonary oedema during resuscitation from thermal injury risks inadequate fluid replacement with resultant acute renal failure which is always fatal.

An early decrease in oxygenation accompanied by a fall in lung compliance can occur with extensive burns in the absence of inhalation injury. This appears to result from changes in the calibre of small airways (Demling et al, 1985).

It is now apparent that there is an inverse relationship between the severity of inhalation injury and the adequacy of fluid resuscitation (Herndon et al, 1986). Several studies have demonstrated significantly higher fluid requirements in patients with inhalation injury than in patients with comparable skin burns but without inhalation injury (Navar et al, 1985). When inhalation injury is present, sufficient fluid should be given to produce but not exceed a urine flow of 0.5–1.0 ml/kg/h.

Tranbaugh et al (1983) studied extravascular lung water (EVLW) during crystalloid resuscitation of patients with inhalation injury. They found increases in EVLW to be uncommon, moderate in degree and present only in the most severe cases of inhalation injury.

The often considerable oedema of unburned soft tissue seen in crystalloid resuscitation also involves soft tissue of the neck and pharynx, aggravating oedema already present from inhalation injury. Extensive cutaneous burns therefore pose a greater threat to the injured upper airway, and intubation may be required when it would be unnecessary in smaller burns with the same degree of inhalation injury. Subeschar oedema of the anterior neck may independently jeopardize the airway, and escharotomies should be performed early when deep burns involve the entire anterior neck. Similarly, extensive chest eschar may severely restrict chest expansion and requires early escharotomies.

Claimed advantages of either initial colloid-containing or hypertonic fluids over isotonic crystalloid resuscitation with respect to the severity of respiratory complications are conflicting and inconclusive.

## Carbon monoxide poisoning

Carbon monoxide (CO) is significant in most fire atmospheres, reaching dangerous concentration in enclosed spaces with inadequate ventilation.

CO poisoning is common following domestic fires. Those at special risk of CO poisoning are victims either trapped, e.g. in burning motor vehicles, or unable to escape because of trauma or drug and alcohol intoxication. In one study of fatalities within 6 h postburn, alcohol was found in the blood in 40% of victims and exceeded 0.15 mg % in 13% (Birky and Clarke, 1981).

CO is colourless and odourless, with an affinity for haemoglobin greater than 200 times that of oxygen, and causes a left shift of the oxyhaemoglobin dissociation curve. The toxicity of CO is due not only to impaired oxygen transport but also to its tissue effects (Dolan, 1985). Up to 15% of total body CO is extravascular, where it binds to myoglobin in both cardiac and skeletal muscle and impairs cytochrome oxidase activity. CO binds more rapidly to cardiac myoglobin than haemoglobin, and COHb% therefore underestimates cardiac myoglobin saturation with CO. The major cause of death in CO poisoning is cardiac arrhythmia.

Clinical presentation is summarized in Table 2. Permanent personality change, mental deterioration, incontinence and gait disturbance may follow severe CO poisoning.

**Table 2.** Symptoms commonly associated with various levels of carboxyhaemoglobin (COHb). From Dolan (1985).

| Level of COHb(%) | Symptoms |
| --- | --- |
| 0–10 | Reduced exercise tolerance in chronic obstructive pulmonary disease. |
| | Decreased threshold for angina. |
| 10–20 | Headache, dyspnoea on vigorous exertion. |
| 20–30 | Throbbing headache, dyspnoea on moderate exertion, difficulty with concentration, weakness. |
| 30–40 | Severe headache, dizziness, nausea, vomiting, visual disturbance. |
| 40–50 | Confusion, syncope on exertion. |
| 50–60 | Collapse, convulsions. |
| 60–70 | Coma, frequently fatal. |
| 70 | Coma, death likely. |

The classical cherry-red colour is rarely seen and diagnosis depends upon clinical suspicion and COHb measurement. A nomogram is available which allows estimation of peak levels of COHb at the time of exposure (Clarke et al, 1981). Arterial $pO_2$ is not affected by CO.

The half-life of COHb is 4–5 h breathing air and 40–60 min breathing 100% oxygen. This reduces to 25 min with 100% oxygen at three atmospheres. Early hyperbaric oxygen (HBO) therapy is recommended when coma or neurological signs are present. However, the logistics of HBO therapy when resuscitation of a major burn and/or transfer to the HBO facility are necessary often preclude its use.

The COHb% is not a reliable marker of the severity of inhalation injury but is suggestive. There is some correlation of COHb% with blood cyanide levels, which may reach lethal levels (Clarke et al, 1981). Whether cyanide poisoning results in deaths not attributable to either CO poisoning or severe inhalation injury is unclear. A low COHb% seems, however, to exclude the possibility of significant blood cyanide concentration (Birky and Clarke, 1981).

## PATIENT EVALUATION

### History

The circumstances of the fire are important as most inhalation injuries are sustained in a closed space, although they are not uncommon in open space injuries, especially with burning petroleum products. A history of unconsciousness at the fire scene should alert one to the possibility of carbon monoxide poisoning, drug or alcohol intoxication or head trauma as a cause of this state, and aspiration of gastric contents as a possible consequence. The occurrence of an explosion increases the likelihood of respiratory injury, from either inhalation or blast.

### Clinical examination

Deep central facial burns denote a significant probability of inhalation injury (Brown, 1978) especially in the presence of massively swollen lips, but facial burns occur in only 66% of victims with inhalation injury. Significant inhalation injury invariably accompanies severe oropharyngeal mucosal damage or heat-affected dentures. The presence of cough with carbonaceous sputum is virtually pathognomonic of inhalation injury.

The presence of wheezing on chest auscultation soon after the burn is ominous, usually denoting a severe lower airways injury. 'Chestiness' in a previously normal individual indicates inhalation injury (Brown, 1978). This may be due to upper or lower respiratory tract involvement. Hoarseness and stridor are cardinal signs of upper respiratory tract involvement. It should be noted that stridor has a soft, snoring quality and inexperienced staff may not recognize the ominous portent of these sounds which may herald total obstruction. Peak swelling usually occurs about 24 h postburn and severe obstruction may develop insidiously in that time. For these reasons most units would consider direct examination of the upper respiratory tract whenever the possibility of inhalation injury is suggested by history or physical findings.

### Investigations

#### Fibreoptic bronchoscopy

This procedure may be both diagnostic and therapeutic. It is best performed via the nose, and if intubation is likely to be needed the bronchoscope is first inserted through the endotracheal tube which can then be passed over the instrument. It is important to precede the examination by instillation of a suitable vasoconstrictor to minimize bleeding which may make the procedure impossible. Topical anaesthesia is used and is often aided by impairment of mucosal sensation due to injury. Anaesthetic solution is instilled into the nose then the nasal cavity is painted with cotton swab sticks dipped in 4% lignocaine. The oropharynx and supraglottis are then sprayed with 10% lignocaine. Lignocaine may also usefully be administered by nebulizer and gargle.

Respiratory complications are uncommon when initial bronchoscopic findings are negative, but a repeat examination should be considered when doubt exists. During the immediate postburn period mucosal ischaemia of the lower respiratory tract may falsely suggest lack of involvement of the trachea unless other signs such as adherent soot are present. For this reason, Hunt et al (1975) caution against diagnostic bronchoscopy until cardiovascular stability is achieved. The procedure should, however, only be delayed when there is no concern whatsoever about the possibility of upper airway obstruction. Repeated bronchoscopies may subsequently be necessary for airway toilet when clearance of mucosal slough is difficult. This is suggested by radiological signs of lobar or segmental obstruction.

*Chest x-ray film*

The initial CXR is usually normal even in quite severe injury, and this must not lead to a presumption of absence of inhalation injury. Attention should be given to signs of possible barotrauma following explosions, or of aspiration of gastric contents if loss of consciousness has occurred. The patient involved in trauma may have signs of rib fracture, lung contusion or pneumothorax. As in other forms of critical illness the supine CXR has no place and all CXR films should be taken in the erect position unless hypotension or spinal injury are prohibitive.

When radiological changes of inhalation injury occur they usually become apparent within 24–48 h. Alveolar or interstitial oedema, especially in peri-hilar regions and upper zones, and lobar or segmental collapse are common findings. Opacities occurring after 48 h are likely to represent pulmonary infection (Teixidor et al, 1983).

*Arterial blood gas analysis*

Serial arterial blood gas analysis is essential, initial values poorly discriminating between presence or absence of inhalation injury (Moylan and Chan, 1978). Transient hypoxaemia may occur in the absence of any inhalation injury. Conversely, hypoxaemia may initially be absent despite inhalation injury. Metabolic acidosis in the first 12–24 h usually reflects tissue hypoperfusion but may occur with the cellular hypoxia of CO and cyanide poisoning.

*Carboxyhaemoglobin and cyanide levels*

Carboxyhaemoglobin levels are usually readily obtained but cyanide levels are difficult to obtain in many centres and often only after considerable delay, making this a research tool only.

*Xenon$^{-133}$ lung scan*

Early detection of inhalation injury is possible using xenon$^{-133}$ lung scan. Delayed excretion of intravenously administered xenon occurs in lung regions with small airways obstruction. This is a useful research tool but is logistically difficult during resuscitation.

### Spirometry

Spirometry has been demonstrated (Whitener et al, 1980) to be a useful test in patients able to co-operate and is as useful as more sophisticated tests of respiratory function.

### Electrocardiogram

An ECG should be performed at admission both as a baseline reference and to detect arrhythmia or ischaemia which may reflect CO poisoning, coronary artery disease or hypoxaemia. Continuous ECG monitoring is then employed.

## MANAGEMENT

Early management postburn should include administration of the highest achievable oxygen concentration whenever the possibility of CO poisoning is present. The optimal duration of this treatment is unknown and it should continue after COHb% has fallen to low levels, especially if signs of poisoning persist. Because of the high incidence of paralytic ileus with discomfort and risk of aspiration, a nasogastric tube is essential in all major burns until gastrointestinal function recovers, and is necessary in intubated patients. Continued use of a gastric tube may be required when the mental state is obtunded, or to allow enteral nutrition and titration of gastric pH to 4 or above to prevent stress bleeding.

### The airway

#### Indications for intubation

The earliest major decision concerns the need for endotracheal intubation. This will be determined by signs of airway obstruction or the presence of certain warning signs, the extent of cutaneous burns and anticipated difficulty of intubation if delayed. The presence of a deep central facial burn with major skin burns (i.e. exceeding 30% TBSA) will usually require intubation. Deep central facial burns with smaller total burn may well require intubation unless repeated direct visualization excludes upper airway swelling. Early major swelling of the lips or neck which threatens to make intubation difficult if delayed demands immediate intubation regardless of burn size. Any degree of hoarseness or inspiratory noise in a patient with a significant skin burn is likely to require intubation, and a safe practice would be to intubate electively all such patients.

Another important consideration is transport of the patient to another medical facility, when the slightest indication makes intubation mandatory. Any error of judgement concerning the need for intubation must favour overtreatment to avoid the disastrous consequences of airway obstruction in transit. This principle is no less important when interhospital transport is not necessary.

## Technique

The technique of intubation deserves comment. This will be determined by the experience of the clinician involved, who may not always be familiar with use of the fibreoptic bronchoscope. Inability to assess directly the airway using this tool does not preclude patient care of the highest quality so long as sound principles are followed.

When upper airway obstruction is present the safest approach is awake intubation using the fibreoptic bronchoscope, direct laryngoscopy or blind nasal intubation. The latter technique, which avoids the intense stimulus of laryngoscopy, is better tolerated and is very useful when the operator has considerable experience of the technique. It does not allow direct visual assessment but this is of little consequence once the need for airway intervention is apparent. Muscle relaxants must not be used unless there is certainty of mask ventilation and ability to intubate.

There is general agreement that initial translaryngeal intubation is preferred to tracheostomy unless the latter is the only possible means of access. Extubation is usually possible within a few days, and as seen in other conditions, early complications are fewer with endotracheal intubation than with tracheostomy (Lund et al, 1985). For prolonged respiratory problems, many centres prefer translaryngeal intubation for 3–4 weeks or even longer before performing tracheostomy. When the need for tracheostomy is anticipated, early excision and grafting of neck burns may be considered to allow the procedure to be performed through healing graft rather than deep burn.

Nasotracheal intubation is for several reasons the preferred route. Fixation of the tube is more secure than with an orotracheal tube. A secure method of fixation must be routine when the use of facial adhesive tape may be impossible. A method using a perforated rubber strip which retains the tube connector is shown in Figure 1. The tube should be cut short to improve fixation and avoid endobronchial intubation. Support of spontaneous breathing of the awake patient, which is preferred, is much more satisfactory using the nasal route.

Choice of an appropriate size of endotracheal tube is especially important in burns patients because of the already injured larynx, which may show vocal cord ulceration and oedema for 3–4 weeks. Posterior laryngeal pressure is greatly increased by increasing tube size from 8.00 mm ID to 9.0 mm ID (Lindholm and Carroll, 1975) and autopsy examination shows the normal male and female larynx to accept 'comfortably' a tube size no larger than 8.0 mm ID and 7.0 mm ID respectively (Mackenzie et al, 1982). Spontaneous breathing and suction are satisfactory through tubes of these sizes, provided that circuit resistance is minimal. It is imperative that intracuff pressure does not exceed 1.7 kPa (30 cmH$_2$O), and cuff pressure measurement should be a routine part of respiratory monitoring.

Peak oedema of the airway usually occurs at about 24 h postburn and subsides over the next 2–3 days. The patient should be positioned with head and trunk elevated to facilitate resolution of head and neck oedema. Extubation can usually be successfully undertaken at about day 3–4, when facial swelling is resolving and direct laryngoscopy shows a parallel decrease in mucosal oedema. Mild supraglottic oedema does not contraindicate a trial of extubation, and provided that lung function is good, signs of mild upper airway obstruction may be accepted in the expectation of steady improvement.

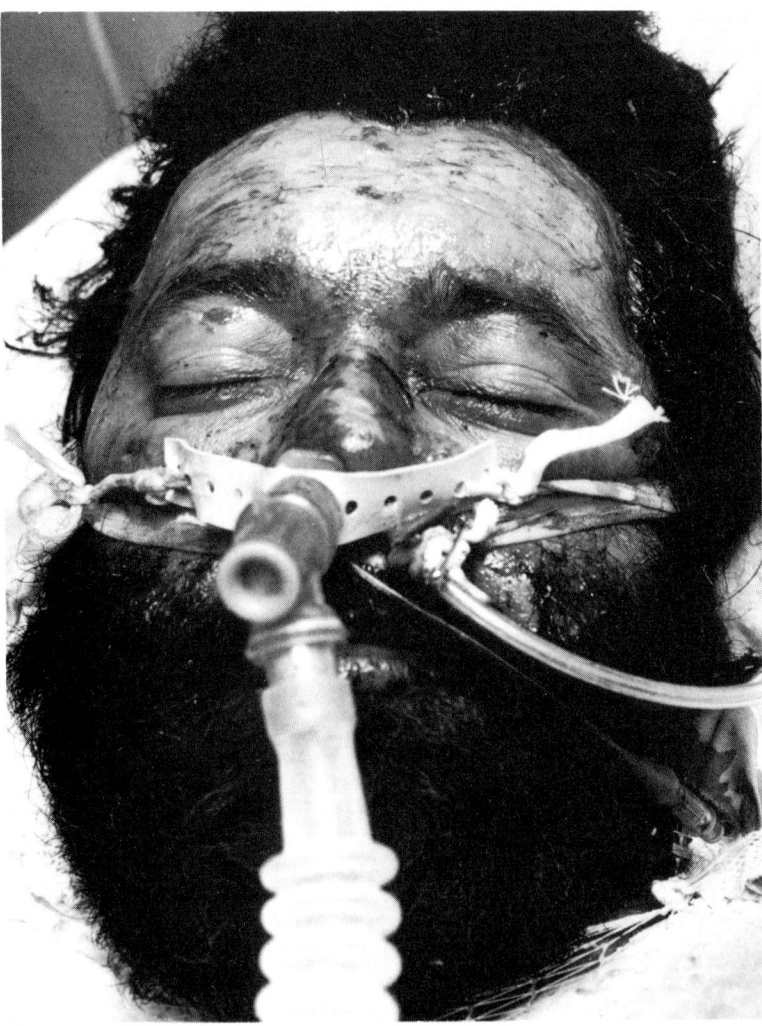

**Figure 1.** Method of fixation of nasotracheal tube using a fenestrated rubber strip which retains the flanges of the connector. The nasogastric tube may also be secured to a separate perforation. Note the Bodai 'Suction-Safe' swivel connector which allows suction without loss of airway pressure, thereby preventing hypoxaemia.

Early tracheostomy is appropriate when mucosal shreds and pseudo-membranes cannot be adequately cleared by endotracheal suction and repeated bronchoscopy including rigid bronchoscopy. Major airway obstruction by casts of such debris with associated secretions can occur in this situation, but their occurrence must also prompt the clinician to ensure adequate humidification by quantification of humidifier performance. During transport of the intubated patient a condenser humidifier should be used.

**Respiratory failure**

Signs of bronchospasm are treated by nebulized salbutamol and intravenous aminophylline. Salbutamol is worth consideration in patients with inhalation injury even when bronchospasm is absent, because of its enhancement of mucociliary transport. It is unknown, however, whether this beneficial effect on ciliary function occurs when diffuse mucosal injury is present.

Respiratory failure is managed along conventional lines. Hypoxaemia requires an appropriate increase in $FiO_2$ and maintenance of lung volume by continuous positive airway pressure (CPAP). CPAP is effective in improving oxygenation and reducing respiratory rate following inhalation injury (Davies et al, 1983) and is the mainstay of treatment of this disorder. In some patients with predominantly smoke inhalation and minor skin burns, management by facemask or nasal CPAP may be possible. More severe injuries will, however, require intubation. There is no evidence that the clinical course is improved by CPAP rather than controlled ventilation, but it is the more logical choice and carries fewer complications (Lawrence, 1986). Pruitt et al (1970) emphasized the possibly disastrous infective consequences of pneumothorax and intercostal drainage in the burned patient, and Lund et al (1985) reported empyema in 3 out of 13 patients with pneumothorax. Avoidance of mechanical ventilation will lessen the incidence of pneumothorax. This author has frequently used, in inhalation injury, CPAP levels of 0.8–1.38 kPa (15–25 cmH$_2$O) and in a few instances 1.7–1.9 kPa (30–35 cmH$_2$O) to achieve a satisfactory $P_aO_2/FiO_2$, without a single instance of clinical or radiological barotrauma. Respiratory acidosis is common, however, following severe injury, and requires adequate additional intermittent mandatory ventilation (IMV).

It is absolutely essential that the circuit used for provision of CPAP and IMV be suitable for that purpose (Lawrence, 1985). Specifically, respiratory work must be reduced, not increased by poor circuit design. This excludes many available ventilators supplying demand flow CPAP. Constant flow CPAP circuits remain the benchmark. Controlled ventilation is certainly preferable to difficult spontaneous breathing through an unsuitable circuit.

*Steroids*

Corticosteroids were once used almost routinely following inhalation injury on the basis of theoretical and anecdotal support. Several animal models have been used to examine their role. Skornik and Dressler (1974) demonstrated decreased lung bacterial clearance and increased mortality following steroid therapy in rats with cutaneous burn but no inhalation injury. In a pure inhalation injury, on the other hand, corticosteroids caused decreased mortality in both rats and rabbits, with unexplained dissociation of lung histopathology and mortality in the rabbit (Beeley et al, 1986). In a goat inhalation model, however, increased small airway obstruction was seen after steroids (Welch et al, 1977). In humans with both isolated inhalation injury (Robinson et al, 1982) and combined inhalation and cutaneous injury (Levine et al, 1978) steroid did not decrease respiratory complications. In one study they were associated with greatly increased infectious complications and mortality (Moylan and Chan, 1978). Without evidence of their benefit it is inappropriate to administer steroids to burned patients when infectious complications may be increased. The only valid indication may be refractory bronchospasm.

### Infection

Antibiotics are used to treat established infection rather than prophylactically. Prophylactic use has not been shown to reduce the incidence of infectious respiratory complications, and selects resistant organisms. Close microbiological surveillance is necessary and daily sputum examination and culture should be routine in inhalation injury. The most common early pathogen is consistently penicillin-resistant *Staphylococcus aureus*. Later infections are usually caused by gram-negative aerobic rods such as *Klebsiella* species and *Pseudomonas* species. Suitable blind treatment while awaiting culture results would be flucloxacillin and an agent active against gram-negatives, such as cefotaxime or an aminoglycoside. It is sensible practice also to administer an oral antifungal agent in the immunocompromised burns patient receiving broad-spectrum antibiotics. When patients are intubated, the mouth can be painted with nystatin several times daily. This could help prevent oesophageal and respiratory tract candidiasis.

Early infection, which is not usually clinically apparent within the first 48 h postburn, is often a tracheobronchitis leading to frank bronchopneumonia. This most commonly develops from the third or fourth day to the seventh day. The onset of purulent sputum accompanied by one or more of rectal temperature above 39°C, toxicity, pulmonary infiltrate, deteriorating oxygenation or increasing leukocytosis, especially above $20 \times 10^9$/l, should prompt careful sputum examination, blood culture and institution of antibiotic therapy. Similarly, any two of the above characteristics should prompt the same actions. The threshold for antibiotic use should be lower following inhalation injury than perhaps is the case in other clinical situations.

## LATE RESPIRATORY PROBLEMS

### Pneumonia

*Incidence*

The single most common respiratory complication after the first 48 h is bacterial pneumonia, which accounts for about 30% of all late burns deaths. Hasleton et al (1983) found evidence of pneumonia in more than half of all patients dying more than 48 h postburn, and the incidence at autopsy increases with time postburn (Sevitt, 1979). The incidence reflects the composition of the patient group at a given institution, and will be influenced by the incidence and severity of inhalation injury, the extent of thermal burns, and age distribution. Robinson et al (1982) reported an incidence of only 1% in isolated smoke inhalation, whereas Eckhauser et al (1974) noted pulmonary sepsis in 36% of patients with burns exceeding 55% TBSA. On the other hand, Linares (1982) found an incidence of pneumonia of only 2.2% in children admitted with burns. Pneumonia is most likely when both inhalation injury and skin burns are present. Tranbaugh et al (1983) found an incidence of pneumonia in these circumstances of 71%.

A factor which may influence the reported incidence of pneumonia is the increased difficulty in making a diagnosis of infection in thermally injured patients. Fever, leukocytosis, altered mentation, altered bacterial flora of the respiratory tract and radiological changes can occur in the absence of infection. A high index of suspicion is required whenever a new or extending pulmonary infiltrate appears on the chest radiograph, and the most likely diagnosis is in fact pneumonia. Good-quality erect chest radiographs using high kilovoltage are essential to detect basal lung consolidation, but in any case clinical examination and auscultation often reveal signs of consolidation prior to obvious radiological change.

*Aetiology*

What are the factors contributing to the high incidence of pneumonia in the burned patient? Pruitt et al (1970) attribute it to improved early survival of patients with inhalation injury, increased use of mechanical ventilatory support as a route of infection, and decreasing burn wound sepsis. The latter was formerly the major cause of death, but with effective topical chemotherapy and earlier excision the balance has swung to pulmonary sepsis. This has resulted in a change in the aetiologies of pneumonia. That study found that prior to the use of topical therapy, two-thirds of pneumonias were haematogenous, but since its introduction only one-third were haematogenous and two-thirds airborne. Haematogenous pneumonia tends to occur relatively late in the clinical course and demands a thorough search for possible primary sites of infection. These include the burn wound, thrombophlebitis of both peripheral and central veins, and endocarditis. Haematogenous pneumonia may present as a nodular pneumonia which then often cavitates but can become confluent and appear similar to the more common airborne bronchopneumonia.

Inhalation injury seriously impairs the lung's ability to respond to infective insults by impairment of mucociliary transport, mucosal damage, alveolar injury and collapse and proteinaceous exudate likely to favour bacterial growth. Impairment of local and systemic immunological mechanisms also occurs in thermally injured patients and favours infection (Alexander et al, 1978). Several weeks after severe inhalation injury the lower airway may still bc covered by squamous epithelium, without the normal protection of mucociliary function (Judkins and Brander, 1986).

Other factors which contribute to bronchopneumonia are impaired laryngeal competence and cough reflex which occur in the sick patient especially during septic episodes, and hypoventilation with lung collapse. Laryngeal incompetence is especially marked in the elderly, but youth is no guarantee against aspiration. Pharmacological suppression of airway reflexes and ventilation may follow excessive analgesia or sedation for dressings, or postoperatively. Supraglottic oedema resulting from both endotracheal and nasogastric intubation will impair swallowing and laryngeal competence, and following prolonged endotracheal intubation it is wise to allow no oral intake for 24 h before cautious trial of water. Episodes of diminished gastric emptying will increase the risk of aspiration, and intensive gastric alkalinization by antacid or histamine antagonist therapy with subsequent bacterial overgrowth may heighten the infective consequences of such events. Published data consistently show a small incidence of major aspiration episodes as a cause of death in burns patients of all ages.

The presence of an endotracheal tube, while allowing beneficial airway pressure therapy and tracheal toilet, increases the infective risk from introduced organisms. Colonization of the lower respiratory tract by those organisms also colonizing the burn wound is almost invariable when artificial airways are present. Thus burn wound surveillance and knowledge of local antibiotic sensitivity patterns will suggest appropriate therapy for new pulmonary infections.

## Pulmonary oedema of sepsis

A significant respiratory problem which occurs after the first few days is that of diffuse interstitial and alveolar infiltrate on CXR with hypoxaemia, the 'adult respiratory distress syndrome'. Large increases in extravascular lung water content in burned patients with or without inhalational injury are usually due to sepsis (Tranbaugh et al, 1983).

### Aetiology

The increased EVLW is due to increased permeability (Adair and Traber, 1979). Wong et al (1985) demonstrated increased sensitivity to endotoxin in the lung of burned animals, with resultant worse lung dysfunction and higher mortality. This condition may occur with extrapulmonary sepsis, with or without bacteraemia, and with pneumonia. It has been suggested but not proven that products of arachidonic acid metabolism and leukocyte activation, which are increased in this disorder, are causally related (Wong et al, 1985).

Aspiration of gastric contents must also be considered as a cause of this syndrome in septic patients. Although initial management of aspiration does not usually include antibiotics, when it occurs as a late complication of burns, intensive therapy for presumed sepsis is usually required.

*Treatment*

The mortality of this condition is high in burns patients, and management must involve a vigorous search for and treatment of extrapulmonary sepsis. Antibiotics should be used even when the source of infection is not immediately identified. Hypoxaemia is corrected by use of CPAP and optimization of cardiac output. The latter is achieved by volume restoration using albumin solutions or blood, inotropic support if indicated and control of supraventricular tachydysrhythmias by digitalization and/or calcium antagonists. Two points regarding these rhythm disturbances, which are very common in the 50+ year age group with sepsis, are worth mentioning. Firstly, dopamine with its high chronotropic activity is relatively contraindicated in the presence of SVT or AF, making adrenaline a better choice when an inotrope is required. Alternatively, dobutamine may be used if significant hypotension is not present. Secondly, when hypotension complicates calcium antagonist therapy, SVT or AF resistant to digitalization may be better controlled with a verapamil infusion of 5–20 mg/h to keep the ventricular rate approximately 100–120 per min.

Renal function is preserved by attention to all these factors and the use of dopamine 0.5–2.0 μg/(kg min). When organ dysfunction is present, be it pulmonary, renal, cardiovascular or other, the overriding concern must be to find and treat sepsis. Excision of infected eschar may improve lung function (Chicarilli et al, 1986).

**Heart disease and failure**

A 'wet' CXR appearance in the burned patient is often attributed incorrectly to cardiac failure or fluid overload, when septic permeability changes or bronchopneumonia are responsible. Administration of a diuretic should not be automatic, nor should it replace a thorough search for sepsis. The correct diagnosis can be extremely difficult and demands careful and repeated clinical and CXR assessment. Echocardiography is useful in assessing left ventricular function and size. When radiological pulmonary oedema is present and LV function appears good on echocardiograph, the diagnosis of non-cardiogenic oedema is likely. Pulmonary artery catheterization only occasionally adds to a careful clinical, radiological and echocardiographic assessment and is an added infection risk.

Echocardiography may demonstrate vegetations on heart valves when endocarditis is present and should be performed routinely when staphylococcal bacteraemia is recurrent or does not rapidly respond to treatment, or when sepsis cannot be explained.

A striking finding in one autopsy study of deaths within 6 h of fire injury was a high incidence of severe coronary artery disease (Birky and Clarke, 1981). Eight of 41 victims younger than 40 had a coronary artery stenosis of greater than 90%, 40% of the entire group had similar lesions and half had in excess of 75% narrowing. Clearly, heart failure and infarction do occur but the former must not be assumed without critical evaluation.

## Pulmonary thromboembolism

Mayou et al (1981) found deep venous thrombosis in 60% and pulmonary embolism in 5.5% of burns autopsies. There is a large variation in reported incidences of pulmonary embolism, from 29% of total admissions and 35% of autopsies (Coleman and Chang, 1975) to only 0.7% of all admissions (Pruitt et al, 1970). It does seem, however, that venous thromboembolism is at least as common following burns as other trauma, although variations in incidence are unexplained.

Immobility and changes in coagulability surely contribute to venous thrombosis, and high utilization of central venous catheters can be a contributing factor. It seems a reasonable but unproven hypothesis that the use of neuromuscular blockers or heavy sedation to facilitate mechanical ventilation may increase venous thrombosis (Lawrence, 1986). This may be an argument for the use of CPAP and IMV in the management of respiratory failure.

Diagnosis requires isotope lung scan and in some instances pulmonary angiography when there is doubt concerning the diagnosis and there are particular risk factors associated with anticoagulation. Significant embolism may occur in the absence of chest pain or haemoptysis, and otherwise unexplained hypoxaemia requires exclusion of an embolic cause. Venography should be considered when central vein thrombosis is suspected clinically, because of the potential for embolization. Anticoagulation imposes special difficulties relating to repeated skin grafting procedures, and a definite need should be established by demonstration of clot.

## Metabolism, nutrition and gas exchange

Metabolic rate is increased after thermal injury, with increased oxygen consumption ($VO_2$), $CO_2$ excretion ($VCO_2$) and minute ventilation. For many years, huge energy loads of 20 800 kJ (5000 kcal) or more, mostly in the form of glucose, were mistakenly administered to fuel this process (Apelgren and Wilmore, 1983). The ability of the burned patient to oxidize glucose is limited (Burke et al, 1979) and excessive glucose intake leads to hyperglycaemia, hepatic dysfunction due to fatty liver and increased cardiovascular stress due to the elevation in $VO_2$. $VCO_2$ also increases excessively and may precipitate ventilatory failure when reserves are poor.

It is now realized that rarely are more than 11 500 kJ/day (2800 kcal/day) required even in the most extensive burns, and by using a daily glucose–lipid mixture the complications of nutritional support can be reduced (Lemoyne and Jeejeebhoy, 1986). During septic episodes, glucose intake should be reduced to 200 g/day or less, and in general a low kJ : nitrogen ratio of 415–500 : 1 (kcal : nitrogen ratio of 100–120 : 1 gram) should be used (Cerra, 1982) until the unhealed burn area is small.

## Influence of respiratory complications on surgery and anaesthesia

Early escharectomy and grafting shortens hospitalization and appears to improve survival in the elderly (Deitch and Clothier, 1983). In a study of 11

American institutions, lower mortality was found with faster burn wound closure (Wolfe et al, 1983). The timing of surgery when inhalation injury or other respiratory complication is present is an important consideration. In the past, lung dysfunction following inhalation injury has been considered a contraindication to surgery, but clearly this can be safely undertaken with careful management (Demling, 1984). We also have found only transiently increased lung dysfunction postoperatively. The chief determinants of whether surgery is appropriate are the ability to oxygenate safely the patient during transport and surgery, and maintain haemodynamic stability. Ventilation with PEEP is often required intraoperatively and during transport. Humidification of inspired gases and heat conservation by warming mattress and blood warmer are essential to maintain ciliary motility and prevent increased postoperative oxygen consumption by shivering. Pulse oximetry is extremely useful when an access site is available and should be considered routine in the daily management, transport and intraoperative care of these patients. Several hours preoperatively the intravenous glucose should be decreased to reduce $VCO_2$, and an intraoperative arterial blood gas determination is desirable in patients with lung dysfunction, especially when pulse oximetry is unavailable. Increased intraoperative minute ventilation is required to excrete the increased $CO_2$ load in the burned patient. Close liaison between anaesthetic and intensive care unit staff is essential to discuss respiratory problems and vascular access and to plan elective postoperative respiratory support. The anaesthetist should maintain strict airway hygiene during intubation and suction, ideally choose a tube of size and design compatible with the unit's protocol, and monitor cuff pressure.

## LATE LUNG FUNCTION AFTER INHALATION INJURY

There have been isolated reports of a variety of respiratory abnormalities following recovery from inhalation injury. These include major airway stenosis, bronchiectasis, endobronchial polyposis, chronic tracheobronchitis, bronchiolitis obliterans and diffusion defect. Squamous metaplasia of tracheobronchial mucosa with bronchiolar stricture formation has been demonstrated at autopsy more than one year after hospital discharge (Chu, 1982).

Unfortunately, the bulk of published follow-up data of respiratory function tests is from firefighters. Detailed follow-up reports of populations of hospitalized fire victims are scarce. Transient hypoxaemia without symptoms is seen in firefighters after smoke exposure, but without adverse lung changes at one month (Tashkin et al, 1977). Longer follow-up of firefighters produced conflicting reports. Loke et al (1980) demonstrated the importance of cigarette smoking as a cause of small airway disease in firefighters, this disorder being present without symptoms in non-smokers only after 25 years of firefighting experience. These authors described one instance of severe obstructive airways disease in a smoker 2½ years after an episode of severe smoke exposure. Peters et al (1974) found conflicting results in Boston firefighters.

Clinical experience is in agreement with the findings of Morris and Spitzer (1973) who found that most survivors of burn injury will usually regain fairly normal lung function. Symptoms such as cough and mild dyspnoea on exertion may occur in the absence of demonstrable abnormality of lung function tests, although clearly there are instances of significant small airways disease which are at times severe. At present such patients cannot be predicted early in the course of the injury. Because of the clear association between cigarette smoking and small airways disease, survivors should be strongly cautioned against smoking.

The effect of different treatment modalities on late lung function is unknown. Steroids have been used to treat bronchiolitis obliterans, although there is no evidence of their efficacy. It is imperative, however, to prevent simple mechanically induced disease such as tracheal stricture and tracho-oesophageal fistula by strict control of intracuff pressure in intubated patients.

## SUMMARY

Inhalation injury occurs in one-third of all burns admissions, with an overall mortality of 50%. Carbon monoxide poisoning, thermal obstructive injury confined to the supraglottic airway, and chemical tracheobronchitis from inhalation of toxic products of combustion may occur. Early severe pulmonary oedema is rare.

The best early clues to inhalation injury are a history of burn in an enclosed space or loss of consciousness, cough with carbonaceous sputum or wheeze and deep central facial burn. Initial CXR films are usually normal, as may be the arterial blood gases. Only the test of time and failure to develop either respiratory symptoms and signs or abnormal investigations can contradict the diagnosis.

Extensive skin burns do not result in increased alveolar-capillary permeability in the lung, but fluid resuscitation of burns aggravate airway but not lung oedema. Inhalation injury significantly increases the volume of resuscitation fluid required.

Great care must be taken to err on the side of overtreatment by intubation (nasotracheal) when there is the slightest indication in major burn injury, unless direct airway inspection suggests otherwise. Respiratory failure is best managed by CPAP and IMV and respiratory toilet of mucosal slough which may obstruct airways. Steroids are of no value and antibiotic use should be therapeutic, not prophylactic.

Respiratory complications occurring after 48 h are most commonly infection-related. Secondary bacterial infection, most commonly with *Staphylococcus aureus*, becomes apparent from days 3–7 postburn. Pneumonia accounts for one-third of all deaths in hospital and occurs in as many as 70% of victims with both inhalation and cutaneous burn injury. Aerobic gram-negative rods are common pathogens. The lung exhibits increased sensitivity to endotoxin after burn injury and large increases in EVLW are usually due to sepsis, often extrapulmonary.

Most survivors of inhalation injury recover normal lung function, but severe small airways obstruction has been reported.


## REFERENCES

Adair TH & Traber DL (1979) Mechanism of pulmonary edema in burn wound sepsis. *Anesthesiology* **51:** S175.

Alexander JW (1986) Burn care: a specialty in evolution—1985 Presidential address, American Burn Association. *Journal of Trauma* **26:** 1–6.

Alexander JW, Ogle CK, Stinnett JD & Macmillan BG (1978) A sequential, prospective analysis of immunologic abnormalities and infection following severe thermal injury. *Annals of Surgery* **188:** 809–816.

Apelgren KN & Wilmore DW (1983) Nutritional care of the critically ill patient. *Surgical Clinics of North America* **63:** 497–507.

Beeley JM, Crow J, Jones JG et al (1986) Mortality and lung histopathology after inhalation lung injury. *American Review of Respiratory Disease* **133:** 191–196.

Birky MM & Clarke FB (1981) Inhalation of toxic products from fires. *Bulletin of the New York Academy of Medicine* **57:** 997–1013.

Brown JM (1978) Inhalation injury and progressive pulmonary insufficiency in a British burns unit. *Burns* **4:** 32–43.

Burke JF, Wolfe RR, Mullany CJ, Mathews DE & Bier DM (1979) Glucose requirements following burn injury. Parameters of optimal glucose infusion and possible hepatic and respiratory abnormalities following excessive glucose intake. *Annals of Surgery* **190:** 274–285.

Cerra FB (1982) Hormonometabolic profiles and the categorisation of surgical stress. *Proceedings of the Metabolic and Nutrition Support for Trauma and Burn Patients Symposium*, 17 July, White Sulphur Springs, West Virginia, pp 29–37.

Chicarilli ZN, Cuono CB, Heinrich JJ, Fichandler BC & Barese S (1986) Selective aggressive burn excision for high mortality subgroups. *Journal of Trauma* **26:** 18–25.

Chu C-S (1982) Burns updated in China: II. Special burn injury and burns of special areas. *Journal of Trauma* **22:** 547–580.

Clarke CJ, Campbell D & Reid WH (1981) Blood carboxyhaemoglobin levels in fire survivors. *Lancet* **i:** 1332–1335.

Coleman JB & Chang FC (1975) Pulmonary embolism. An unrecognised event in severely burned patients. *American Journal of Surgery* **130:** 697–699.

Davies LK, Poulton TJ & Modell JH (1983) Continuous positive airway pressure is beneficial in treatment of smoke inhalation. *Critical Care Medicine* **11:** 726–729.

Deitch EA & Clothier J (1983) Burns in the elderly: an early surgical approach. *Journal of Trauma* **23:** 891–894.

Demling RH (1984) Effect of early burn excision and grafting on pulmonary function. *Journal of Trauma* **24:** 830–834.

Demling RH, Wong C, Li-Juan J et al (1985) Early lung dysfunction after major burns: role of edema and vasoactive mediators. *Journal of Trauma* **25:** 959–966.

Dolan MC (1985) Carbon monoxide poisoning. *Canadian Medical Association Journal* **133:** 392–399.

Eckhauser FE, Billote J, Burke J & Quinby WC (1974) Tracheostomy complicating massive burn injury. A plea for conservatism. *American Journal of Surgery* **127:** 418–423.

Harms BA, Bodai BI, Kramer GC & Demling RH (1982) Microvascular fluid and protein flux in pulmonary and systemic circulation after thermal injury. *Microvascular Research* **23:** 77–86.

Hasleton PS, McWilliam L & Haboubi NY (1983) The lung parenchyma in burns. *Histopathology* **7:** 333–347.

Herndon DN, Thompson PB & Traber DL (1985) Pulmonary injury in burned patients. *Critical Care Clinics* **1:** 79–96.

Herndon DN, Traber DL & Traber LD (1986) The effect of resuscitation on inhalation injury. *Surgery* **100:** 248–251.

Hunt JL, Agee RN & Pruitt BA (1975) Fiberoptic bronchoscopy in acute inhalation injury. *Journal of Trauma* **15**: 641–649.

Judkins KC & Brander WL (1986) Respiratory injury in children: the histology of healing. *Burns* **12**: 357–359.

Lawrence PJ (1985) Alternatives to intermittent positive pressure ventilation (IPPV). *Clinics in Anaesthesiology* **3**: 849–875.

Lawrence PJ (1986) The end of the IPPV era. *Intensive Care World* **3**: 40–41.

Lemoyne M & Jeejeebhoy KN (1986) Total parenteral nutrition in the critically ill patient. *Chest* **89**: 568–575.

Levine BA, Petroff PA, Slade CL & Pruitt BA (1978) Prospective trials of dexamethasone and aerolosized gentamicin in the treatment of inhalation injury in the burned patient. *Journal of Trauma* **18**: 188–193.

Linares HA (1982) A report of 115 consecutive autopsies in burned children: 1966–80. *Burns* **8**: 263–270.

Lindholm C-E & Carroll RG (1975) Evaluation of tube deformation pressure in vitro. *Critical Care Medicine* **3**: 196–199.

Loke J, Matthay RA, Putman CE & Walker-Smith CJ (1980) Acute and chronic effects of fire fighting on pulmonary function. *Chest* **77**: 369–373.

Lund T, Goodwin CW, McManus WF et al (1985) Upper airway sequelae in burn patients requiring endotracheal intubation or tracheostomy. *Annals of Surgery* **201**: 374–382.

Mackenzie CF, Hallisey J, Clark D, Steinberg S & Helrich M (1982) Adult tracheal and laryngeal dimensions as an indicator for correct tracheal tube size. *Anesthesiology* **57**: A500.

Mayou BJ, Wee J & Girling M (1981) Deep vein thrombosis in burns. *Burns* **7**: 438–440.

Moritz AR, Henriques FC & McLean R (1945) The effect of inhaled heat on the air passages and lungs. An experimental investigation. *American Journal of Pathology* **21**: 311–331.

Morris AH & Spitzer KW (1973) Lung function in convalescent burn patients. *American Review of Respiratory Disease* **108**: 989–993.

Moylan JA & Chan C-K (1978) Inhalation injury—an increasing problem. *Annals of Surgery* **188**: 34–37.

Navar PD, Saffle JR & Warden GD (1985) Effect of inhalation injury on fluid resuscitation requirements after thermal injury. *American Journal of Surgery* **150**: 716–720.

Peters JM, Theriault GP, Fine LJ & Wegman DH (1974) Chronic effects of fire fighting on pulmonary function. *New England Journal of Medicine* **291**: 1320–1324.

Pruitt BA, Flemma RJ, DiVincenti FC, Foley FD & Mason AD (1970) Pulmonary complications in burn patients. A comparative study of 697 patients. *Journal of Thoracic and Cardiovascular Surgery* **59**: 7–20.

Purser DA & Buckley P (1983) Lung irritance and inflammation during and after exposures to thermal decomposition products from polymeric materials. *Medicine Science and the Law* **23**: 142–150.

Robinson NB, Hudson LD, Robertson HT et al (1981) Ventilation and perfusion abnormality after smoke inhalation injury. *Surgery* **90**: 352–363.

Robinson NB, Hudson LD, Riem M et al (1982) Steroid therapy following isolated smoke inhalation injury. *Journal of Trauma* **22**: 876–879.

Sevitt S (1979) A review of the complications of burns, their origin and importance for illness and death. *Journal of Trauma* **19**: 358–369.

Skornik WA & Dressler DP (1974) The effects of short-term steroid therapy on lung bacterial clearance and survival in rats. *Annals of Surgery* **179**: 415–421.

Tashkin DP, Genovesi MG, Chopra S, Coulson A & Simmons M (1977) Respiratory status of Los Angeles firemen. One month follow-up after inhalation of sense smoke. *Chest* **71**: 445–449.

Teixidor HS, Rubin E, Novick GS & Alonso DR (1983) Smoke inhalation: radiologic manifestations. *Radiology* **149**: 383–387.

Thompson PB, Herndon DN, Traber DL & Abston S (1986) Effect on mortality of inhalation injury. *Journal of Trauma* **26**: 163–165.

Tranbaugh RF, Lewis FR, Christensen JM & Elings VB (1980) Lung water changes after thermal injury. The effects of crystalloid resuscitation and sepsis. *Annals of Surgery* **192**: 479–490.

Tranbaugh RF, Elings VB, Christensen JM & Lewis FR (1983) Effect of inhalation injury on lung water accumulation. *Journal of Trauma* **23:** 597–604.

Welch GW, Lull RJ, Petroff PA et al (1977) The use of steroids in inhalation injury. *Surgery, Gynecology and Obstetrics* **145:** 539–544.

Whitener DR, Whitener LM, Robertson KJ, Baxter CR & Pierce AK (1980) Pulmonary function measurements in patients with thermal injury and smoke inhalation. *American Review of Respiratory Disease* **122:** 731–739.

Wolfe RA, Roi LD, Flora JD, Feller I & Cornell RG (1983) Mortality differences and speed of wound closure among specialised burn care facilities. *Journal of the American Medical Association* **250:** 763–766.

Wong C, Wenger H & Demling RH (1985) Effect of a body burn on the lung response to endotoxin. *Journal of Trauma* **25:** 53–59.

Zikria BA, Weston GC, Chodoff M & Ferrer JM (1972) Smoke and carbon monoxide poisoning in fire victims. *Journal of Trauma* **12:** 641–645.

# 4

## Anaesthesia for grafting procedures

### CONSTANCE C. M. HOWIE

Anaesthesia for skin grafting of a burned patient may be requested either in the immediate days following the injury in association with primary surgical or tangential excision, or later for grafting on granulation tissue when a burn has been treated conservatively. The requirements for anaesthesia differ sufficiently that the two techniques must be considered separately; the reader will no doubt forgive any necessary repetition that this involves.

## PRIMARY EXCISION AND GRAFTING

### Indications

Primary excision may be indicated for the treatment of small deep burns, thereby achieving early healing, shorter hospitalization, and better cosmetic and functional results. A good example is tangential excision of deep or partial thickness burns of the hand. The burn is shaved with a grafting knife until punctate bleeding indicates that all the dead tissue has been removed. Grafts are then applied to the shaved surface.

In more extensive injuries the object of primary excision is to reduce the total percentage of the injury and diminish the subsequent metabolic upset. There is some evidence (Wolfe et al, 1983) that primary excision achieves a reduction in ultimate mortality. It must, however, be remembered that patients' lives could be put immediately at risk in the operative and postoperative period by this type of surgery. In all but the smallest burns this is major surgery. It causes massive rapid blood loss and is time consuming. The creation of a large donor area increases the heat and fluid loss and the metabolic stress. If the grafts are meshed, as in the bigger burn they commonly would be, this is not counterbalanced by any immediate reduction in the skin defect due to the burn. The patient's condition is not immediately improved. Indeed, in the 48 h following surgery the patient's condition may be more precarious than it would have been had he not been operated on.

Primary excision demands large quantities of blood for transfusion, a team of skilled surgeons, anaesthetists, and nurses, and a high standard of postoperative care. This is no place for an inexperienced surgeon, or an anaesthetist or nurses unfamiliar with the problems. It demands a patient in the optimum possible condition for surgery. If these requirements cannot be met it should be remembered that, whatever its drawbacks, conservative treatment remains an acceptable, and for some patients the only, alternative treatment.

### Timing of surgery

The optimum time for primary excision is from the 3rd to the 5th day postburn. The wound at this time should not be infected, and in the more extensive injuries the patient's condition should have stabilized after the initial 48 h resuscitation period.

Primary excision may commonly be done up to the 8th day postburn. It is generally accepted that by the 10th day postburn the wound will be infected and surgical intervention contraindicated. Surgery of an infected burn is likely to cause increased bleeding which is difficult or impossible to control, and may precipitate invasive infection. The question is occasionally raised whether even earlier excision during the initial resuscitation period might benefit the patient with an extensive burn. However, on present evidence, the addition of sudden blood loss to the continuing colloid loss from the burned surface and the massive fluid shifts taking place would seem to be potentially very hazardous.

### Problems of primary excision

The major problem is the loss of large volumes of blood rapidly during the excision. Added to this is the blood loss from the donor areas. While the greater part of this blood loss will occur during the operation, oozing into the dressings will continue in the postoperative period. In a retrospective study Spijker (1975) found that an average of 100 ml of blood had to be transfused for every 1% of body surface area excised. This is a most useful figure to bear in mind both preoperatively, when assessing the severity of the surgery contemplated and the patient's fitness for it, and intraoperatively as a guide to the volume of blood transfusion required. In this author's hands this has proved to be a very accurate guide. It is very rarely that less blood than this has been required, and occasionally a greater volume has been necessary. The volume of blood needed is more a reflection of the selection of patients for surgery, the timing of the surgery, and the skill and speed of the surgeon than of the anaesthetic technique used.

Heat loss during surgery is also considerable and measures have to be taken to prevent a serious fall in body temperature. Large areas of the body surface have to be exposed at any one time. Wet swabs are usually applied to prevent the burn surface from drying out, and evaporation from these produces further cooling.

The distribution of the burn and the chosen donor areas may make positioning on the operating table difficult or necessitate changes in position. If the face and neck are burned there may be problems with intubation. Access to the vascular bed for transfusion or monitoring is likely to be limited. Postoperative problems may include continued oozing. The fluid balance must be accurately maintained, and blood loss replaced, and the body temperature restored.

### Selection of patients for primary excision

The selection of patients for this type of surgery must be very careful. Many patients admitted to burn units are elderly or suffering from other diseases. These may indeed have been the primary or a contributory cause of the injury. Chronic or acute cardiorespiratory disease, neurological disease, chronic renal impairment, or anaemia may be found to be present. A number of patients may be in poor general condition due to chronic alcoholism or drug addiction, and some may be psychologically or psychiatrically disturbed. A few will be on multiple drug therapy. While some of these patients may be improved sufficiently within the limit of eight days to allow primary surgery, in others this is not possible and conservative treatment has to be the method of choice.

In other patients there may be problems directly related to the burn injury. The presence of pulmonary damage or renal complications are considered by some to be absolute contraindications to immediate surgery (see below, and Chapter 3). In those who have suffered a burn from high-voltage electricity the myocardium is likely to be irritable; there may be irregularities of the pulse, or ECG evidence of myocardial damage. The risks of anaesthesia in these patients are increased.

Patients should not be accepted for anaesthesia for primary excision unless, or until, their general condition is stable. The hourly urinary output should be steady and adequate (between 50 and 100 ml/h in the adult), the pulse, blood pressure and peripheral circulation good, the haemoglobin percentage over 11 g, and the haematocrit and electrolytes normal. In the smallest burns, i.e. those under 5%, there is no more difficulty in assessment than in any other surgical patient. Hypovolaemia would be very unlikely and the surgery is relatively minor.

Burns of between 5% and 15% can be a dangerous trap for the unwary. These are the 'marginal' burns. Excision of a burn of this size is not minor surgery and it should never be contemplated against a background of hypovolaemia, which occurs more commonly than it ought to in this group of patients. The fluid balance, electrolytes and haemoglobin level should be carefully checked. Indeed, if a decision has been taken initially that the patient is likely to be an early candidate for primary excision it may be preferable to give intravenous fluids during resuscitation, rather than relying on oral fluids. This is particularly so in two groups of patients. The elderly, especially if they live alone, are commonly chronically dehydrated on admission to hospital. The dehydrating effects of alcohol must be remembered in those who have sustained their injuries while under the influence of drink. Surgery must be delayed until dehydration has been corrected, and this, particularly in the elderly, may take several days.

The partial early excision and grafting of an extensive burn reduces the total size of the injury, the size of burned surface open to infection and the consequent toxic and metabolic disturbance. It clearly should be beneficial to the patient to reduce a burn of over 50% by 10–25%. This is a common surface area to excise. It may make an almost certainly lethal injury salvageable. Rarely, as much as 40% may be excised but this may create difficulty in obtaining enough donor skin to achieve skin cover. In recent years artificial skins have been developed but they are not yet generally available. These may be invaluable, or even lifesaving, in the future. The use of lyophilized pigskin as a biological dressing is common practice in some centres at this stage.

The presence of renal or pulmonary complications, as mentioned at the beginning of this section, is considered by many to contraindicate early excision. These, as well as pre-existing illnesses, greatly increase the risks involved. While some workers have suggested that early excision results in a lower mortality overall (Wolfe et al, 1983), this should not be seen as giving the all-clear to proceed in the presence of life-threatening complications. Great care, and close liaison within the burns team, are needed. The anaesthetic team should be well-versed in handling this type of patient. Chapter 3 considers briefly the special requirements for early excision in a respiratorily injured patient. The risks of surgery in these gravely ill patients must be balanced by clear evidence of more benefit than would be provided by conservative management—benefit which is not so evident in the literature for these patients as it is for the uncomplicated burn. The presence of infection in the burn wound or cellulitis around it, as evidenced by its appearance or by microbiological report, will also influence the decision for or against early excision.

Once a decision in favour of early excision has been taken, it must be clearly understood by all involved that no firm, irreversible decision can be taken preoperatively about its extent. Greater than average bleeding, difficulty in obtaining haemostasis, or deterioration in the patient's condition which does not respond to treatment, may necessitate curtailing the procedure. The situation should be reassessed after excising approximately 10% surface area. A marked fall in body temperature will also be an indication for caution.

**Intraoperative requirements**

*Duration of surgery*

The operation should be performed in the minimum time possible. The scrub staff should have all the necessary equipment ready, tested, and in working order. Delay while an instrument or a dressing which has been forgotten is obtained is unacceptable. Even the final dressings can be prepared to some extent before the operation starts. It used to be said that the time of surgery should not exceed 1 h. This is a difficult, or even impossible, target for many of the bigger excisions. The longer the operation, the greater is the blood loss and the temperature fall. Thus it may be more possible for a speedy surgeon to excise a larger area safely than one of his slower colleagues. For bigger excisions more than one team of surgeons is required. At least a second team cutting, preparing and if need be, meshing the skin grafts, is necessary, so that time under anaesthesia is not wasted.

### Maintenance of body temperature

The theatre temperature has to be higher than in a standard operating theatre. A temperature of 27–30°C is necessary. This is uncomfortable for the working staff, and a facility for boosting the theatre temperature quickly is an advantage. The theatre can then be kept at an acceptable working temperature for the greater part of the procedure and boosted if the patient's temperature falls, or towards the end of the surgery, to restore body temperature. There should be a warming blanket on the operating table. A circulating water blanket is probably the commonest type in use. All areas of the patient not being operated on at any time should be covered with sterile gamgee. All transfused fluids should be warmed.

### The maintenance of circulating volume

For all but the smallest excisions a freely running drip established prior to the surgery commencing is vital. While in the more extensive excisions two drips may be desirable, it is better to have one good drip than two indifferent ones. The transfusion of blood should start simultaneously with the surgery and if possible keep pace with the loss. Surgery may have to be halted occasionally to achieve this. All transfusions should be filtered and put through a blood warmer. The blood used should be as fresh as possible.

The estimation of blood loss is very difficult. Of necessity it has to be by subjective estimation, which of course is untrustworthy. Almost inevitably the loss is likely to be underestimated. A high proportion of the blood loss will not be on swabs but on the surgeons, the drapes, the operating table, or even on the theatre floor. Wet swabs are extensively used to prevent the excised surface drying out. Gravimetric methods of assessment are therefore contraindicated. Colorimetric assessment of blood loss of this magnitude is unsatisfactory. In our experience the washing machine cannot cope with large blood clots. The final answer will not be available until after the surgery has ended. Either method will give a gross underestimate of the total blood loss. There seems at the present time to be no satisfactory or more accurate alternative to subjective estimation of blood loss together with assessment of the patient's clinical condition. This author again recommends transfusion, on average, of 100 ml of blood for every 1% body surface area excised.

### Monitoring

The distribution of the burn and the chosen donor areas create considerable difficulties in achieving the scientific monitoring to which we have become accustomed in other major surgical cases.

*ECG and pulse monitoring.* These will normally have been established early in the resuscitation period. Usually, enough intact skin can be found to attach adhesive electrodes, but trailing cables to limbs can get in the way of the surgeon and can be easily displaced. Our own preference is to insert stranded stainless steel surgical sutures, either through intact skin or burn eschar, on the chest wall. The sutures are then attached either to a subtrode cable or to the metal clips of the ordinary leads. If the chest wall is to be excised, new sutures can be inserted immediately into the bed of the excision.

### Blood pressure

In the more extensively burned patients it is rare to have a limb available for a sphygmomanometer cuff. Even in burns of about 25% the limbs spared by the injury will commonly be required as donor sites. Invasive arterial monitoring is desirable but may be very difficult to achieve. Its potential value will have to be weighed against the difficulties and dangers of inserting the line through burned oedematous tissue and the effects on the patient of prolonged and possibly unsuccessful attempts to establish it.

*Central venous pressure.* The same problems arise as with arterial lines, though finding a large vein may be slightly easier than finding an artery. As with all drips and lines, surgical manipulations, e.g. elevation of a limb, may interfere with the readings, and the risk of the line becoming dislodged is increased. Good fixation to a burned surface is not easy. If invasive lines are used they may be maintained into the postoperative period. The risk of infective complications in burned patients is high (Warden et al, 1973) and these lines should be removed as soon as the patient's condition is stable.

### Clinical assessment

Even in the presence of sophisticated monitoring aids, the value of clinical assessment of the circulation should not be underestimated. On rare occasions this may be almost the only assessment possible. A peripheral or temporal pulse can usually be found and felt even through burn eschar. The patient's colour and capillary refill can be assessed. With practice, any anaesthetist can acquire skill in assessing capillary refill, which is a very sensitive measure of the state of the circulation. A delay in capillary refill precedes a rise in the pulse rate, which in turn precedes a fall in the blood pressure. These changes precede a fall in the CVP, which is an indication of gross underinfusion and failure of the compensating mechanisms.

### Urinary output

In all but the smaller excisions the patient should be catheterized and an adequate urinary output maintained. Major injuries will already have a catheter in place. If haemaglobinuria occurs, the patient should be given 200 ml of 15% mannitol to produce a diuresis.

*Temperature*

The core temperature should be monitored continuously. Rectal probes usually become displaced early in the procedure, so we have abandoned their use. Oesophageal probes are satisfactory but our own preference is for a tympanic ear probe.

The tympanic temperature is about 0.5 of a degree centigrade lower than the oesophageal. If a satisfactory skin probe can be attached it may be of value, but a core–peripheral difference may be more an indication of cooling than of peripheral circulatory failure.

**Anaesthetic techniques**

There is no one specific technique applicable to these patients. Virtually every anaesthetic technique has been used successfully. The smaller primary excisions present no different problems from any other minor emergency or semi-elective case. With more extensive excisions one is dealing with a patient who has suffered major trauma and who is to undergo major surgery. He may have had a previous anaesthetic for the initial toilet and dressing of the burn wound. A smooth induction of anaesthesia, good oxygenation, and the avoidance of any factors likely to increase bleeding are essential. Muscle relaxation is not necessary other than to achieve intubation. A smooth recovery of consciousness and good analgesia in the postoperative period should be ensured.

*Premedication*

The use of sedative or tranquilizing premedication and the use or omission of antisialogogues is a matter of personal preference. Many of these patients will be having potent analgesics for pain relief and this may influence the choice. If inhalational induction is likely to be used, it may be best to avoid respiratory depressant drugs.

*Induction and intubation*

An intravenous induction with any of the usual agents is acceptable. At this early stage, the use of muscle relaxants, including suxamethonium, is also acceptable and can be a considerable aid to intubation. If the face or neck are involved in the injury, the resultant oedema may make intubation very difficult. In these circumstances an inhalational induction maintaining spontaneous respiration is safer. Halothane will achieve the necessary depth in a reasonable time. Enflurane is a weaker agent, and if it is to be used for intubation the availability of a vaporizer able to give up to 7% is a considerable help. In the author's experience, isoflurane is not a useful agent for intubation nor is trichlorethylene.

A burned face can be protected by swabs or a ring of thin foam. The normal anatomical contours are lost and the face becomes flattened. A soft cuffed non-anatomical face mask will produce a better fit and cause less damage. In the smallest injuries, intubation may not be necessary. In the majority of cases it is indicated because of the duration of surgery and the need at all times to maintain a clear airway, good oxygenation, and no carbon dioxide retention.

## Maintenance of anaesthesia

Many anaesthetists prefer to use a controlled ventilation technique with nitrous oxide and oxygen (Bush, 1972) and supplemental narcotics or neuroleptanalgesics. The use of the closed circuit may help to conserve body temperature. A technique using the inhalational agents and spontaneous respiration is also acceptable. Halothane and more recently enflurane have been widely used. The addition of trichlorethylene, or its use alone in less muscular patients, provides good analgesia which continues into the postoperative period, ensures a smooth recovery, and does not depress the blood pressure or the respiration (Howie, 1972). If it is to be used in combination with one of the other volatile agents as a form of balanced anaesthesia, it is vital that it is not used with soda-lime, and that the trichlorethylene vaporizer is last in line to the patient, to prevent contamination of the other vaporizers with trichlorethylene.

Ketamine causes tachycardia, raises the blood pressure, and increases intraoperative bleeding. Local anaesthetic techniques in other than the smallest injuries have little application for surgery. The burn and the donor area are usually in two completely different anatomical areas.

## Reduction of intraoperative bleeding

The volume of blood lost largely depends on the speed of the surgeon in excising the dead tissue and obtaining haemostasis. A minority of surgeons will excise burns of the distal parts of limbs under tourniquet. The use of gravity to aid venous drainage is of considerable value. Limbs should be elevated during excision. Hypotensive anaesthesia in this group of patients is not popular. In Spijker's cases (Spijker, 1975) the volume of transfusion required in the operative and postoperative periods was the same regardless of the anaesthetic technique used. Hypotensive anaesthesia appeared to alter the timing but not the total blood loss. Szyfelbein (1982), using ganglion blockade or sodium nitroprusside, achieved a reduction in blood loss of 30%, still leaving a massive transfusion requirement. Both he and Brown (1985) feel that this moderate reduction in blood loss has to be weighed carefully against the practical difficulties of monitoring blood pressure. The dangers of a hypotensive technique are obvious in a situation where blood loss is going to be rapid and large in spite of the lowered blood pressure. Some surgeons use swabs impregnated with adrenaline to reduce bleeding from donor areas. This may influence the choice of anaesthetic technique. Relatively new donor area dressings manufactured from seaweed appear to have a haemostatic effect. One gram of ethamsylate given intravenously can reduce capillary oozing from the donor area or from a surface which has been tangentially excised (Richmond and Sutherland, 1986).

*Postoperative care*

Recovery from anaesthesia should be smooth. Good analgesia should be ensured. Donor areas are very painful. Analgesia should be started before the patient recovers consciousness and maintained for the first 48 h postoperatively. Regimes are discussed in Chapter 5.

The intravenous infusion must be maintained for at least 48 h. Urinary output, fluid balance, circulatory state and temperature must be regularly assessed. If bleeding occurs the blood clotting mechanisms should be checked and the blood loss replaced. Even if there is no obvious bleeding, the patient's condition may indicate the need for further transfusion of blood. Even in the most experienced hands, it is not uncommon to have underestimated the intraoperative loss. The haemoglobin and haematocrit should be checked, but the results may be difficult to interpret in the immediate postoperative period. The electrolytes should also be regularly checked. In addition to the normal requirement of free water, allowance will still have to be made for the extra evaporative loss.

Initially the patient should be returned to a well-warmed room. Following rewarming, the temperature may overswing and indicate the need to lower the room temperature or even, on occasion, to use fans or other measures to reduce the pyrexia. Burn dressings can make the patient very warm. A remarkable degree of control of body temperature can be achieved by varying the physical conditions in the environment. Oral and, if necessary, nasogastric tube feeding should be started as early as possible in the postoperative period.

## LATE GRAFTING ON GRANULATION TISSUE

In young patients, if a burn has been treated conservatively the eschar will have separated and granulation tissue grown in 3–4 weeks from injury. The time to the development of healthy granulation tissue increases with age. These patients cannot be 'selected' for surgery and anaesthesia in the same way as patients chosen for primary excision. Donor skin has got to be obtained and the burn wound closed. Smaller burns may be well, but the patient with an extensive injury will be suffering the resultant metabolic disturbance. The burned surfaces will have been infected and the patients will be toxic with a swinging pyrexia and a tachycardia. Their condition will not improve greatly until skin cover is achieved. Many will be very sick indeed and a poor anaesthetic risk may have to be accepted. While the need to obtain skin cover as early as possible is accepted, there is no requirement to accept a patient for anaesthesia who is anaemic, or in fluid or electrolyte imbalance, or who has had above average weight loss and is still losing weight. Not only would the risks of anaesthesia be unacceptably high but a good take of skin grafts would be unlikely. These risks can be considerably reduced by good general management from the time of injury by maintenance of adequate nutrition, a good haemoglobin level, and proper fluid and electrolyte balance. It is vital to have the patient in the optimum condition for surgery.

The presence of an acute chest infection, anaemia, or intestinal disturbance affecting the fluid and electrolyte balance may temporarily contraindicate surgery and anaesthesia. The more extensively burned will require multiple grafting procedures. Occasionally one may have to accept a patient who is on a ventilator or on renal dialysis.

### Problems of surgery and anaesthesia

Many of the problems encountered in the patient having primary excision will continue to be present. Some will be different. The patient's general condition will have deteriorated compared to his condition in the immediate days postburn. During the operative procedure massive blood loss should not occur, the main loss being from the donor areas. Stripping a whole thigh donor area requires a replacement of 500 ml of blood to restore the pre-operative physiological status. A donor area which is being re-used will bleed more than one being used for the first time.

Heat loss during surgery is, if anything, even more marked, as some body fat and its insulating properties has been lost. Granulation tissue is a large capillary bed which, for much of the procedure, is inevitably exposed.

The burned face and neck will no longer be oedematous but contractures may have developed, making intubation increasingly difficult. Friable burns around the lips will bleed readily on even minor trauma.

The available veins will have been used many times for blood sampling and transfusions. Paradoxically, venous access may occasionally be made easier by the diminution of body fat. A selection of cannulae should be available, as relatively small veins and unusual drip sites may have to be used. The largest cannula which can be successfully inserted should be chosen. It is a wise practice to use the most peripheral drip sites first, preserving the more proximal and bigger veins for blood sampling and for use in the future when cannulating the smaller vessels may have become more difficult. Occasionally, the cannula may have to be inserted through burned tissue.

### Preoperative assessment

Some degree of tachycardia and pyrexia may have to be accepted. The haemoglobin percentage should be above 11 g. If it is not, a transfusion should be given and the surgery delayed until 48 h after the transfusion, when the circulation should have stabilized. The electrolytes should be within normal limits. Particular attention should be paid to potassium and sodium levels, which are commonly low in the extensively burned.

Hypovolaemia is an ever-present threat to the burned patient and the biggest single cause of deterioration under anaesthesia. The risk of negative fluid balance continues until skin cover has been achieved. It can develop insidiously. There is continuing loss of water by evaporation from the burned surface. There is increased respiratory loss, and intestinal disturbances are not uncommon. Both the intake and output should be checked. Burned patients have an inevitable osmotic diuresis and may maintain what appears to be a more than adequate urinary output even in the presence of an inadequate intake. If a burned patient's condition deteriorates with the induction of anaesthesia, a degree of hypovolaemia should be suspected. A response to the rapid infusion of 200 ml of Hartmann's solution will confirm the diagnosis and indicate the need for further infusion.

The preoperative assessment of these patients cannot be adequately done by one preoperative visit. The patient should be seen repeatedly over a period of days. In the more seriously ill, the final assessment and decision whether to proceed may only be taken in the hours immediately prior to surgery.

## Intraoperative requirements

### Maintenance of circulating volume

The maintenance of a normal circulating volume should be ensured by a freely running drip. It is commonly said that this should be established prior to the induction of anaesthesia, but this may be unnecessarily unkind to the patient who has already suffered much, especially because gaining venous access in the extensively burned can be very difficult indeed. It is much easier to establish a good drip once the patient is anaesthetized. These patients do not tolerate even minor changes in circulating volume. All but the smallest grafts will require blood transfusion.

### Maintenance of body temperature

Maintaining the body temperature continues to be important. The same precautions should be taken as during primary excision. Most graftings on granulation tissue can be done within approximately 1 h.

If the body temperature is allowed to fall, the patient's condition will give rise to anxiety and will be difficult to assess in the postoperative period. The peripheral circulation will be reduced, and the recovery of consciousness and return to oral feeding delayed. Shivering in an attempt to restore body temperature creates a sudden metabolic demand which puts an unnecessary stress on these often very ill patients.

### Monitoring

The pulse and ECG should be monitored throughout. No limb may be available for a sphygmomanometer cuff. There is little justification for invasive monitoring for this procedure, as blood loss is not likely to be massive; the ultimate morbidity and mortality from invasive lines in burned patients are above average. The core temperature should be monitored continuously. Capnography may be helpful in assuring adequate minute ventilation.

Clinical assessment is all-important. The presence of visible granulation tissue is an added advantage. This is a large capillary bed which will give early indication of the pallor of shock or of poor oxygenation. There may also be recently healed burn in which to assess capillary refill time. The response to the anaesthetic agents can be helpful.

## Anaesthetic techniques

### Premedication

This is a matter of individual preference. The patient by now will be familiar with his surroundings and the staff of the unit. Sedative premedication may not be necessary. The presence of tachycardia may make it desirable to reduce or omit preoperative atropine.

### Induction and intubation

If veins are plentiful then intravenous induction can be used. Caution should be exercised with newer induction agents until their effects on blood pressure and respiration and on repeated exposure are well established. An inhalational induction may have to be used.

Intubation may be indicated because of the distribution of the injuries, the operating position, or difficulties in maintaining a clear airway. Suxamethonium is contraindicated because of the increased risk of cardiac arrest (Bush et al, 1962; Gronert et al, 1969). If a controlled ventilation technique is to be used for maintenance, the longer acting non-depolarizing muscle relaxants may be used. Burned patients become resistant and require an above average dose (Martyn et al, 1980; and see Chapter 6). The exact requirement is difficult to predict, but may be as high as 2½ times normal. D-Tubocurarine and alcuronium have been widely used. It may be best to avoid the muscle relaxants altogether in the more seriously ill patients. If intubation has to be achieved using the inhalational agents, then it should be ensured that the depth of anaesthesia is adequate to block reflexes from the larynx before intubation is attempted.

### Maintenance of anaesthesia

The alternatives are a controlled ventilation technique using muscle relaxants and analgesic supplements or a technique using one of the inhalational agents and maintaining spontaneous respiration. Muscle relaxation is not required by the surgeon. Whichever technique is used, it must be remembered that the patient's metabolic rate is high and so is the alveolar ventilation requirement. Good oxygenation must be ensured and the inhaled oxygen percentage should not be less than 50%. Carbon dioxide retention should be avoided. Minute volume requirement may be as high as twice normal. Multiple anaesthetics may be needed, which may influence the individual anaesthetist's choice of agents.

Ketamine may be of value in the very sick patients, in patients on ventilators, or in the elderly. Following premedication with atropine and pethidine, Sage and Laird (1972) described the use of a 0.1% solution of ketamine in 5% dextrose. 2 mg/kg body weight was administered over a period of 30–60 s for induction. The rate of infusion thereafter was regulated according to the patient's reaction.

Local anaesthetic techniques are again of little value. Local infiltration may be used for smaller grafts in unfit patients. Occasional nerve blocks may be acceptable. Because of the presence of gross infection, epidural or spinal anaesthesia would carry an unacceptable risk; even if the burn does not involve the back, handling a burned patient causes a large increase in the bacterial count in the atmosphere surrounding the patient. Local refrigeration of donor areas has been repeatedly used in very poor-risk patients requiring larger grafts than would be possible under local infiltration (Howie, 1971). At the present time, some success has been claimed for the epicutaneous application of local anaesthetic creams (Ohlsen et al, 1985). These may prove useful in the future. While it may be acceptable in the very poor risk patient to provide only anaesthesia for the donor area, it must be remembered that the granulation tissue itself can be very painful. The patient's comfort will be considerably improved by the simultaneous administration of a carefully titrated dose of a narcotic or benzodiazepine intravenously.

### Postoperative care

A smooth recovery of consciousness without shivering, restlessness or vomiting should be ensured. This is desirable for all patients but vital for the patient with exposed grafts. The patient should again be returned to a well-warmed room. Good analgesia is essential.

The intravenous drip should be discontinued as soon as possible to minimize the risk of infective complications and preserve veins for future use, usually as soon as the necessary blood has been given, unless fluids are needed in patients with exposed grafts, or intravenous analgesia is to be used (see Chapter 5). Respiratory physiotherapy, which should be part of the routine care from the time of injury, will have to be increased in the perioperative period.

### CHILDREN

All the above considerations apply at least equally to children as to adults. It is therefore unnecessary to go into detail on the care of children presenting for burns surgery. The reader is referred to texts of paediatric anaesthesia, or see Sumner and Hatch (1985).

It must, however, be emphasized that all margins for error are smaller in children, and particular attention must be paid to adequate advance preparation. Care in assessing the ease for airway control during anaesthesia, and in assessing and correcting blood loss, are essential. The circulating volume should be estimated prior to anaesthesia (85 ml/kg in infants, 75 ml/kg in children is a useful rule of thumb) and blood carefully replaced as lost. The potential for concealed loss is much greater, as small volumes, say less than 100 ml, are significant.

Major excisions in one procedure will probably require invasive monitoring. They should not be contemplated in a unit which is not very familiar with the problems that can arise. Total or near-total escharectomy such as is carried out in the Shriner's Burns Institutes in the USA is heroic surgery for a highly experienced and specialized paediatric burns team. It is beyond the scope of the average, all-ages burns unit and beyond the scope of this review.

## SUMMARY

The burned patient may require anaesthesia for skin grafting either in the immediate days post-injury in association with primary excision or later for grafting on granulation tissue. Multiple procedures may be required. The distribution or extent of the injury may cause difficulties with gaining venous access, with intubation, and with sophisticated monitoring. Primary excision causes rapid blood loss. Patients should be carefully selected for this type of surgery and their condition stabilized prior to surgery. The timing and duration are of vital importance.

Burned patients requiring later grafting on granulation tissue will have suffered the metabolic and infective consequences of the injury. Their general condition will inevitably have deteriorated and some may be very ill. It should be ensured that they are in the optimum condition for surgery. The ever-present risks of hypovolaemia, electrolyte imbalance, anaemia, and unacceptable weight loss must be remembered. The risks of anaesthesia can be reduced by good basic care from the time of injury and by careful preoperative assessment and preparation. Intraoperatively, during either primary excision or later grafting procedures, the maintenance of circulating volume, the prevention of heat loss, and the clinical skills of an experienced anaesthetist are more important than the actual technique used. Virtually every anaesthetic technique and agent, with the exception of suxamethonium, has been used successfully in burned patients. Postoperatively, the fluid and electrolyte balance should be maintained and good analgesia ensured.

## REFERENCES

Brown JM (1985) Aspects of thermal injury. *Recent Advances in Analgesia and Anaesthesia* **15:** 155–172.
Bush GH (1972) Problems of anaesthesia in the burnt child. *Postgraduate Medical Journal* **48:** 148–151.
Bush GH, Graham HAP, Littlewood AHM & Scott LB (1962) Danger of suxamethonium and endotracheal anaesthesia for burns. *British Medical Journal* **ii:** 1081–1085.
Gronert GA, Dolin LN, Ritchey CR & Mason AD (1969) Succinylcholine induced hyperkalaemia in burned patients, II. *Anaesthesia and Analgesia* **48:** 152–155.
Howie CCM (1971) Refrigeration anaesthesia for donor areas. *British Journal of Anaesthesia* **43:** 616–619.
Howie CCM (1972) General anaesthesia in the adult burned patient. *Postgraduate Medical Journal* **48:** 152–155.
Martyn JAJ, Szyfelbein SK, Ali HH, Matteo RS & Savarese JJ (1980) Increased D-tubocurarine requirements following major thermal injury. *Anaesthesiology* **52:** 352–355.

Ohlsen L, Englesson S & Evers H (1985) An anaesthetic Lidocaine/Prilocaine cream (EMLA) for epicutaneous application tested for cutting split skin grafts. *Scandinavian Journal of Plastic and Reconstructive Surgery* **19**: 201–209.

Richmond JD & Sutherland AB (1986) A new approach to the problems encountered with opsite: systemic ethamsylate. *British Journal of Plastic Surgery* **39**: 516–518.

Sage M & Laird SM (1972) Ketamine anaesthesia for burns surgery. *Postgraduate Medical Journal* **48**: 156–161.

Spijker RE (1975) Anaesthesia for early excision of extensive full thickness burns. *Research In Burns*. Proceedings of the Symposium for Treatment of Burns, Prague 1973, 55–57.

Sumner E & Hatch DJ (eds) (1985) Paediatric anaesthesia. *Clinics in Anaesthesiology*, **3**(3).

Szyfelbein SK (1982) Large burns—a transatlantic view. *Journal of Royal Society of Medicine* **75**(supplement): 26–32.

Warden GD, Wilmore DW & Pruitt BA (1973) Central venous thrombosis: a hazard of medical progress. *Journal of Trauma* **13**(7): 620–626.

Wolfe RA, Roi LD, Flora JD, Feller I & Cornell RG (1983) Mortality differences and speed of wound closure among specialised burn care facilities. *Journal of the American Medical Association* **250**: 763–766.

# 5

# Pain control in burns

## KEITH C. JUDKINS

'Reflection tells me that I am so far from being able satisfactorily to define pain, . . . that the attempt could serve no useful purpose. Pain, like similar subjective things, is known to us by experience and described by illustration.'

So wrote Thomas Lewis in 1942 in the preface to his monograph on pain (Lewis, 1942). His comment sets the scene for any review of pain, pinpointing as it does the central challenge in its study and treatment, that it is a highly subjective and often emotive experience. This is especially true for pain in the burned patient, for whom the fact of being burned may be so devastating that to try to separate psychological from physical pain is unhelpful. The need to be involved in the patient's pain and to try to understand it is paramount.

The aim in this chapter will be to examine the causes of pain in burn injury, whether the result of the injury directly or inflicted necessarily in its treatment; to look briefly at methods of measuring the pain experience; and then to review therapies for pain in different circumstances.

## FACTORS AFFECTING THE PAIN EXPERIENCE

The physical pain felt by a burned patient is influenced by several factors having their origins both within and external to the patient. Anxiety, depression and a sense of helplessness are all seen and these contribute to suffering. Repeated surgical debridement and grafting, wound dressings and infection add to the physical pain and to the destruction of morale.

### Anxiety and depression

It is probably more surprising that depression is not a universal consequence of a serious burn than that it occurs at all. Anxiety about the outcome of the burn, about social status after recovery, about future employment or sexual competence, especially in large burns or burns of the face, hands or genitalia, is inevitable. The seemingly never-ending round of treatments and dressings, the debilitating effects of infection and the lack of freedom from pain or discomfort for several weeks or months, magnify this anxiety so that patients not infrequently become more demanding and irritable as time goes by. The patient has little control over the outcome of his or her anxieties, and so a sense of helplessness can develop.

It cannot help that, according to the available evidence (e.g. Perry and Heidrich, 1982), we do not actually succeed in relieving pain as often or as well as we would like. This accords with this author's experience, although Perry and Heidrich make the valid point that documentation of pain and pain relief is poor.

Nevertheless, in one study using several detailed measures of pain, anxiety and depression, and examining all the above-mentioned factors (Charlton et al, 1983), only one-third of patients were identified as having progressed from these understandable anxieties to depression. The role of medical and nursing communication in minimizing these responses is discussed later.

### Medically inflicted factors

These will be considered in detail along with the methods used to measure, prevent and treat the pain they generate. They include all the necessary but painful things we do to the patient, such as surgery, dressings changes and physiotherapy. Here too, reassurance and communication have a major part to play.

### Infection

The presence of infection in a burn wound will lead to inflammation in the surrounding tissues, the extent of which will vary according to the organism and the degree of colonization. Infection and its treatment are considered in detail in Chapter 8. The treatment of pain from this source is the same as for other pain in burns. The main point to be emphasized here is that a change in the character or severity of the patient's pain may be one of the first indications that infection has become established in the burn wound. Care must then be taken to confirm the diagnosis and institute appropriate antibiotic therapy as well as to provide increased analgesia.

### MEASURING PAIN

The patient's perception of pain is usually a synthesis of all the factors causing distress at the time, pain being predominant. It is important therefore to separate as far as possible the elements that make up the pain experience when measuring how much pain is being suffered and especially when comparing the efficacy of analgesic regimes. These additional factors include the side-effects of the analgesic drugs, some possibly desirable such as euphoria or amnesia, and some undesirable such as nausea, dizziness, undue sedation or psychomimetic effects.

Fuller accounts of methods used are given in textbooks on the treatment of pain. They include descriptive scales: 'none—mild—moderate—severe', and visual analogue scales using a 10 cm line. In assessing the benefit of treatment a 'pain intensity difference' can be derived from the pain assessed before and after treatment. These methods have found wide acceptance as being easy to do, reliable and reproducible. The linear analogue has been well tested in this regard by Revill et al (1976); discussion since then has centred around whether the scale gives best results when drawn vertically or horizontally! A practical snag, easily overcome with imagination, is that when conventionally used it requires the patient to write, which may be impossible if the hands are burned.

The McGill Pain Questionnaire has been used with good effect in burned patients (Charlton et al, 1983). Its particular merit is that it attempts to discriminate between words that describe the sensory element of pain, words that describe affective qualities such as fear and emotion, words that describe the intensity of pain, and other assorted words used by the patient but which do not fit easily into the other three categories. This feature would appear to make it especially suitable for the study of pain in burns, although this author has no personal experience of its use.

Measures of other factors influencing the pain would appear to be important. The visual analogue scale has been used for this purpose (Charlton et al, 1983), as well as for pain. A variety of sophisticated scales for affective experience are to be found in the psychology literature, but it may be thought more prudent to enlist the help of a clinical psychologist if these are to be investigated seriously.

In contrast to the measurement of pain in adults, pain in children has usually been assessed by observers, or, more often, children have been excluded from analgesia studies. An interesting 'pain thermometer' has been described by Szyfelbein et al (1985) which in essence is just a 10-point severity scale which can be held up to view beside the patient's bed. It can be used for any child old enough to understand and to count. The assessment of the affective component of burn pain in children is unlikely to be achieved quite so neatly, however, and the assistance of a child psychologist would probably need to be sought; observation of behaviour may be a worthwhile indicator (Beales, 1982). Szyfelbein et al (1985) have also identified an inverse correlation between the pain experienced by children and plasma $\beta$-endorphin levels, which after more investigation may prove a useful tool for measuring pain in very small children or patients on ventilators.

## THE ACUTE BURN

That the acute burn can be extremely distressing is illustrated by a story told by Ambroise Paré in his 'Apologia and Treatise' (quoted by Murray, 1972). Three French soldiers were found standing against a wall following an assault on Turin, burned from head to toe by a gunpowder explosion. An old soldier, on being told by Paré that nothing could be done for them, gently slit their throats. The soldier, in response to Paré's outrage, declared that if the same thing were to happen to him he prayed to God that someone would treat him likewise.

It would be unwise to attribute all of a patient's distress on being burned to physical pain (Noyes et al, 1971). Initially, a strong psychological reaction to the fact of being burned and to the horrifying accident in which it occurred forms part of the distress.

Physical pain is dependent on the area and the depth of the burn: large-area burns will be more painful than small-area burns; partial thickness burns will be paradoxically more painful than deep full thickness burns, since in the latter many of the nerve endings in and under the dermis have been destroyed; superficial burns can be excruciatingly painful. This rather simplistic categorization must be qualified by the voice of experience, which shouts that few burns fit a single pattern, and that large burns will have some superficial, some deep and some partial thickness areas. Further, there is some evidence, albeit experimental, that destruction of nerve endings as in burned skin leads to hyperalgesia in adjacent areas (Srinivasa et al, 1984; Coderre and Melzack, 1985). Careful assessment of each patient's pain is necessary, with no preconceptions by the clinician. The practice of assuming that a large, full-thickness burn is pain-free, and therefore dressing without analgesia is, I hope, dead and buried.

## First aid

There is no doubt that prompt first aid by cooling can diminish the severity and extent of a burn (reviewed by Davies, 1982). The beneficial effect of cooling in reducing pain has been understood for a very long time. The cutaneous threshold for pain is about $43\,^{\circ}C$, but the risks of hypothermia or frostbite preclude the use of ice-water. Ordinary tap water (usually around $10\,^{\circ}C$) is best and readily available. Steady application of tap water for a period of at least 15 min is now recommended as standard first aid by the British Burn Association (Lawrence, 1987) in its advice to the general public through the voluntary organizations.

## During resuscitation

The priority in this phase is to assess and treat the patient for life-threatening conditions such as fluid loss and respiratory injury, and the treatment of these is considered elsewhere in this volume. The anaesthetist, who uses intravenous analgesics more frequently than most other clinicians and has a lively sense of their problems, can be of great assistance in providing confident pain relief in the acute phase as well as assisting in the resuscitation and monitoring.

Pain relief during resuscitation must be immediate, reliable and safe, and for these reasons opiate analgesia by the intravenous route, titrated against the patient's complaint of pain, is usually given. Sir Cecil Wakeley, in 1944, is reported to have advocated the use of morphine ad lib. in burned patients as 'morphine will never kill a patient in severe pain' (Murray, 1972). His comment carries a grain of truth, as pain is a powerful respiratory stimulant, but the difference between enough and too much is probably very small, so caution is required. Care must also be exercised in that the shocked patient may become more shocked under opiate analgesia, from the hypotensive effect of the drug. General anaesthesia may be the only means of achieving adequate analgesia for this initial dressing, especially in children, and the total oblivion this brings may often be a great kindness for a patient with a large burn.

The intramuscular route for analgesia is inappropriate because the shock of injury and its associated fluid deficit will seriously impair peripheral blood flow in an unpredictable manner. Absorption of the opiate will be impaired initially, making it ineffective; as the circulation improves, the drug may be absorbed much later than intended with detrimental consequences for the patient.

When the respiratory system is injured, any degree of respiratory depression is probably undesirable. It may then be appropriate to use a partial agonist analgesic such as nalbuphine (Fahmy, 1983), in which the extent of respiratory depression is limited. It has a reputedly lower incidence of nausea than conventional opiates, but a small incidence of psychomimetic symptoms similar to those seen with pentazocine has been reported. In the author's experience, this latter symptom may be related to the rate of injection, which should therefore be carried out cautiously over 1 or 2 min. Slow, careful administration should in any case be the norm when intravenous narcotics are being used.

Time spent reassuring the patient that all help is to be given, that painkillers will be administered in adequate doses, that his family is being looked after, that we will keep him informed of all that is to happen to him (and then keeping our promises!), is time well spent. The reduction of tension and anxiety cannot but have a beneficial effect on the total distress and hence on the pain suffered. This is certainly true of the pain of dressing changes (see below).

## MORE CHRONIC PAIN

The moment by moment experience of pain outside the acute phase or the day or two immediately after surgery is probably not very great, although little work is evident in the literature to verify or deny this remark. The sum total of this more chronic element of the burned patient's pain may well be large and potentially demoralizing. In this respect, it probably resembles in character and effect the pain of osteoarthritis or even of terminal cancer. Some of the treatment attitudes applicable to these types of pain may therefore be appropriate (for a review of this approach, see Twycross, 1975), although of course in the burned patient the final prognosis is usually much more optimistic. In particular, the use of regular prophylactic analgesia, supplemented by as required medication, may be of value. In the author's unit, slow release oral morphine (MST) is often effective in patients whose pain is not relieved by as required medication alone. Titration of the dose over a couple of days may be needed, as there is great patient variation in the requirement. A peripherally acting prostaglandin antagonist such as aspirin or paracetamol is usually effective supplementation.

More intractable pain is uncommon. It should be treated vigorously, using if necessary parenteral opiates by infusion or by a patient-controlled syringe driver (see below). The patient who is severely ill with a large burn presents a complex problem of assessing both severity of pain and adequacy of relief; if he is on a ventilator, assessment is even harder, but the solution is easier as generosity with opiates carries fewer risks.

Attention to other details such as anxieties, depression (which may be very difficult to assess by clinical observation), tightness or otherwise of dressings, posture in bed or chair, and generally making a fuss of the patient may well help in reducing the distress voiced in response to pain. It is here that psychological support is of paramount importance, in minimizing helplessness and in teasing out the often hidden anxieties that destroy morale and hence aggravate the subjective attitude to pain. Administrative statistical analysis of staffing levels in a burn unit must take adequate account of this supportive element in nursing, which is difficult to quantify. Access to the services of a clinical psychologist may be helpful (Klein and Charlton, 1980).

## DEBRIDEMENT AND GRAFTING

It goes without saying that surgical procedures are painful. That we inflict several of these on burned patients in as many weeks with hardly a second thought should not blind us to the magnitude of this for the patient. The effect of poorly controlled pain on morale is a problem to be avoided as far as possible. Donor sites may be extremely painful, which will come as a severe surprise to a patient whose burn has not given much pain.

The use of intramuscular opiates on demand is traditional practice for the treatment of any postoperative pain, including that due to skin grafting in burns. Their absorption is, however, unpredictable and involves a delay between administration and effect, so they are not ideal. Demands on nursing time mean that there may also be a significant delay between request for pain relief and its provision, so the relief of pain by this means is inevitably intermittent. Further, the dose required varies considerably from patient to patient (Austin et al, 1980), and even in the same patient at different times, so the response is difficult to predict and impossible to titrate. In contrast with an intravenous infusion, if signs of overdosage occur the injection cannot be switched off so that further absorption and a worsening clinical situation can ensue, although the problem of overdosage is miniscule compared to the inadequate analgesia more usually associated with intramuscular administration.

The handling of opiates by burned patients is not clearly worked out (Martyn, 1986). There may be changes in the pharmacokinetic or the pharmacodynamic responses to these drugs, or the endogenous opioids released in response to injury may alter the responses to exogenous opiates. The need to titrate dose against effect is again emphasized, making the advantage of intravenous administration even more apparent.

### Infusions

Short-acting opiates, such as fentanyl and alfentanil by infusion, provide excellent background pain relief and can be topped up with smaller doses of intramuscular morphine. Fentanyl infusions have been used in the author's unit for patients in whom pain after grafting has been a problem; the syringe driver is set at a starting rate of 0.1 mg/h and adjusted according to the response. An initial bolus of 0.1 to 0.2 mg over a minute may be required if the patient awakes from the anaesthetic in severe pain. Careful observation for respiratory depression is needed. The use of opiates by infusion is described by Church (1979) and Fry (1979). For a more detailed review of the pharmacological background to the use of infusions for analgesia, see Mather (1983).

### Patient-controlled analgesia

Patient-controlled analgesia (PCA) using opiates intravenously has its advocates in the postoperative general surgical patient (Chakravarty et al, 1979). The practical difficulty in applying this method with existing apparatus to patients with burned hands is obvious, but otherwise the use of PCA in burns has not been described. As with any patient-controlled system, inhalational or intravenous, several safety criteria must be met (Evans et al, 1976): the system must be incapable of accidental or half-hearted activation (such as by a drowsy, disorientated patient); the dose and the minimum interval between doses must both be set so that undue sedation or respiratory depression are avoided; personnel supervising the patient must on no account 'help' him or her take a dose (PCA is therefore unsuitable for any patient who cannot activate the machine during a dummy run prior to surgery). If these criteria are fulfilled, PCA may be a potentially very useful tool in burns once the initial cost of the apparatus has been met. PCA syringe drivers are now being marketed that allow a basal continuous infusion which can then be topped up on demand by the patient. Their use in burned patients needs evaluating.

## CHANGE OF DRESSINGS

Exposure treatment of burns is now uncommon so that frequent changes of dressings that have become stuck to large, raw areas of the body are a normal part of the experience of patients in a burns unit. The importance of this aspect of care and the difficulties encountered in trying to minimize the discomfort are emphasized by the observation that the vast majority of papers on treatment of pain in burns address this problem.

Dressing changes are undertaken at varying intervals according to the policy of the particular centre and the treatment regime applied. When antibiotic creams are applied, the effective life of the active ingredient may be as little as 8 h, so that dressing changes every nurse shift change are not uncommon in the USA. More commonly, dressings are changed every 24–48 h (Lowbury, 1974). In many centres, particularly when topical prophylaxis is not used, dressings are left in place for several days on the grounds that bacterial contamination is more likely the more often a dressing is disturbed; when established infection has been demonstrated, dressing changes are undertaken more frequently thereafter. The less frequently a dressing is changed, the more adherent and so the more painful to remove it is likely to be.

## General anaesthesia

If pain is likely to be very severe, general anaesthesia may be the only adequate means of achieving freedom from pain. All the considerations described in Chapter 4 apply; in particular, the strong likelihood of multiple anaesthesia being needed brings into question the use of halothane with its attendant risk of inducing hepatitis. Total intravenous anaesthesia may have a place in this context but its use has yet to be evaluated.

Ketamine has a place, but in the author's experience psychomimetic reactions occur too often for it to be a very useful drug in adults, even when a benzodiazepine is given as well. In children, however, it is very valuable (Ward and Diamond, 1976), and it has even been given orally in subanaesthetic dose with reported good analgesic effect (Morgan and Dutkiewicz, 1983). Ideally, when venous access is possible, it should be given intravenously in a dose of 2 mg/kg, *preceded* by atropine 0.015 mg/kg; the consequences of omitting the atropine have only to be seen once to be never repeated! Alternatively, and less acceptably, a dose of 6–10 mg/kg may be given intramuscularly, again with atropine. Unreliable absorption means that dose control is less certain, and relative overdosage requiring airway support and risking aspiration of gastric contents is more likely. The patient should be starved before ketamine, as for a conventional GA (Diamond, 1982), so disruption of food intake occurs. By whatever means it is given, profound analgesia can persist for a long while after the anaesthetic effect is worn off.

## Mild analgesics and opiates

At the other end of the scale are the patients with small burns for whom reassurance and lots of tender loving care during the dressing procedure are all the analgesia required. Even these patients are often better served by the prior administration of a mild analgesic such as aspirin, if tolerated, or paracetamol. In between these extremes come the vast majority of patients for whom some potent means of providing analgesia is required.

Intramuscular opiates such as papavaretum are sometimes used, and may be all that is necessary for a fairly small burn, or for dressing a donor site, or in the later stages when healing is well under way. Alternatively, they can be used as a background for inhalational analgesia. The disadvantages are as stated elsewhere in this chapter, namely delayed and unpredictable absorption and interference with appetite. These problems are not insurmountable, and may be no problem at all in the minor situations where this method of analgesia is appropriate.

## Neuroleptanalgesia

As for the relief of acute pain, opiate analgesics can be given intravenously. This achieves controlled, potent analgesia with a shorter half-life than intramuscular. The addition of a neuroleptic agent such as droperidol enhances the analgesia and may also help by modifying the affective response to the procedure. Smith and Hollis (1966) describe this technique using droperidol 10 mg intramuscularly or intravenously followed by intravenous phenoperidine 1 mg plus increments of 0.5–1 mg. Baskett (1972) refined the technique by using lower doses of phenoperidine, thus reducing greatly the main problem, respiratory depression; inhalational analgesia was used (Entonox) as a supplement, and the method was successfully adapted for use in children. The main criticism of both these studies is that the assessment of pain, and therefore of the success of the method, is based entirely on the subjective observations of the investigators.

### Demand analgesia

Either on its own or on a background of intramuscular opiate or neuro-leptanalgesia, inhalational demand analgesia has several attractions: it is self-administered, and therefore inherently safe (if the patient gets too much, he drops the device and cannot take more until some has worn off); it is easy to use and does not require an anaesthetist when used alone; analgesia can be increased and decreased to cope with peaks and troughs in pain stimulus, by simply breathing more or less; and it wears off very quickly when the procedure is over. A mask can be used, or a mouthpiece, depending on whether the face is involved in the burn or if the patient does not like masks. There is a strong temptation in practice to try and 'help' the patient whose hands are burned; this must be resisted or at least done with great care because the inbuilt safety of self-administration is bypassed.

Trichlorethylene (Trilene) has been used but has never found favour. Entonox (pre-mixed oxygen and nitrous oxide 50:50) has already been mentioned (Baskett, 1972) in use with neuroleptanalgesia. It is also used on its own in this author's unit for smaller dressings. Methoxyflurane (Laird and Gray, 1971) was effective at 0.3% but is now not used since its toxicity to the kidney has been recognized. More recently, enflurane has been tried with good success (Firn, 1982) using 1% ± 0.25% in air through a drawover vaporizer (Cyprane). There is no experience recorded in the literature of isoflurane used in this way.

The safeguards necessary for the use of demand inhalational analgesia in Britain are well set out in the regulations of the Central Midwives Board, and similar guidelines exist in other countries. They include the provisions that within the error limits laid down the apparatus should deliver the set concentration of agent no matter what attitude the machine is in, and that the apparatus should be incapable of delivering liquid agent to the patient even after complete inversion. These criteria are met by the standard Entonox apparatus and by the Trilene and Penthrane demand vaporizers, but not by the enflurane apparatus. Until this problem is dealt with, an anaesthetist will have to be present when enflurane is used.

## PHYSIOTHERAPY

It is well said, usually by physiotherapists, that the physiotherapist is the person in the burns unit most hated by the patient! Their necessary ministrations can be frequent, demanding and stressful, and may generate much discomfort and frank pain.

Extreme analgesic measures such as general anaesthesia are inappropriate, since co-operation is required. Passive physiotherapy during 'tanking' or saline bathing is less painful than at other times. Otherwise, measures to relieve pain are largely the same as for change of dressings, considered above.

Motivation plays a part here, and the establishment of a good working relationship between patient and physiotherapist is vital. The understanding that he has some control over how much pain he induces in himself, and that the therapy is designed to improve function and hence to get him out, independent and hopefully working, can go a long way to minimizing pain, improving morale and establishing self-confidence.


**CHILDREN**

Children deserve a mention for themselves, as they present subtle but real differences in their perception of pain (Klein and Charlton, 1980). In particular, the presence of pain may be seen indirectly through behavioural changes rather than by direct complaint, especially in very small children. Also, the inability to understand why painful things are done to them can result in them seeing their therapists as ogres (Beales, 1972). There has been relatively little separate investigation of their needs (Elliott and Olson, 1983).

Most treatment of pain in children is woefully inadequate and merely a scaled-down version of adult therapy (Perry and Heidrich, 1982). Behavioural therapies have been used successfully in some centres (Elliott and Olson, 1983; Beales, 1972), including the imaginative use of cartoon films (Kelley et al, 1984). In most centres, the value of time spent with the patient, simple explanation when appropriate, and involvement of parents whenever possible, cannot be overstated (Beales, 1972).


**MISCELLANEOUS**

Other therapies that have been tested include stress inoculation (Wernick et al, 1981), acupuncture (Jichova et al, 1983) and hypnosis (Hammond et al, 1983). The authors claim success but admit that these methods are time-consuming. They will probably find little place in the average burns unit, but are mentioned here so that interested readers may enquire further.


**NUTRITION**

So far in this chapter, no mention has been made of the need to maintain the nutritional intake of the patient. The importance of this is elaborated in Chapter 7 of this volume, but it behoves us here to examine the effect of pain and the measures used to relieve it on the success or otherwise of maintaining adequate dietary intake.

## Control of nausea

Low morale, the presence of hand or face burns making normal feeding difficult, and the presence of even a small amount of background pain, can all impair the appetite. More specifically relevant in this context is the problem of nausea and vomiting induced by the agents used to relieve pain, as these symptoms will mitigate against adequate feeding even by the nasogastric route, the mainstay of nutritional provision in burned patients.

Even slight nausea or loss of appetite is a hindrance to normal eating. If the nausea and vomiting are severe or resist treatment, a gastrointestinal cause should be excluded and the influence of medication examined. The choice of analgesic agents with lower nausea potential is important, especially for oral medication. Aspirin or paracetamol, if adequate, are usually well tolerated. Mixtures containing codeine often provoke nausea and are probably best avoided. Oral opiates such as MST given regularly seem to have a surprisingly low incidence of emetic side-effects (Leslie et al, 1980).

When nausea is apparent from any cause, the administration of an antiemetic such as metoclopramide or, better, prochlorperazine, or a small dose of droperidol, usually helps to minimize the problem. If intravenous opiates are to be used, it may be beneficial to give these agents prophylactically, as anticipation of nausea can be shown to be more effective. Haloperidol 5 mg given with premedication was found to provide potent anti-emesis for up to 24 h postoperatively in abdominal surgery (Judkins and Harmer, 1982).

In one study, the adequate relief of pain was associated with a lower incidence of nausea than partially relieved pain, even though the total dose of opiate was greater, in a group of post-surgical patients (Andersen and Krohg, 1976). Although this work has not been followed up, it reinforces the common subjective clinical observation that the relationship between nausea and dose when using opiates may be anything but linear. The rate of injection of an opiate may also be important for the generation of symptoms such as nausea.

## Dressing changes

Dressing changes, especially when general anaesthesia is used, present special difficulty as the obligatory pre-anaesthetic starvation encroaches significantly on the time available to achieve the required high nutritional intake. There may then be a further loss of time due to drowsiness after an anaesthetic, or after opiate analgesia. Vigilance pays dividends in ensuring that food is presented at other times to make up, and the fine-bore nasogastric tube enables intake to be maintained during the night hours as well as by day in patients in whom appetite is poor or nutritional requirements are high. The importance of meticulous attention to this factor is amply stressed in Chapter 7.

The use of patient-controlled inhalational analgesia as described above for changes of dressings is usually associated with a faster recovery time than anaesthesia or opiates, and so, where appropriately employed, it can benefit the ease of nutritional control for the patient.

## SUMMARY AND CONCLUSION

The pains experienced by a burned patient are complex in origin, very variable in degree but often severe, occur over long periods of time, and can be demoralizing and difficult to treat adequately.

Effective therapies are available, but can be as varied and complex as the pain experience. They require tailoring to the source and type of pain and to the individual patient. Research into improved pain control is taking place and can never be overdone. Meanwhile, personal effort to understand, reassure and control an individual's pain requires time and patience, commodities that are sometimes in short supply in a busy burns unit. Behavioural therapies, whether formal or the informal spin-off of caring attitudes by staff from consultant to cleaner, are at least as important as pharmacological remedies. The importance of maintaining a good nutritional intake in the burned patient must never be forgotten.

## REFERENCES

Andersen R & Krohg K (1976) Pain as a major cause of postoperative nausea. *Canadian Anaesthetic Society Journal* **23:** 366–369.

Austin KL, Stapleton JV & Mather LE (1980) Multiple intramuscular injections: a major source of variability in analgesic response to meperidine. *Pain* **8:** 47–62.

Baskett PJF (1972) Analgesia for burns dressing in children. *Postgraduate Medical Journal* **48:** 138–142.

Beales JF (1982) Factors influencing the expectation of pain among patients in a children's burns unit. *Burns* **9:** 187–192.

Chakravarty K, Tucker K, Rosen M & Vickers MD (1979) Comparison of buprenorphine and pethidine given intravenously on demand to relieve post-operative pain. *British Medical Journal* **ii:** 895–897.

Charlton JE, Klein R, Gagliardi G & Heimbach DM (1983) Factors affecting pain in burned patients—a preliminary report. *Postgraduate Medical Journal* **59:** 604–607.

Church JJ (1979) Continuous narcotic infusions for relief of postoperative pain. *British Medical Journal* **i:** 977–979.

Coderre TJ & Melzack R (1985) Increased pain sensitivity following heat injury involves a central mechanism. *Behavioural Brain Research* **15:** 259–262.

Davies JWL (1982) Prompt cooling of burned areas: a review of benefits and the effector mechanisms. *Burns* **9:** 1–6.

Diamond AW (1982) Analgesia for burns dressing. *Journal of the Royal Society of Medicine* **75**(supplement 1): 33–35.

Elliott CH & Olson RA (1983) The management of children's distress in response to painful medical treatment for burn injuries. *Behavioural Research and Therapy* **21:** 675–683.

Evans JM, Rosen M, MacCarthy J & Hogg MIJ (1976) Apparatus for patient-controlled administration of intravenous narcotics during labour. *Lancet*, Jan., 17–18.

Fahmy NR (1983) Nalbuphine hydrochloride. *Clinics in Anaesthesiology* **1:** 164–167.

Firn S (1982) Enflurane analgesia. *Journal of the Royal Society of Medicine* **75**(supplement 1): 36–39.

Fry ENS (1979) Aspects of anaesthesia: postoperative analgesia using continuous infusion of papavaretum. *Annals of the Royal College of Surgeons of England* **61:** 371–372.

Hammond DC, Keye WR & Grant CW (1983) Hypnotic analgesia with burns: an initial study. *American Journal of Clinical Hypnosis* **26**(1): 56–59.

Jichova E, Konigova R & Prusik K (1983) Acupuncture in patients with thermal injuries. *Acta Chirurgiae Plasticae*, February, 102–108.

Judkins KC & Harmer M (1982) Haloperidol as an adjunct analgesic in the management of postoperative pain. *Anaesthesia* **37:** 1118–1120.

Kelley ML, Jarvie GJ, Middlebrook JL, McNeer MF & Drabman RS (1984) Decreasing burned children's pain behaviour: impacting the trauma of hydrotherapy. *Journal of Applied Behavioral Analysis* **17:** 147–158.

Klein RM & Charlton JE (1980) Behavioral observation and analysis of pain behavior in critically burned patients. *Pain* **9:** 27–40.

Laird SM & Gray BM (1971) Intermittent inhalation of methoxyflurane and trichlorethylene as analgesics in burns dressings procedures. *British Journal of Anaesthesia* **43:** 149–159.

Lawrence JC (1987) British Burn Association recommended first aid for burns and scalds. *Burns* **13**(2): 153.

Leslie ST, Rhodes A & Black FM (1980) Controlled release morphine sulphate tablets—a study in normal volunteers. *British Journal of Clinical Pharmacology* **9:** 531–534.

Lewis T (1942) *Pain*. London: The MacMillan Press Ltd.

Lowbury EJL (1974) Recent advances in controlling infections of burns. *Annali Italiani di Dermatologia Clinica et Sperimentale* **28:** 137–148.

Martyn J (1986) Clinical pharmacology and drug therapy in the burned patient. *Anesthesiology* **65:** 67–75.

Mather LE (1983) Pharmacokinetic and pharmacodynamic factors influencing the choice, dose and route of administration of opiates for acute pain. *Clinics in Anaesthesiology* **1:** 17–40.

Morgan AJ & Dutkiewicz TWS (1983) Oral ketamine. *Anaesthesia* **38:** 293 (letter).

Murray JF (1972) The history of analgesia in burns. *Postgraduate Medical Journal* **48:** 124–127.

Noyes R, Andreasen NJC & Hartford CE (1971) The psychological reaction to severe burns. *Psychosomatics* **12:** 416–442.

Perry S & Heidrich G (1982) Management of pain during debridement: a survey of U.S. burn units. *Pain* **13:** 267–280.

Revill SI, Robinson JO, Rosen M & Hogg MIJ (1976) The reliability of a linear analogue for evaluating pain. *Anaesthesia* **31:** 1191–1198.

Smith GB & Hollis DA (1966) The use of dehydrobenzperidol and phenoperidine for repeated burn dressings. *British Journal of Anaesthesia* **38:** 471–475.

Srinivasa NR, Campbell JN & Meyer RA (1984) Evidence for different mechanisms of primary and secondary hyperalgesia following heat injury to the glabrous skin. *Brain* **107:** 1179–1188.

Szyfelbein SK, Osgood PF & Carr DB (1985) The assessment of pain and plasma beta-endorphin immunoactivity in burned children. *Pain* **22:** 173–182.

Twycross RG (1975) The use of narcotic analgesics in terminal illness. *Journal of Medical Ethics* **1:** 10–17.

Ward CM & Diamond AW (1976) An appraisal of ketamine in the dressing of burns. *Postgraduate Medical Journal* **52:** 222–223.

Wernick RL, Jaremko ME & Taylor PW (1981) Pain management in severely burned adults: a test of stress inoculation. *Journal of Behavioural Medicine* **4:** 103–109.

# 6

## Altered pharmacology in burned patients

CHUNGSOOK KIM
JEEVENDRA MARTYN

A burn injury that covers over 15% of the total body surface area can cause many pathophysiological alterations in the cardiovascular, pulmonary, renal and hepatic systems, as well as fluctuations in plasma protein concentrations. These changes may be due to direct damage to the skin itself or the result of the pathophysiological response of the body to injury. The combined effect induces significant changes in the pharmacokinetics and pharmacodynamics of drugs. This chapter gives an overview of the altered pathophysiology and its influence on pharmacology.

### PATHOPHYSIOLOGICAL CHANGES OF BURN INJURY

#### Cardiovascular factors

The changes in the vascular system of burned patients can be classified into two phases. In the acute (or resuscitative) phase immediately after injury, blood flow to the organs and tissues is decreased (Aikawa et al, 1978). This diminution in blood flow occurs as a result of hypovolaemia, increased viscosity, depressed myocardial function and increased vasoconstriction. In the second phase, the so-called hypermetabolic or recovery phase, the well resuscitated patient usually experiences increased blood flow to the organs and tissues (Goodwin et al, 1980; Martyn et al, 1980).

Decreased blood flow to the organs and tissues can cause altered drug kinetics, especially for high extraction ratio drugs for which the clearance rates are almost exclusively dependent on blood flow through the clearing organ (Wilkinson and Shand, 1975). Moreover, hypovolaemia can result in higher than normal plasma concentrations and effect for a given dose. This situation can be confounded by another element, namely the increased loss of drug through the burn wound, which can effectively decrease plasma concentration and possibly effect (Ziemniak et al, 1984). Except for intravenous administration, absorption (e.g. from gastrointestinal, intramuscular and subcutaneous administrations) may be decreased because of the decreased local blood flow. This can lead to decreased bioavailability and non-linearity of drug absorption, all of which can result in a decreased therapeutic concentration. Another effect of decreased blood flow is an altered clearance rate in the eliminating organs.

In contradistinction, the hypermetabolic phase, in which there is increased blood flow to the organs and tissues, is associated with high total body oxygen consumption, glucose, and protein turnover (Wilmore et al, 1980). The increase in systemic and local blood flow can potentially increase systemic and individual organ clearance rates. Intramuscularly administered drugs may have a rapid absorption. The efficacy and rate of absorption via the gastrointestinal tract is not clear. Finally, changes in circulating and extracellular volume have received little attention but probably are quite variable.

**Protein binding**

Plasma protein concentrations either increase or decrease, depending on the particular protein, the time after burn, and the magnitude of burn (Daniels et al, 1974). The alterations are attributable to various factors, including increased capillary permeability, loss of protein through the burn wound, and/or increased protein synthesis or catabolism (Demling, 1985). Kramer et al (1982) have demonstrated a sharp decrease in total plasma protein concentration after burn, although they did not measure concentrations of specific proteins. Relative to altered pharmacology in burns, two important drug binding proteins have been identified, albumin and alpha$_1$-acid glyco-protein, the latter a component of alpha$_1$-globulin (Martyn et al, 1984). Bloedow et al (1986), studying burned patients with mean body surface burns of 20%, divided their subjects into two groups; the acute stage 6–8 days after burn, and the convalescent stage, about one month after burn. Total protein levels in the first group of burned patients were about 30% lower than normal values. Although the second group also showed lower than control levels, the values did not reach significance. Albumin levels, however, in both groups were about 50% of control, but alpha$_1$-globulin levels in both groups were increased 2–3-fold over control. In the acute phase, gamma-globulin was about 70% of control. The alpha$_1$-acid glyco-protein in the acute phase was about 3-fold higher than the control, but in the later phase it had decreased to 2.3-fold.

The effect of changes in concentrations of the drug binding proteins albumin and alpha$_1$-acid glycoprotein on the plasma binding properties of drugs has also been studied. Using two model drugs, diazepam and imipramine, which bind to albumin and alpha$_1$-acid glycoprotein respectively, it has been documented that the free fraction increases for diazepam while for imipramine the free fraction decreases (Martyn et al, 1984). Therefore, depending on individual binding proteins and time after burn, free drug concentrations in the blood can be increased or decreased. These changes in drug binding have important implications in terms of clearance, volume of distribution, and interpretation of measured plasma concentrations (Greenblatt et al, 1982).

## Apparent volume of distribution

The generalized increase in cell membrane permeability causes continued plasma water loss which results in intracellular swelling and worsening of the hypovolaemia (Harms et al, 1981). The increased microvascular permeability of burned tissues, together with changes in protein components, plays an important role in oedema formation (Kramer et al, 1982; Mullins and Bell, 1982). Although the rate of early fluid loss far exceeds that which would be expected from increased permeability alone, it is suggested that an increase in the interstitial osmotic pressure of burn due to products of tissue destruction aggravates the already present oedema (Leape, 1970). These changes in fluid flux and protein concentration can increase or decrease the apparent volume of distribution, depending on whether the drug is highly bound to protein or if the drug is distributed only in the extracellular fluid. For example, the increased protein binding of d-tubocurarine results in a decreased total volume of distribution of the drug (Martyn et al, 1982b), while the decreased protein binding of diazepam results in an increase in total volume of distribution (Martyn et al, 1983).

## Metabolic rate

The increase in generalized metabolic rate (oxygen consumption) that begins in the second phase of burn is far higher than with other traumas (Wilmore et al, 1978). This hypermetabolic state is associated with protein catabolism, ureagenesis, lipolysis and accelerated gluconeogenesis (Wilmore et al, 1978). Skeletal muscle protein is the principal site of proteolysis. An important contributor to the hypermetabolic state is the increased heat loss occasioned by the impaired barrier of burned skin (Wilmore and Aulick, 1975). Excess hormones, including hydrocortisone, glucagon, and epinephrine constitute another aetiological factor in the hypermetabolic phase (Bessey et al, 1984). For example, a direct correlation can be made between plasma catecholamine concentrations, burn severity and oxygen consumption (Wilmore et al, 1974). The increased proteolysis of skeletal muscle in burn may be due to the increase in protease activity caused by either enhanced enzyme synthesis, or activation or removal of endogenous inhibitors. Odessey (1985) showed that burn may increase the activity of lysosomal or non-lysosomal proteases, change the protease inhibitors, or alter substrate susceptibility. There is little correlation, however, between lysosomal protease activity and increased protein breakdown in muscle. The importance of these changes in skeletal muscle in relation to the altered pharmacodynamics observed for the neuromuscular blocking drugs is unclear.

## Hepatic changes

Major thermal burn injury causes impairment of liver function. Microscopic evidence of congestion, fatty degeneration, and focal necrosis of the liver has been reported (Chen et al, 1985). Czaja et al (1975) showed that 58% of 81 burned patients had acute liver injury, evidenced by abnormal transaminase elevation, with or without bilirubinaemia and jaundice within the first week after burn. The liver damage was observed to occur as early as 24 hours after burn. Hepatic aryl hydrocarbon hydroxylase is another enzyme which has been used clinically as an indicator of hepatic drug metabolizing capacity. After a 15% burn injury, the levels of this enzyme decreased to 62% of control 26 hours after burn, and then decreased further to 43% of control after this period (Ciaccio and Fruncillo, 1979). Similarly, the enzyme p-nitroanisole O-demethylase has been used in conjugation with pento-barbital sleeping time as in vitro and in vivo parameters, respectively, of liver metabolizing capacity (Fruncillo and DiGregorio, 1983). While the enzyme was depressed, the sleep times were prolonged even after a 16% burn injury in the rat. Whether or not changes in this enzyme reflect the clinical activity of both phase I and phase II reactions is unclear. Phase I reactions include oxidation, reduction, hydroxylation and demethylation reactions. The metabolites of phase I reactions can be active (e.g. chloral hydrate) or inactive (e.g. theophylline). If phase I is depressed then in the previous examples the onset of effect of chloral hydrate will be prolonged since only the metabolite is active, while the effect of the theophylline parent compound will last longer because conversion to inactive metabolite is prolonged. Phase II reactions are the conjugation reactions and include acetyl, sulphate, glucuronide and methyl conjugations. The products of conjugation are usually less active (e.g. morphine vs morphine glucu-ronide). As mentioned above, it is evident that consequent to burn-induced hepatic disease the drug clearance can be decreased or increased in com-parison with normal (Williams, 1983).

**Renal changes**

Endogenous creatinine clearance in the kidney, a reflection of glomerular filtration, is increased in burned patients beginning approximately 48 hours after burn and lasting probably until the time when the hypermetabolic state subsides (Loirat et al, 1978). The increase may be due to elevated prosta-glandin and glucagon release (Martyn, 1986). In addition, renal blood flow in burned patients has been shown to be 80% higher than that of normal and the kidney itself about 60% heavier (Goodwin et al, 1980). The increase in renal weight is primarily related to cellular hypertrophy and hyperplasia. Thus, drugs that are filtered in the glomerulus may exhibit enhanced excretion, while tubularly secreted drugs may or may not be dynamically altered.

### THEORETICAL FACTORS AFFECTING PHARMACOKINETICS IN BURN INJURY

Clearance is one of the more important parameters in pharmacokinetics, especially in altered pathophysiological states, because it can be used to characterize drug disposition in patho-physiological context (Gibaldi and Perrier, 1982). Clearance also lends itself to examination by either compartmental or non-compartmental analysis. The old method of compartmental analysis, where individual flow to organs (as a proportion of cardiac output) is taken into account in clearance calculations, is not commonly used at present. All of the pharmacokinetics described below are based on linear, non-compartmental kinetics.

## Clearance

Clearance of a drug from the body usually involves many organs. By definition, total (or systemic) clearance $(Cl_s)$ is the sum of all organ clearances. Therefore, systemic clearance of a drug can be defined as:

$$Cl_s = \frac{dx/dt}{C} = \frac{\int_0^\infty (dx/dt)dt}{\int_0^\infty C_t\,dt} = \frac{D_{iv}}{AUC} \tag{1}$$

where $dx/dt$ is the overall elimination rate of the drug, $C$ is the drug concentration in the blood, $\int_0^\infty (dx/dt)dt$ is the total amount of drug eliminated from time 0 to infinity, which is also equal to the administered dose by intravenous bolus injection $(D_{iv})$, and $\int_0^\infty C_t$ is the total area under the drug concentration in blood versus the time curve $(AUC)$, from time 0 to infinity.

The organ clearance of a drug is defined as the product of the extraction ratio and the blood flow:

$$Cl = Q \cdot \left(\frac{C_a - C_v}{C_a}\right) = Q \cdot ER \tag{2}$$

where $Cl$ is the organ clearance of a drug, $Q$ is the blood flow across the organ, $C_a$ is the drug concentration in the arterial blood entering the organ, $C_v$ is the drug concentration in the venous blood leaving the organ, and $ER$ is the extraction ratio which quantifies the efficiency of the organ with respect to drug elimination under fixed conditions of flow.

If the extraction ratio of the organ does not change before and after burn, clearance of the drug in the organ depends on blood blod. For most drugs, the major elimination organs are liver and kidneys. These two are shown below as examples of organ clearance.

*Hepatic clearance*

Hepatic clearance, $Cl_h$, is the product of the hepatic extraction ratio and the total hepatic blood flow (portal and arterial). It can also be defined as the clearance capacity or intrinsic clearance, $Cl_i'$, of the drug in the liver (Wilkinson and Shand, 1975).

$$Cl_h = Q_h \cdot ER_h = Q_h \cdot \frac{(f_B \cdot Cl_{i,h}')}{(Q_h + f_B \cdot Cl_{i,h}')} \tag{3}$$

where $f_B$ is the fraction free in blood and $Cl_{i,h}'$ is the intrinsic hepatic clearance of free drug. If $Q_h \gg f_B \cdot Cl_{i,h}'$, equation (3) can be expressed as:

$$Cl_h \simeq f_B \cdot Cl_{i,h}' \tag{4}$$

Many drugs, such as antipyrine, most barbiturates, anticonvulsants, hypoglycaemic agents, benzodiazepines, and coumarin anticoagulants, follow equation 4. These drugs are also called restricted or low extraction drugs in respect to their hepatic metabolism because the hepatic clearance of these drugs depends on free fraction of drug found in blood and the intrinsic ability of the liver to eliminate the drug.

In burned patients, changes in hepatic blood flow contribute little to the hepatic clearance of the above drugs listed. However, induction or inhibition of the metabolizing enzymes in the liver do significantly affect the hepatic clearance of these drugs. As indicated previously, there is in vitro evidence of the inhibition of drug metabolizing capacity in burn (Ciaccio and Fruncillo, 1979). Burned patients also experience fluctuations in the free fraction of drugs in the blood (Martyn et al, 1984; Bloedow et al, 1986). Therefore, as shown in equation 4, hepatic clearance of low extraction ratio drugs can be influenced by a change in the free fraction. These changes in metabolizing enzyme capacity and protein binding can be synergistic or antagonistic in their effect on clearance. In burned patients, changes in red blood cell mass may also contribute to clearance by their effect on haematocrit and plasma volume (Davies, 1964).

All of the above examples concern situations in which $Q_h \gg f_B \cdot Cl_{i,h}'$. There are other circumstances in which $Q_h \ll f_B \cdot Cl_{i,h}'$. In such instances the latter equation can then be rewritten as:

$$Cl_h \simeq Q_h \tag{5}$$

Hepatic clearance of the drug now depends mainly on hepatic blood flow. Factors such as enzyme metabolizing capacity and free fraction do not play a role. In other words, the intrinsic ability of the liver to clear drugs is working at maximum level while the limiting factor in the clearance process is the blood flow. Changes in hepatic blood flow in both hypodynamic and hyperdynamic phases of burn injury can therefore contribute significantly to hepatic clearance. Examples of flow-dependent drugs include propranolol and lidocaine, but clinical studies in burned patients have not been performed.

*Renal clearance*

Quite unlike hepatic clearance, renal excretion of a drug can be influenced by three factors; filtration, active secretion, and reabsorption. Therefore, the model for renal clearance is more complicated.

Renal clearance, $Cl_r$, can be defined as:

$$Cl_r = (Cl_{rf} + Cl_{rs})(1 - FR) \tag{6}$$

where $Cl_{rf}$ is clearance due to renal filtration, $Cl_{rs}$ is clearance due to renal secretion, and $FR$ is the fraction of drug filtered and secreted that is reabsorbed. When one considers individual physiological factors that can affect these clearance rates, equation 6 can be described as:

$$Cl_r = f_B \cdot \left( Cl_{cr} + \frac{Q_k \cdot Cl'_{i,k}}{(Q_k + f_B \cdot Cl'_{i,k})} \right) (1 - FR) \tag{7}$$

where $Cl_{cr}$ is creatinine clearance, $f_B$ is the fraction free in blood, $Q_k$ is blood flow to the kidney, and $Cl'_{i,k}$ is the intrinsic renal tubular secretion clearance.

If $Q_k \gg f_B \cdot Cl'_{i,k}$, the renal clearance becomes

$$Cl_r + f_B \cdot (Cl_{cr} + Cl'_{i,k})(1 - FR) \tag{8}$$

In this case, changes in kidney blood flow do not play a role in the renal clearance; rather, renal clearance is a function of the free fraction in the blood; creatinine clearance or rate of filtration in the glomerulus ($GFR$), intrinsic renal tubular secretion clearance, and the fraction of drug filtered and secreted that is reabsorbed. Thus in burned patients, changes of $GFR$, $f_B$, and induction or inhibition of metabolizing enzymes in the kidney may contribute significantly to the renal clearance of the drug.

If $Q_k \ll f_B \cdot Cl'_{i,k}$, renal clearance is expressed as:

$$Cl_r = f_B \cdot (Cl_{cr} + \frac{Q_k}{f_B})(1 - FR) = (f_B \cdot Cl_{cr} + Q_k)(1 - FR) \tag{9}$$

In this case, changes of kidney blood flow, $f_B$ and $Cl_{cr}$ are major contributors to renal clearance in burned patients. However, induction of metabolizing enzymes in the kidney does not affect renal clearance.

**Apparent volume of distribution**

Another important parameter contributing to altered pharmacokinetics is the apparent volume of distribution, defined as *the proportionality constant*, relating drug concentration in blood or plasma to the amount of drug in the body (Gibaldi and Perrier, 1982). The apparent volume of distribution is calculated after some assumptions are made, including instantaneous distribution into vascular space after intravenous administration and first-order elimination at a rate that is proportional to the free drug concentration.

$$Vd = \frac{D_{iv}}{C_o} \tag{10}$$

where $Vd$ is the apparent volume of distribution in a one-compartment model and the apparent volume of distribution of the central compartment in a multicompartment model is $V_c$; $D_{iv}$ is the dose given by intravenous administration; and $C_o$ is the initial drug concentration immediately after intravenous bolus injection. $C_o$ is not useful for other routes of administration. Therefore, the volume of distribution can be calculated from:

$$Cl_s = Vd \cdot K \tag{11}$$

$$\text{or } Cl_s = Vd \cdot \beta \tag{12}$$

where $K$ and $\beta$ are the first-order elimination constants in one-compartment and two-compartment models, respectively. A more useful volume term in a multicompartment model is the apparent volume of distribution at steady state, $Vd_{ss}$, which is independent of drug elimination.

$$Vd_{ss} = \frac{D_{iv}\,[A/\alpha^2) + (B/\beta^2)]}{[(A/\alpha) + (B/\beta)]^2} \tag{13}$$

where A, B are constant values and $\alpha$, $\beta$ are elimination rate constants from curve fitting of the drug concentration–time data after intravenous bolus injection in a two-compartment model,

$$C_t = A \cdot e^{-\alpha t} + B \cdot e^{-\beta t} \text{ or } C_t = \frac{D_{iv}(\alpha - k_{21}) \cdot e^{-\alpha t}}{V_c(\alpha - \beta)} + \frac{D_{iv}\,(k_{21} - \beta) \cdot e^{-\beta t}}{V_c(\alpha - \beta)}$$

The model independent estimation of $Vd_{ss}$ is

$$Vd_{ss} = \frac{D_{iv} \cdot \left[\int_0^x t \cdot C_t \, dt\right]}{\left[\int_0^x C_t \, dt\right]^2} = \frac{D_{iv} \cdot [AUMC]}{[AUC]^2} \tag{14}$$

where $AUMC$ is the area under the first moment, a numerical integration using the trapezoidal rule from concentration–time data, following drug administration of the drug concentration in the blood or plasma curve. In the acute (or resuscitative) phase, water loss through damaged stratum corneum, hyperventilation and fluid resuscitation may cause rapid fluctuations in the apparent volume of distribution.

Under the assumptions described previously, as in equation 10, the volume of distribution can also be expressed simply in a multicompartment model, taking protein binding into consideration (Wilkinson and Shand, 1975):

$$Vd = V_B + \frac{f_B}{f_T} \cdot V_T \tag{15}$$

where $V_B$ is blood volume, $V_T$ is volume of the tissues which combines the volume of the extravascular space plus the erythrocyte volume, $f_B$ is the fraction of free (unbound) drug concentration in blood, and $f_T$ is the fraction of free drug concentration in the tissue space.

From equation 15, the smallest apparent volume of distribution of a drug is blood volume. However, the apparent volume of distribution depends on the ratio of free fractions in the blood and tissues and the volume of tissues when it is larger than the blood volume.

Burned patients may have decreased intravascular albumin levels (as much as 50% of control) and increased alpha$_i$-acid glycoprotein levels (2–3-fold of control). These changes in protein binding can have tremendous influences on the apparent volume of distribution and clearance, especially for drugs that are highly protein bound. We cannot, however, exclude other potential influences, such as pathophysiological alterations in capillary permeability and partition coefficients between drug and proteins.

If a drug with a low extraction ratio is eliminated through the liver only, the systemic clearance $(Cl_s)$ of the drug follows equation 8. Therefore, from equations 1, 3, and 15,

$$\beta = \frac{f_B \cdot Cl'_{i,h}}{V_B + \dfrac{f_B}{f_T} \cdot V_T} \tag{16}$$

Since plasma volume is only about 40 ml/kg, some drugs have an apparent volume of distribution greater than 400 ml/kg, equation 16 becomes

$$\beta \approx \frac{f_T \cdot Cl'_{i,h}}{V_T} \tag{17}$$

Therefore, its half-life becomes

$$t_{1/2} = \frac{0.693 \cdot V_T}{f_T \cdot Cl'_{i,h}} \qquad (18)$$

Equation 18 shows that the half-life of the drug is a function of $V_T, f_T$, and the intrinsic ability to eliminate the drug in the liver. When burn causes changes in tissue volume, tissue binding and activities of metabolizing enzymes, then it is not surprising that the half-life of a drug changes.

## CLINICAL PHARMACOLOGY IN BURNS

As described earlier, pathophysiological changes in burned patients can affect the pharmacokinetics and pharmacodynamics of many therapeutic agents. The aetiology of altered pharmacological responses can be broadly classified into pharmacokinetic and pharmacodynamic changes. Some of these changes in pharmacology are described below.

### Pharmacokinetic changes

#### Antibiotics

Antibiotics are a key therapeutic agent ubiquitous in burned patients because of the common complication of sepsis after the trauma. It is known that dosage requirements for antibiotics (tobramycin, gentamycin, amikacin) in burned patients are usually higher than normal (Loirat et al, 1978; Zaske et al, 1980). Normal doses do not result in adequate therapeutic concentrations because the clearance of antibiotics is increased in burned patients. There are many possible causes for the increased clearance described above. In general, most antibiotics have very low (<10%) protein binding in plasma and are mainly eliminated through the kidneys (Gilman et al, 1980). Thus changes of renal blood flow, creatinine clearance, and the intrinsic clearance of the kidney are key factors to the altered kinetics (see equation 7). Although loss of drug through the burn wound has been documented, loss of drug via this route is not significant compared to the changes in organ clearance.

The study of Loirat et al (1978) of tobramycin in burned patients is a good example of altered pharmacokinetics. Although they did not measure renal clearance of the drug directly, the half-life of the drug was significantly, but inversely, correlated with creatinine clearance. In the study the apparent volume of distribution was increased 1.25-fold but did not reach statistical significance. That is, the decreased half-life is entirely explicable on the basis of increased systemic clearance ($t_{1/2} = 0.693 \cdot Vd/Cl_s$) which occurs mainly via renal elimination. This is confirmed by the fact that these patients had a mean increase of 38% in the rate of glomerular filtration.

#### Cimetidine

The incidence of Curlings ulcer is very high in burned patients and some have life-threatening gastrointestinal haemorrhage. These acute stress ulcers are more common in children than in adults. The antisecretory drug, cimetidine, is extensively used to ameliorate this sequel of burn. In healthy people, the bioavailability of an oral dose is approximately 62%, with 19% binding to the plasma proteins. The normal dose has a high volume of distribution and is eliminated mainly (about 78% of the dose given) as parent drug via the kidney. Because of the relatively low plasma protein binding of the drug, the changes in protein binding are not critical to the pharmacokinetics, but changes in renal function can significantly affect the elimination kinetics. Systemic clearance of the drug is about five times that of the glomerular filtration rate. This finding indicates that renal secretion is an important step in the elimination process (following equation 7).

The dosage requirement and pharmacokinetics of cimetidine in adult burned patients are related to the time after burn and burn size. In the early stage, about 18 hours after burn, urinary tubular excretion of the drug is decreased (Ziemniak et al, 1984). Non renal (or metabolic) clearance, however, is increased about 2-fold over control. The creatinine clearances in these subjects during the first 48 hours were normal ($126 \pm 46$ ml/min in burned patients and $108 \pm 22$ ml/min in control). Despite this, the urinary excretion of cimetidine was impaired in burned patients because of impaired tubular secretion related to blood flow (equation 9), as indicated by a ratio of renal cimetidine clearance to creatinine clearance of about 2.2 compared with 4.2 in healthy subjects, suggesting impairment of tubular secretion after burn injury.

In the hyperdynamic phase of burn, cimetidine elimination is increased and the usual doses are less effective. The mean renal clearance of cimetidine in burned patients is increased about 2-fold. The increase in clearance was directly proportional to the burn size. A gastric pH greater than 4 is maintained, however, as long as the plasma concentration of cimetidine is kept above 0.5 µg/ml, the therapeutic concentration in normals (Martyn et al, 1985). Thus for cimetidine, the pharmacokinetics are altered but the pharmacodynamics are not. The clinical implications are that the dose, renal function and response have to be closely monitored.

## Diazepam

Benzodiazepines such as chlordiazepoxide, diazepam and lorazepam are commonly used in burned patients. All have high plasma protein binding properties ($>90\%$), are eliminated mainly by hepatic metabolism, and have low metabolic restricted clearances (Gilman et al, 1980). The pharmaco-kinetics of benzodiazepine drugs are dependent on both protein binding (mostly to albumin) and intrinsic clearance in the liver. First, protein binding is an important factor since an increase in the free fraction can lead to enhanced re-uptake by the metabolizing enzymes. The increase in free fraction can also increase the effect of the drug at target organs. The second factor, the intrinsic clearance of the drug, can be measured in vitro and can be used to predict the hepatic extraction ratio (Rane et al, 1977), which depends not only on the quantity of enzyme but also on the affinity of the enzyme for the drug. Intrinsic clearance can be influenced by pathophysio-logical changes of burn on the liver and by other factors, including drugs which might cause enzyme induction or inhibition (Klotz and Reimann, 1980).

The pharmacokinetics of diazepam serve as a representative example of the benzodiazepines. Martyn et al (1983), studying pharmacokinetics of diazepam, documented an increased half-life and apparent volume of distribution in burned patients while systemic clearance was unchanged. The free fraction was also increased 2.8-fold in burned patients. Despite the increase in free fraction, the intrinsic clearance was decreased. That suggests an impairment of the metabolizing enzyme capacity either due to burn or to concomitantly administered drugs.

## Pharmacodynamic changes

### Muscle relaxants

Muscle relaxants are used in burn patients, both in the intensive care setting and in the operating room. The aberrant pharmacological responses to both depolarizing and non-depolarizing relaxants in burned patients have been reported by many investigators (Gronert and Theye, 1975; Martyn et al, 1986). Administration of depolarizing relaxants such as succinylcholine (suxamethonium) in burned patients can induce a massive potassium release from the muscle cell that may result in lethal hyperkalaemia. The ensuing hyperkalaemia is related to the dose of succinylcholine, time after burn, and degree of burn injury (Martyn et al, 1986). Similar patterns of hyperkalaemia have also been reported in denervated and paraplegic patients (Gronert and Theye, 1975).

With non-depolarizing muscle relaxants such as d-tubocurarine, metocurine, pancuronium and atracurium, however, burned patients show hyposensitivity (Martyn et al, 1986). The $ED_{95}$ dosage requirement is increased from 2.5- to 5-fold in burned patients. The shift in the dose-response curve for the non-depolarizing muscle relaxants is correlated to both time after burn and the magnitude of burn injury. The resistance to non-depolarizing muscle relaxants reaches a maximum about 2 weeks after burn, continues for many months in patients with major burn, and decreases gradually with healing of the burn wound. The resistance in some patients has persisted for over a year after complete healing of the burn (Martyn et al, 1982a).

The aetiology of the altered response is probably multifactorial, but mainly points to changes in target organ sensitivity. As indicated previously, there is an increase in plasma binding of drugs, which includes the muscle relaxants (Leibel et al, 1981). This component can only partly explain the hyposensitivity to non-depolarizing muscle relaxants, but more importantly cannot account for the lethal hyperkalaemia following succinylcholine. The pharmacokinetics of d-tubocurarine also cannot completely explain the hyposensitivity response, since the urinary excretion increases only at 24 hours and not at 6 hours, and the volume of distribution in the central compartment is only minimally elevated (Martyn et al, 1982b). The other pharmacokinetic parameters are comparable in both controls and burned patients.

Kim et al (1986), in the rat burn model, have now reported that there is an increase in the number of nicotinic acetylcholine receptors in the diaphragm following a cutaneous burn, and that the receptor number decreases to control levels with healing of the burn wounds. The increase in acetylcholine receptors is not as high as in denervated animals (Merlie and Sanes, 1985). Quite unlike the denervated situation, however, where only the affected muscle expresses an increase in acetylcholine receptors, with burn there appears to be a generalized increase in acetylcholine receptors. Kim et al (1986) have also documented a decrease in the slope in burned animals compared with controls in the dose-response curve of d-tubocurarine. This finding is suggestive of change also in the type or nature of the receptors at the muscle membrane. The increase in receptor number, which is similar to denervation has been confirmed clinically by the use of electromyography. Mills et al (1986) have confirmed evidence of denervation-like changes in the muscle beneath burn areas. The increase in acetylcholine receptors (denervation-like syndrome) can explain both the hypersensitivity to succinylcholine and the hyposensitivity to non-depolarizing relaxants.

## SUMMARY

Pathophysiological alterations in burned patients result in many pharmaco-therapeutic difficulties. The major responsible factors include changes in cardiovascular dynamics, protein binding, volume of distribution, and altered intrinsic clearance. First, changes in blood flow to organs and tissues result in altered clearance, especially for high clearance drugs, which are dependent on blood flow. Also affected are drug absorption and bioavailability of intramuscular, oral, or subcutaneously administered drugs. Secondly, changes in protein binding can affect clearance of restricted drugs as well as the volume of distribution. Thirdly, intrinsic clearance may be changed by hepatotoxic or nephrotoxic effects of burn or by the administration of exogenous substances used in the therapy of burns. Finally, the changes in intrinsic clearance play a key role, especially in the renal and hepatic biotransformation of low-clearance drugs.

In addition to the altered pharmacokinetics, altered pharmacodynamics complicate and confound drug therapeutics in burned patients. Although some recent evidence suggests changes in target organ receptors, the mechanisms which induce these changes at distant sites are unknown. Neuronal and hormonal mediators may be involved. The state of nutrition also affects pharmacodynamics and pharmacokinetics. Pharmacotherapy in burns is complicated and should be closely monitored both in terms in toxic effects and adequacy of response.

## REFERENCES

Aikawa N, Martyn JAJ & Burke JF (1978) Pulmonary artery catheterization and thermo-dilution cardiac output determination in the management of critically burned patients. *American Journal of Surgery* 135: 811–817.

Bessey PQ, Watters JM, Aoki TT & Wilmore DW (1984) Combined hormonal infusion simulates the metabolic response to injury. *Annals of Surgery* **200:** 264–280.

Bloedow DC, Hansbrough JF, Hardin T & Simons M (1986) Postburn serum drug binding and serum protein concentrations. *Journal of Clinical Pharmacology* **26:** 147–151.

Chen Y, Li N, Shi J, Li Y & Davies JWL (1985) Histopathological and ultrastructural changes in liver tissue from burned patients. *Burns* **11:** 408–418.

Ciaccio EI & Fruncillo RJ (1979) Decreased aryl hydrocarbon hydroxylase after a 15% burn injury. *Biochemical Pharmacology* **28:** 3151–3152.

Czaja AJ, Rizzo TA, Smith WR & Pruitt BA (1975) Acute liver disease after cutaneous thermal injury. *Journal of Trauma* **15:** 887–894.

Daniels JC, Larson DL, Abston S & Ritzmann SE (1974) Serum protein profiles in thermal burns: I. Serum electrophoretic patterns, immunoglobulins, and transport proteins. *Journal of Trauma* **14:** 137–162.

Davies JWL (1964) Blood volume changes in patients with burns treated with either colloid or saline solutions. *Clinical Science* **26:** 429–444.

Demling RH (1985) Burns. *New England Journal of Medicine* **313:** 1389–1398.

Fruncillo RJ & DiGregorio GJ (1983) The effect of thermal injury on drug metabolism in the rat. *Journal of Trauma* **23:** 523–529.

Gibaldi M & Perrier D (1982) *Pharmacokinetics*, 2nd edn. New York: Marcel Dekker. 477 pp.

Gilman AG, Goodman LS & Gilman A (1980) *The Pharmacological Basis of Therapeutics*, 6th edn. New York: Macmillan publishing. 1843 pp.

Goodwin CW, Aulick LH, Becker RA & Wilmore DW (1980) Increased renal perfusion and kidney size in convalescent burn patients. *Journal of the American Medical Association* **244:** 1588–1590.

Greenblatt DJ, Sellers EM & Koch-Weser J (1982) Importance of protein binding for the interpretation of serum or plasma concentrations. *Journal of Clinical Pharmacology* **22:** 259–263.

Gronert GA & Theye RA (1975) Pathophysiology of hyperkalemia induced by succinylcholine. *Anesthesiology* **43:** 89–99.

Harms BA, Bodai BI, Smith M et al (1981) Prostaglandin release and altered microvascular integrity after burn injury. *Journal of Surgical Research* **31:** 274–280.

Kim C, Fuke N & Martyn J (1987) Burn injury in the rat causes increased nicotinic acetylcholine receptors and hyposensitivity to d-tubocurarine. *Clinical Pharmacology and Therapeutics* **41:** 193.

Klotz U & Reimann I (1980) Delayed clearance of diazepam due to cimetidine. *New England Journal of Medicine* **302:** 1012–1014.

Kramer GC, Harms BA, Bodai BI, Demling RH & Renkin EM (1982) Mechanisms for redistribution of plasma protein following acute protein depletion. *American Journal of Physiology* **243:** H803–H809.

Leape LL (1970) Initial changes in burns: tissue changes in burned and unburned skin of rhesus monkeys. *Journal of Trauma* **10:** 488–492.

Leibel WS, Martyn JAJ, Szyfelbein SK & Miller KW (1981) Elevated plasma binding cannot account for the burn related d-tubocurarine hyposensitivity. *Anesthesiology* **54:** 378–382.

Loirat P, Rohan J, Baillet A et al (1978) Increased glomerular filtration rate in patients with major burns and its effect on the pharmacokinetics of tobramycin. *New England Journal of Medicine* **299:** 915–919.

Martyn J (1986) Clinical pharmacology and drug therapy in the burned patient. *Anesthesiology* **65:** 67–75.

Martyn JAJ, Snider MT, Szyfelbein SK, Burke JF & Laver MB (1980) Right ventricular dysfunction in acute thermal injury. *Annals of Surgery* **191:** 330–335.

Martyn JAJ, Matteo RS, Szyfelbein SK & Kaplan RF (1982a) Unprecedented resistance to neuromuscular blocking effects of metocurine with persistence after complete recovery in a burned patient. *Anesthesia and Analgesia* **61:** 614–617.

Martyn JAJ, Matteo RS, Greenblatt DJ, Lebowitz PW & Savarese JJ (1982b) Pharmacokinetics of d-tubocurarine in patients with thermal injury. *Anesthesia and Analgesia* **61:** 241–246.

Martyn JAJ, Greenblatt DJ & Quinby WC (1983) Diazepam kinetics in patients with severe burns. *Anesthesia and Analgesia* **62:** 293–297.

Martyn JAJ, Abernethy DR & Greenblatt DJ (1984) Plasma protein binding of drugs after severe burn injury. *Clinical Pharmacology and Therapeutics* **35:** 535–539.

Martyn JAJ, Greenblatt DJ & Abernethy DR (1985) Increased cimetidine clearance in burn patients. *Journal of the American Medical Association* **253:** 1288–1291.

Martyn J, Goldhill DR & Goudsouzian NG (1986) Clinical pharmacology of muscle relaxants in patients with burns. *Journal of Clinical Pharmacology* **26:** 680–685.

Merlie JP & Sanes JR (1985) Concentrations of acetylcholine receptor mRNA in synaptic regions of adult muscle fibres. *Nature* **317:** 66–68.

Mills A, Schriefer T & Martyn JAJ (1986) Electromyographic studies in patients with thermal injury. *Anesthesiology* **65:** A294 (abstract).

Mullins RJ & Bell DR (1982) Changes in interstitial volume and masses of albumin and IgG in rabbit skin and skeletal muscle after saline volume loading. *Circulation Research* **51:** 305–313.

Odessey R (1985) Characteristics of burn-induced proteolysis in skeletal muscle. *Progress in Clinical and Biological Research* **180:** 615–617.

Rane A, Wilkinson GR & Shand DG (1977) Prediction of hepatic extraction ratio from *in vitro* measurement of intrinsic clearance. *Journal of Pharmacology and Experimental Therapeutics* **200:** 420–424.

Wilkinson GR & Shand DG (1975) A physiological approach to hepatic drug clearance. *Clinical Pharmacology and Therapeutics* **18:** 377–390.

Williams RL (1983) Drug administration in hepatic disease. *New England Journal of Medicine* **309:** 1616–1622.

Wilmore DW, Long JM, Mason AD, Skreen RW & Pruitt BA (1974) Catecholamines: mediator of the hypermetabolic response to thermal injury. *Annals of Surgery* **180:** 653–668.

Wilmore DW, Mason AD, Johnson DW & Pruitt BA (1975) Effect of ambient temperature on heat production and heat loss in burn patients. *Journal of Applied Physiology* **38:** 593–597.

Wilmore DW & Aulick LH (1978) Metabolic changes in burned patients. *Surgical Clinics of North America* **58:** 1173–1187.

Wilmore DW, Goodwin CW, Aulick LH et al (1980) Effect of injury and infection on visceral metabolism and circulation. *Annals of Surgery* **192:** 491–502.

Zaske DE, Cipolle RJ & Strate RJ (1980) Gentamicin dosage requirements: wide interpatient variations in 242 surgery patients with normal renal function. *Surgery* **87:** 164–169.

Ziemniak JA, Watson WA, Saffle JR et al (1984) Cimetidine kinetics during resuscitation from burn shock. *Clinical Pharmacology and Therapeutics* **36:** 228–233.

# 7

## Nutrition of the burn patient

ANNE B. SUTHERLAND

Since Cuthbertson (1934) first described the metabolic changes subsequent to trauma, many investigators have studied and described their effect on the patient with burn injury. It soon became evident that because of these changes nutritional care would be an important part of total care and could influence both morbidity and mortality. It was apparent that the magnitude of the changes was greater and of longer duration following burning than in almost any other situation.

### THE BURN PROBLEM

As the extent and depth of the burn increases, its metabolic effects become progressively more severe. In practice the patients at risk will be adults with over 15–20% of the body surface involved, while in children a burn of 10% of the body surface or less may have nutritional significance.

#### Significant effects of the response to the injury

*Nitrogen*

There will be a prolonged period of negative nitrogen balance during the catabolic phase following injury. If a protein-containing solution is used in resuscitation there will be a very short period of positive balance followed rapidly by a strongly negative balance, the degree and duration of which will increase with the severity of the burn both in its extent and depth. Commonly this will continue for 3–4 weeks, even in those for whom a high nitrogen intake is provided. Over such a period there will be a net loss of protein. Thereafter the balance becomes strongly positive as the anabolic phase takes over and this too is maintained for several weeks (Figure 1).

*Sodium and potassium*

The initial infusion will provide a large sodium load and for about one week the balance is strongly positive, often in the face of a low serum sodium. Thereafter sodium losses are high and may require replacement. The potassium balance follows the pattern of the nitrogen.

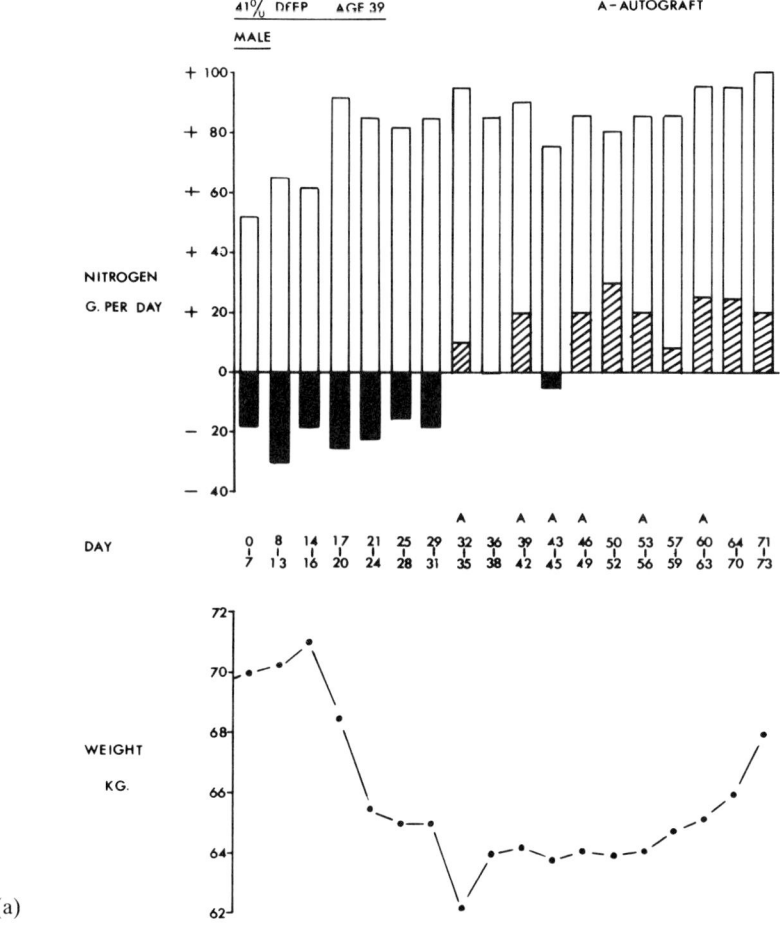

**Figure 1.** Typical nitrogen balance and weight curve following moderately severe burn injury. (a) Adult. (b) Child.

## Calories

Studies of metabolic rate in the major burn show a dramatic increase. This rise has not been shown to be related to increased thyroid activity and its aetiology is not fully understood. Wilmore et al (1974) consider that the catecholamines are in part the calorigenic mediators responsible for the hypermetabolic response. Barr et al (1968) and Arturson (1978) consider it is due to the large evaporative losses from the burn wound. Whatever the cause, the increased metabolism will impose high energy demands, to meet which sufficient calories must be provided.

Weight loss will accompany these changes and is greatest over the first 2–3 weeks. Thereafter it should level out and show a slow but continuing rise during anabolism to reach pre-injury level (Figure 1).

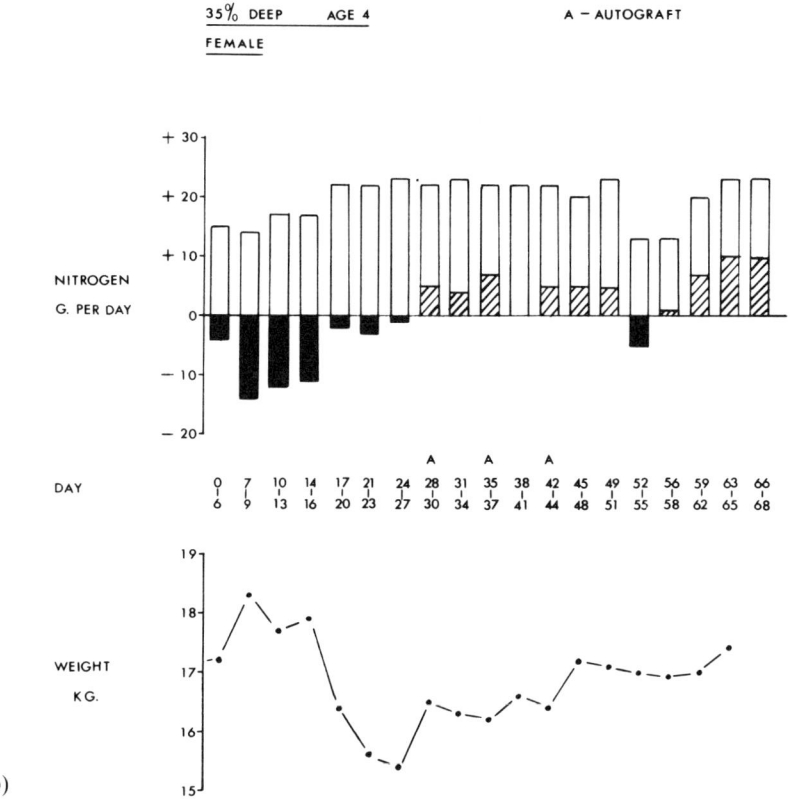

**Figure 1** *(cont.)*

## Other factors affecting nutrition

### Reduction in intake

Intake will be reduced for the first few days after injury but this period of relative starvation should not be prolonged. There may be diminished intestinal activity for 2–3 days at the most, but thereafter oral intake can be established quickly. Appreciation of the difficulties in eating and drinking for patients with burns around the mouth and, less commonly realized, for those with burns of both hands, avoids a poor intake in these groups.

A very important cause of reduced intake is associated with the provision of pain relief for treatment of the burn wound. Depending on the unit, dressing changes will range from daily to weekly. Adequate analgesia can often leave a patient reluctant to eat or drink for some hours. Inadequate analgesia leaves a patient exhausted. General anaesthesia can provide excellent pain relief, but the repeated fall in intake from preoperative and postoperative 'starvation' can also reduce *average* daily intake, as measured over a week, to unacceptable levels.

*Increased losses*

In addition to the nitrogen deficit imposed by the prolonged negative nitrogen balance there is additional loss from the burned surface. This loss will increase as the dead tissue separates, and will only reduce as the raw areas are covered by autograft skin. Infection will aggravate this loss, and, in addition to nitrogen, surface loss of sodium and potassium can be significant.

The insensible loss from large raw areas imposes a need for high fluid intakes if dehydration is not to occur. The high urinary nitrogen losses can have a diuretic effect and can make the urine output figure a misleading guide as to the adequacy of fluid intake. Insensible loss from the *uninvolved* skin will increase with the higher body temperatures produced by infection.

Further losses can occur from an injudicious feeding regime, diarrhoea and vomiting giving yet another source of loss of nitrogen, calories, electrolyte and water. On occasion the use of broad-spectrum antibiotics can have similar effects.

## MODIFICATION OF ADVERSE FACTORS

### Provision of an adequate intake of protein, calories, electrolytes, vitamins, trace elements and water

From our own studies of nitrogen balance, surface losses and weight patterns, a formula was devised which was shown to provide an adequate intake of the important factors in the uncomplicated burn (Sutherland, 1976). Recently, other improvements and advances in total patient care have allowed modification of the original formula. Over the past three years the following has proved satisfactory for the vast majority of patients.

Protein:    1 k/kg of body weight + 2 g/% burn
Calories:   20 (0.08 MJ)/kg + 50 (0.21 MJ)/% burn

In the child under 12 years of age, we have used the intake for the same child in health using standard tables but have ensured that this was the average intake obtained despite possible daily fluctuation.

Many feeding programmes are available commercially, but have, of course, not been devised specifically for the burned patient. Clinifeed 400 (Roussel), Fortison Standard (Cow & Gate), Isocal (Mead Johnson) are all suitable, but in our hands Fortison Standard has given good results in the vast majority of patients. These feeds will provide sufficient vitamins and trace elements, although on occasion supplementary sodium and potassium may be required, mainly in those with very extensive injury or high surface losses. None will provide enough free water. This need is in the range of 4–6 litre/24 h, depending on the size of the patient and the size of the burn, and is adjusted if necessary to produce a urinary output in the adult of not less than 1.5–2 litre/24 h. The amount required in the younger child will be dependent on body weight.

*Means of administration*

Most burn patients will have a normally functional gastrointestinal tract, and therefore the enteral route should be chosen for provision of the required intake. Introduction of infection through a central catheter line is a major risk in a patient who already has an extensive source of infection in the burn wound. Parenteral feeding is therefore undesirable and unnecessary except in rare instances. For example, a gram-negative septicaemia is usually accompanied by paralytic ileus and the parenteral route will be required but should be used for as short a time as possible.

The detailed arrangements for intravenous feeding are not described here, as they are no different from those used in most intensive care units. It needs stressing, however, that when a central feeding line is required it should be set up under strict aseptic conditions, in theatre if possible. It should be handled as little as possible; a 24 h sterile feeding system using 3-litre bags is ideal; all other fluids and drugs such as intravenous antibiotics should be given via a peripheral line if possible, and if not they should pass through bacterial filters.

Close observation of the patient for signs of systemic sepsis should be routine in a burns unit, or intensive care unit handling burned patients; when they arise, any central line should be removed and if necessary resited as it will inevitably have become colonized even if it was not the original source of the infection. The use of occlusive dressings such as Op-site allows insertion site sepsis to be seen and decreases handling of the site. The possibility must, however, be realized that the fluid and other material which inevitably collects under such dressings may be an ideal bacterial culture medium.

The use of tunnelled parenteral feeding lines is popular with intensive care doctors and may generally reduce the incidence of new sepsis in or caused by the line. Caution is required before they are used in burns, however, for two reasons: (1) the tunnel is more likely to become infected in the burned patient, either from colonized skin or by haematogenous spread from established bacteraemia, and will then be a nidus for life-threatening sepsis; and (2) areas of unburned skin are at a premium for graft donor material in large burns and should not be wasted for subcutaneous tunnels.

Further comment on patients with septicaemia or respiratory injury requiring nutritional support is to be found in Chapter 3.

Patients with smaller injuries are adequately treated by the addition of one of the high-protein high-calorie milk-shake type of preparations available commercially and given with a high-protein high-calorie diet. Patients with injuries of over 30% body surface area, and especially if there is a major full thickness component, are unlikely to maintain the high levels of intake required over a prolonged period of time.

A fine-bore nasogastric feeding tube should be passed on the second or third day after injury and the necessary intake introduced slowly in step-ladder fashion over the next 10 days or so. An attempt to do this more quickly will almost certainly give rise to problems with diarrhoea and vomiting. Because of the high water intake required, feeds can be diluted and tolerance achieved more readily, especially in the early stages. Interrupted feeding is the method of choice, either 3- or 4-hourly, leaving a gap between midnight and 6 a.m. This gap can be used on days when anaesthesia or surgery interfere with the normal pattern of intake. Interrupted feeding also allows the patient more freedom, physiotherapy can be carried out more effectively between feeds, and the position of the feeding tube can be checked regularly. Continuous feeding can be considered in the rare instances when tolerance is difficult to achieve. Delivery of the feed is by simple gravity drip, a feeding pump being unnecessary in this situation. The patient is allowed to eat what he wishes in addition to the feed, and a considerable amount of the free fluid is usually taken by the oral route.

## Control of environmental temperature

It has been shown that if heat loss is controlled the high metabolic rate can be reduced although not eliminated. Higher environmental temperatures of around 28–30°C are recommended. Because this temperature can be unpleasant for attendants, a warm 'micro-climate' can be produced by the use of special beds including the Clinitron bead bed, the Mediscus low air loss bed and the Rotaire warm air bed. In addition, Arturson et al (1978) have shown that the provision of overhead infra-red heaters adjusted by the patient to keep him comfortable can produce a significant reduction in metabolic rate and weight loss. The same authors stress and demonstrate the rise in metabolic rate where pain is not controlled. This emphasizes the need for adequate analgesia during dressing change or other manipulation of the burn wound.

Cold will also increase the metabolic rate, and it is extremely important that heat loss is prevented in wards, in operating theatres and in dressing rooms. Operating table water blankets and the covering of areas not being treated with an insulating layer (e.g. gamgee tissue) will give additional protection. In more prolonged procedures, temperatures should be monitored throughout.

## Care of the burn wound

Surgically the aim must be to close the burn wound as soon as possible. Excision and autografting of areas of deep burn within the first week following injury is common policy, thereby reducing the total size of the injury. This is not always possible due to poor general state or lack of available skin graft donor sites. Even in these patients the availability of homograft, heterograft and synthetic skin allows temporary closure of large raw areas until autografting can be undertaken. These materials will also be of use in the patient who has had early excision of part of his burn, the remainder having to be treated conservatively until the original donor sites can be re-used. The use of mesh grafting which allows expansion of a strip of skin to three times its original width or more also allows rapid cover when skin graft donor sites are limited.

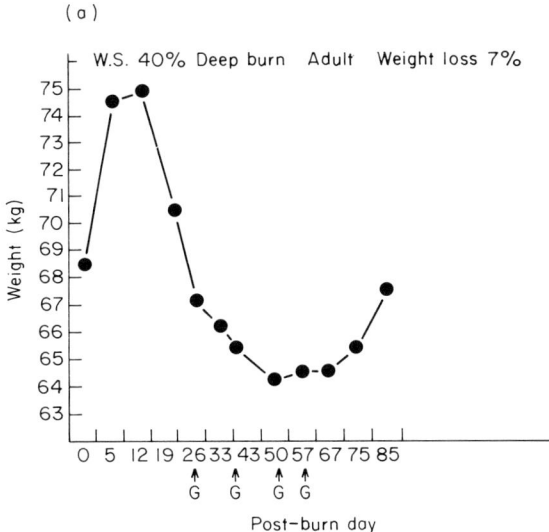

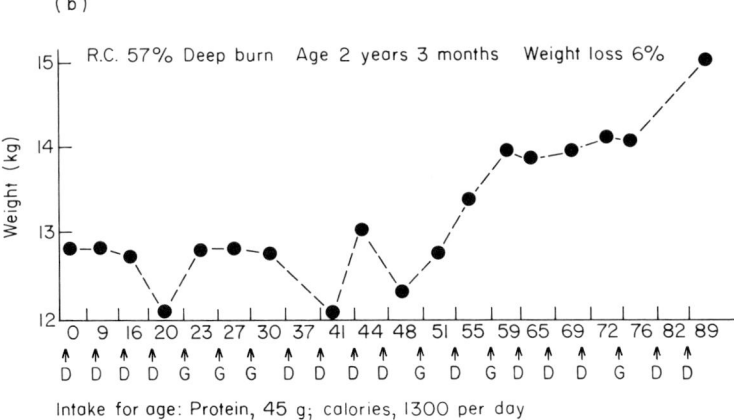

**Figure 2.** Satisfactory weight curve. (a) Adult—intake using formula. (b) Child—intake for age.

### Early recognition of problems

Accurate intake–output recording is mandatory. The levels of intake achieved can then be calculated by the dietician to ensure that the estimated requirement is being obtained over long periods of time. When progress is satisfactory, spot checks may be all that are required. Accurate recording of naked body weight (at the time of dressing change) should be made weekly and recorded on a chart placed in a position *where it can be seen*. Such information probably serves as the most reliable single measurement of success or otherwise of the regime adopted, provided there are no gross abnormalities of fluid balance.

A weight loss of 10% or less of admission body weight is acceptable. More than this suggests that a detailed reassessment is urgent and a loss of more than 20% is of grave significance and associated with high mortality (Figure 2).

Laboratory measurements are not particularly helpful, but weekly estimation of serum protein levels may show significant trends, although usually in the low normal range with a reversed albumin globulin ration. Similarly, twice-weekly measurement of urea and electrolytes with routine haematology will allow earlier recognition of developing problems. Maintenance of a good nutritional state can only be achieved if the whole burn team understands the problem and its significance. Difficulties are more likely to arise through ignorance, apathy or insufficient attention being paid to established routines. Adequate nutritional support does make a real contribution to a successful outcome by helping to maintain a good general condition throughout the long and often complicated course of the patient with major burn injury.

### SUMMARY

The reasons for development of nutritional problems in patients with extensive burn injury are presented. Suggestions are made regarding treatment which may modify some of the adverse factors. These include a possible formula for calculation of the intake of protein and calories, a regime for feeding with emphasis on the use of the enteral route, and the provision of additional care which can have beneficial effect on nutritional needs. The value of frequent measurement of body weight as an index of success or otherwise of the regime adopted is discussed.

### REFERENCES

Arturson MGS (1978) Metabolic changes following thermal injury. *World Journal of Surgery* 2: 203–213.
Arturson G, Danielsson U & Wennberg L (1978) The effects on metabolic rate and nutrition of patients with severe burns following treatment with infra-red heat. *Burns* 5: 164–168.
Barr PO, Birke G, Liljedahl SO & Plantin LO (1968) Oxygen consumption and water loss during treatment of burns with warm dry air. *Lancet* 1: 164–168.

Cuthbertson DP (1934) Certain aspects of metabolic response to injury. *Glasgow Medical Journal* **121:** 41.

Wilmore DW, Long JM, Mason AD, Skreen RW & Pruit BA (1974) Catecholamines/Mediator of the hypermetabolic response to thermal injury. *Annals of Surgery* **180:** 653–659.

Sutherland AB (1976) Nitrogen balance and nutritional requirement in the burn patient: a re-appraisal. *Burns* **2:** 238–244.

# 8

## Infection control in burns

J. C. LAWRENCE

### INTRODUCTION

Burns, by definition, contain devitalized tissue. The burn wound is surrounded by damaged and oedematous tissue continually kept moist by a constant flow of serous exudate at near body temperature, thus an excellent nutrient medium is available readily to support the growth of a wide variety of micro-organisms. Consequently, until about 40 years ago, bacterial colonization of burns was regarded as inevitable and, in fatal burns at least, septicaemic complications were common. As Lowbury (1985) pointed out, prior to the 1950s burns did not seem to be amenable to Listerian antisepsis, so the infective problem was largely ignored.

Since then it has become increasingly widely recognized that infection is the major cause of death in patients with burns—Artz and Reiss (1957) reported that at least half the deaths following burning injury were attributable to bacterial infection. Such infection remains a major factor in the mortality and morbidity associated with burns (Pruitt, 1984).

Despite the failure during the first half of this century to recognize bacterial complications following burning, the problem of 'burn suppuration' was recognized by very early civilizations and, ever since, these wounds have been accorded a wide variety of treatments such that in 1832 Baron Dupuytrens stated 'Burns have always been subject to the most bizarre forms of empiric treatment'. Topical therapy over the centuries has included tea, alcohol, phenol, mercuric chloride, picric acid and dyestuffs (Cason, 1981).

The nature of the bacteria detected in burns depends on a wide variety of factors. The treatment accorded is clearly important but other factors also play a role. These include the workload of the treatment centre, the number and expertise of the staff available to manage the workload, and the arrangement of the treatment unit. This chapter records the experience of the West Midlands Regional Burns Unit situated within Birmingham Accident Hospital, but it is likely that much of the information is applicable to other centres.

### THE EPIDEMIOLOGY OF BURNS AND SCALDS

In England and Wales burns and scalds account for about 6% of all accident and emergency cases (Home Accident Surveillance System); the annual total is over 120 000 casualties provided that burns sustained at work are included. Estimates given by The Hospital In-Patient Enquiry suggest that at least 10% of these burns are admitted to hospital for treatment. Analysis of burns arising within the City of Birmingham (with a population 1 006 527 in 1983) during 1981 to 1985 inclusive shows an annual admission rate of 298 cases. Their distribution by percentage body surface burned is shown in Table 1. The numbers may well reflect the national pattern. Information on causation and their distribution by age and sex is published elsewhere (Lawrence and Wilkins, 1987) but 85% of the casualties were classified as

**Table 1.** Burns and scalds from Birmingham during 1981 to 1985; their distribution by extent of injury.

| Extent of burn (%) | Total cases | Mean annual cases, Birmingham | Estimated number, England and Wales | Estimated national number |
|---|---|---|---|---|
| Below 10 | 1240 | 248.0 | 12 301 | 13 640 |
| 10–19.9 | 203 | 40.6 | 2014 | 2233 |
| 20–29.9 | 49 | 9.8 | 486 | 539 |
| 30–39.9 | 24 | 4.8 | 238 | 264 |
| 40–49.9 | 21 | 4.2 | 208 | 231 |
| 50–59.9 | 11 | 2.2 | 109 | 121 |
| 60–69.9 | 6 | 1.2 | 60 | 66 |
| 70–79.9 | 3 | 0.6 | 30 | 33 |
| 80–89.9 | 4 | 0.8 | 40 | 44 |
| Above 90 | 10 | 2.0 | 99 | 110 |
| All cases | 1571 | 314.2 | 15 584 | 17 281 |

non-industrial; apart from a few road traffic accidents and assaults most of the injuries arose from accidents in and around the home. About half of the victims were children and two thirds of these children were below school age. Extensive burns, i.e. 'shock cases', numbered 48 per annum and deaths 13. Nationally there are about 700 deaths from burns and scalds every year including victims who died before reaching hospital. The death rate has more than halved since Colebrook reviewed the causes of burns in 1950 but, in Birmingham at least, burns admissions and deaths have varied little since 1970 (Lawrence, 1985; Lawrence and Wilkins, 1987). The causes of domestic burning injury have also been investigated by the Department of Trade (Domestic Thermal Injuries, 1983).

It is likely that the number of burns and scalds in countries having a living standard comparable to that of the UK experience a similar burns epidemiology. Scandinavia may be better and recent reports show a downward trend (Lyngdorf et al, 1986) but the German Democratic Republic has a higher incidence than the United Kingdom (Roding, 1978). There is concern in the USA with the incidence of burns and scalds (MacKay et al, 1979), in South Africa (deKock, 1978) and in Australia (Pegg et al, 1979; Phillips et al, 1986). Socioeconomic circumstance is an important factor in burn causation.

The incidence and severity of burns is high in less well developed countries such as Algeria (Agha and Benhamia, 1978), Libya (Akhtar and Gang,

1980) and India (Keswani, 1986). Apart from poor living conditions national culture and dress are important factors.

## BACTERIOLOGICAL TECHNIQUES

Because burns readily acquire bacteria it is essential that an efficient bacteriological service is provided in order to advise on therapy and to maintain infection control. The latter is also one reason that most developed societies recognize that burns are best managed in designated centres, preferably purpose built.

In Birmingham, which has a 40 bedded unit in old accommodation, it is standard practice to sample all main wound sites on admission and at each dressing change (or daily if the wound is left exposed) using cotton tipped swabs moistened with peptone water. The laboratory is close to the burns unit so delays are minimal. Out-of-hours specimens are stored at 4°C; in situations where the laboratory is remote from the treatment unit it is preferable to place swabs in a suitable transport medium.

A modified standard system is used such that all initial cultures from wound swabs are made using blood agar 4% rather than the more usual 2% to prevent *Proteus* spp. swarming (Lowbury, 1960)—a major advantage since this bacterium occurs in 10–15% of specimens. The use of 4% agar results in a reduction in colony size of most organisms but does not cause practical disadvantages. Initial wound swabs are also made on improved cetrimide agar to facilitate prompt detection of *Pseudomonas aeruginosa* (Lilly and Lowbury, 1972). In recent years an antibiotic ditch, usually containing gentamicin, has also been included to enable prompt detection of resistant strains (Lawrence, 1985). A further initial culture is made onto mannitol–salt agar to confirm rapidly the presence of *Staphylococcus aureus*; this also reduces laboratory work (Lawrence, 1985).

Until three years ago routine anaerobic cultures were also made but, although *Clostridium perfringens* can be detected in 2% wound swabs and *Bacteroides* spp. in a high proportion of burns involving the lower trunk and lower limbs, anaerobic complications are rare (Cason, 1981) and the organisms tend to be transient (Lawrence, 1985). This experience may not be universal, Wang de Wang et al (1985) reported an appreciable incidence of anaerobic sepsis in burns. Therefore, although it may not be necessary to examine routinely specimens for anaerobes, it is essential that the burns unit maintains a close liaison with the laboratory so that normal routine can be tailored to clinical requirement and special investigation initiated promptly according to clinical need.

Fungi, particularly *Candida* spp., are detected in about 12% of patient's wounds (Kidson and Lowbury, 1979) but, apart from oral or urinary tract infection, fungi seldom cause clinical problems, so wound swabs are not routinely examined for such organisms. By contrast, some American units report that wound infection and septicaemia attributable to *Candida* spp. (MacMillan et al, 1972; Pruitt, 1984) or other fungi (Spebar and Lindberg, 1979) are not uncommon.

Brief training enables most persons with a basic microbiological knowledge to report on such cultures. The presence of *Staph. aureus* and *Ps. aeruginosa* can be promptly reported with certainty as can the presence of non-pathogens such as micrococci, skin diphtheroid bacilli and aerobic sporing bacilli. The presence of streptococci and gram-negative bacilli can also be reported; an experienced Medical Laboratory Scientific Officer can distinguish β-haemolytic streptococci of Lancefield Group A from other haemolytic streptococci with about 80% certainty and can also distinguish *Klebsiella* spp. and *Acinetobacter* spp. from other coliform bacilli. Reports concerning the previous day's specimens are made by a microbiologist in person by 9.30 a.m. every day. This is considered necessary since burn admissions and dressing changes are not restricted to weekends nor are infective complications. The system creates an excellent relationship between the burns unit and laboratory and almost certainly enhances infection control. It may not be possible to establish this system in many units and compromises will have to be made; nevertheless, it is essential that wounds are sampled regularly and results promptly reported.

Antibiotic sensitivities also need prompt reporting, but because of the number of specimens involved (10 000 wound swabs and 2500 nose and throat swabs annually) it is impractical to screen all isolates. One *Staph. aureus* isolate per patient per week is checked unless there is a specific reason for increasing this. All *Ps. aeruginosa* are investigated for gentamicin sensitivity and, if resistant, they are then tested against other antibiotics. For other gram-negative bacilli one isolation of each species detected per patient per month is tested against a range of antibiotics. It is important that all antibiotics that may be deployed are included in these tests and that the frequency of testing is increased according to local need.

Coliform bacilli are distinguished into species by subculture on urea agar, maltose and eosin-methylene blue agar. This readily distinguishes the majority of isolations of common species and the small remainder are typed using the API system.

## QUANTITATIVE BACTERIOLOGY

Surface swabs only sample the surface and there is no reason to suppose that the distribution of bacteria within colonized tissues is uniform. Moreover, there may be organisms in the deeper wound layers that are not present on the surface or superficial tissue (Lawrence, 1983a; 1985). This limitation can be overcome by removing biopsies and suitably processing these in the laboratory. What risk is associated with this surgical intervention is unknown; the technique is common practice in the USA (Pruitt and Foley, 1973; Neal et al, 1981; Pruitt, 1984). Crude quantitation is readily achieved with swabs and culture plates using a standard plating technique (Lawrence, 1983a). Swabs from burns covered with dressings yielding greater than ± growth, i.e. more than 30 colony forming units (CFU), reliably indicate more than $10^5$ CFU per g tissue. Correlation between swabs and biopsies is excellent (Figure 1). The need for regular wound sampling is also demon-

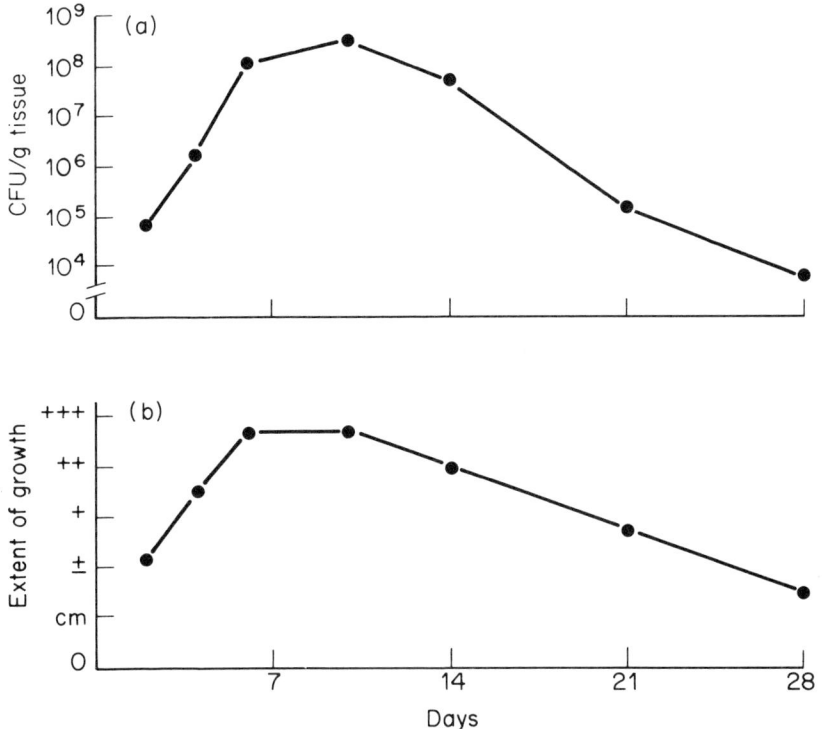

**Figure 1.** Variation of numbers of *Staph. aureus* in burns over a 28 day period. (a) CFU in biopsied time; (b) quantitation of swabs. From Lawrence, 1983a.

strated, since samples taken at either day 2 or day 20 would yield a ± result, about $10^5$ organisms per g tissue (Figure 1), but provide no indication whether the bacterial count was rising or declining. It is generally accepted that $10^5$ CFU per g tissue is the threshold for a potentially infective level in burns (Pruitt, 1984) and other wounds (Bornside and Bornside, 1979) but, in burns at least, the presence of small numbers of pathogenic bacteria requires further monitoring. A technique for quantifying bacteria present in swabs (Nathan et al, 1978) appears to be useful for evaluating antimicrobials for which standard discs are not available but offers no advantages for estimating the bacterial content of burned tissues.

Burns treated by exposure in which surface drying tends to minimize bacterial growth do not always show a good correlation between surface swab results and quantitation. On occasion a surface swab yields scant bacterial growth yet tissue deep to the burn may be purulent (Lowbury et al, 1954). In such circumstances quantitation of biopsies may be useful but the simple technique described by Selwyn and Ellis (1972) which works well for moist tissue such as that obtained from dressed burns often underestimates bacterial numbers in dry burns. Suitable techniques are described by Lawrence and Lilly (1972) and can also be applied to difficult specimens such as burned bone (Groves et al, 1981).

## OTHER BACTERIOLOGICAL SAMPLING

Urinary and respiratory tract infections are not uncommon complications of extensive burns; the former is particularly associated with the use of catheters and the latter is more likely to occur if the victim has inhaled smoke or noxious gas; such inhalation injuries appear to have increased in recent years (Settle, 1986). Such infections are frequently caused by bacteria that have colonized the burn wound so regular monitoring of specimens from 'at risk' patients is necessary; normal standard bacteriological procedures are adequate. It is to be remembered that an appreciable proportion of patients are elderly and may be admitted with pre-existing respiratory or other infective complications not related to the burn injury. Standard medical

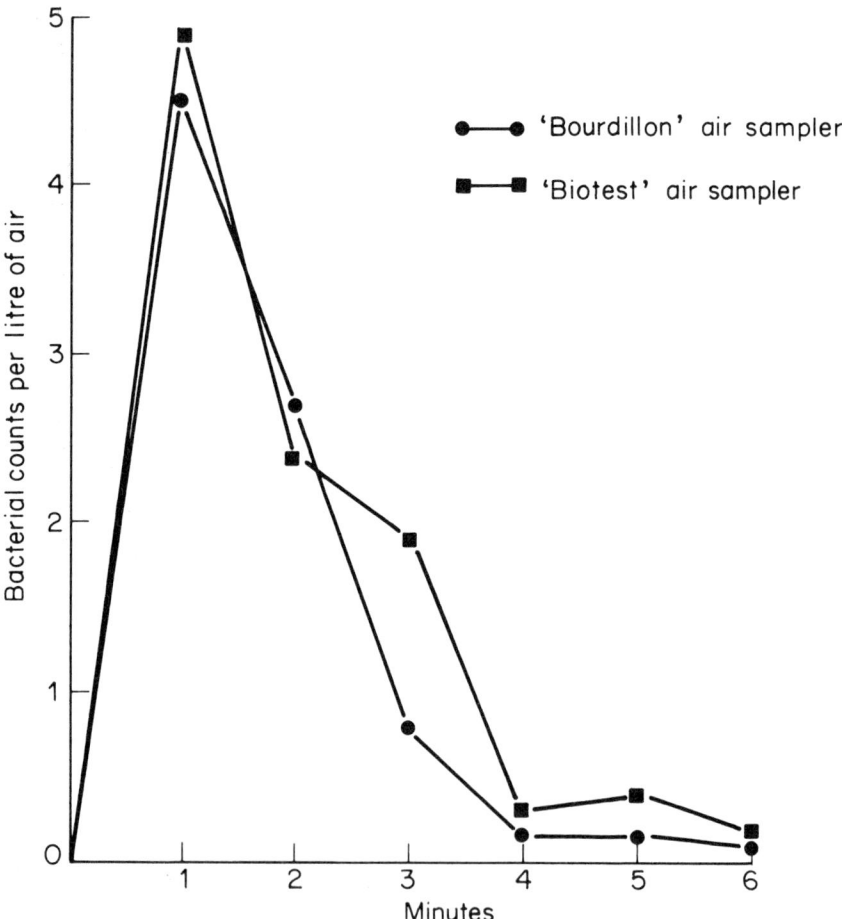

**Figure 2.** Bacterial numbers in the air of a plenum-ventilated dressing station measured with two different air samplers while dressing a 10% burn heavily colonized with *Staph. aureus*, *E. coli* and *Ps. aeruginosa*.

microbiology handbooks (e.g. Sleigh and Timbury, 1986) give adequate information.

Intravenous lines provide portals for entry of bacteria, moreover on occasion these may have to be inserted through dead tissue. Although catheter tips are only monitored on request, a proportion yield bacteria, usually only in small numbers, but, nevertheless, some may well enter the bloodstream and occasionally cause septicaemia.

The presence of an artificial airway increases the risks of pulmonary infection and many burned patients requiring respiratory support will also have burns on prospective tracheostomy sites. Early excision and grafting of such areas is recommended in order to provide reasonably clean areas for tracheostomy; endotracheal intubation will often suffice until such an area is available (Thomas, 1987). Similarly Lund et al (1985) favour use of naso-tracheal tubes to avoid the complications of early tracheostomy in burns.

*Streptococcus pyogenes* of Lancefield Group A is a notorious burn pathogen (Cason, 1981) but fortunately reasonably easily controlled (Lowbury, 1979). As part of such control it is our standard practice to take nose and throat swabs from all patients on admission and then at weekly intervals; cultures are examined specifically for *Strep. pyogenes* and *Staph. aureus*. Although carriage of *Staph. aureus* in the noses of burned patients on admission does not significantly differ from that of a normal population the incidence in burned patients significantly increases during their hospital stay (Lawrence, 1985).

Other bacteriological monitoring can be employed as considered neces-sary. Colonized burns readily disperse bacteria into the air especially if dressings are disturbed so it is recommended that all dressing changes are carried out in a specially designed room with positive pressure plenum ventilation. Modern air samplers are compact and easy to use (Lawrence et al, 1981); results compare favourably with those obtained using more cumbersome equipment (Figure 2). It is not always appreciated that com-paratively small wounds shed many bacteria during a dressing change (Figure 3) and the practice of performing any dressing in a ward or a non-ventilated cubicle is to be avoided. Rooms reserved for dressing even minor wounds tend to accumulate bacteria in their environment (Lowbury et al, 1981).

Although they are less sophisticated than mechanical air samplers judicious use of settle plates can be rewarding and can provide an indication of potential bacterial problems in areas where there may be much movement. Settle plates should not be exposed for more than 4 h, to avoid undue drying of the agar.

Low air loss beds such as the 'Mediscus' or 'Clinitron' are increasingly being used in burns units and it is pertinent to query whether the extra air movement creates any hazard. A comparison of management of patients with extensive colonized wounds on such beds with a standard hospital bed showed that neither type of low air loss bed presented any extra hazard (Lawrence and Lilly, to be published).

Unsuspected problems can arise; Lilly et al (1982) found that waterproof mattresses could deteriorate after prolonged contact with certain topical

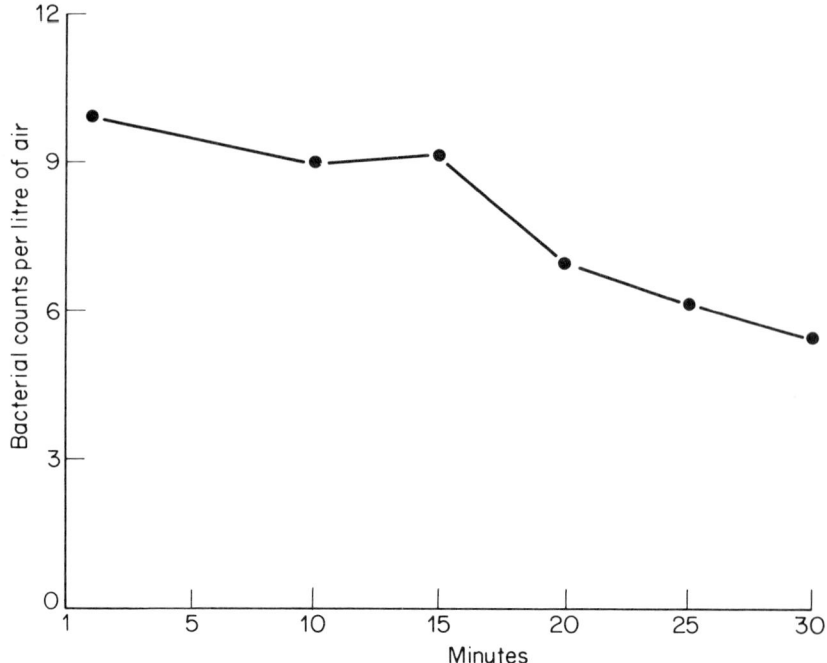

**Figure 3.** Bacteria liberated into the air on removing the dressing of a 1% burn colonized with *Staph. aureus* in a non-vented cubicle.

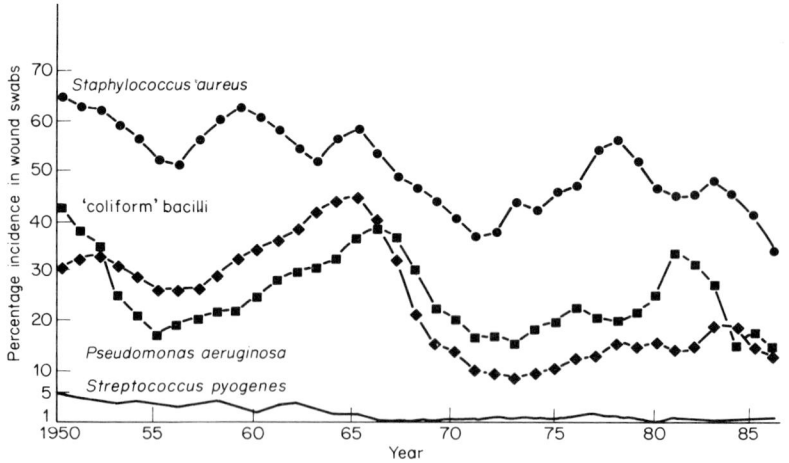

**Figure 4.** The incidence of bacteria detected in burn wound swabs of patients treated at Birmingham Accident Hospital 1950–1986 (three point moving average).

preparations especially those containing silver nitrate. The resultant loss of permeability provided a source of cross-infection for gentamicin-resistant *Ps. aeruginosa* and other bacteria. The mattress problem affords an example of the need to assess regularly equipment and procedures, especially if wound colonization or infection rates increase since unlikely sources of bacteria can arise. The problem of cross-infection in burns units is discussed by Ayliffe and Lilly (1985).

Little information on virus infection in burns is available but it is likely that some burns are admitted with respiratory problems of viral origin, and this could account for some of the pyrexic episodes early after burning which can only rarely be attributed to bacterial complications. In order to protect staff it is prudent to check certain types of patient, such as known intravenous drug abusers, for carriage of hepatitis B antigen. At present, human immunodeficiency virus is thought to be carried by 1 person in 1500 and this incidence is rising. At what point screening may be desirable is debatable; it is now accepted that this should be done for potential organ donors, and no exception should be made for homologous skin. Homografts are potential vectors of both viruses and bacteria.

## THE INCIDENCE OF BACTERIA IN BURNS

Forty years ago, *Strep. pyogenes* of Lancefield Group A could be isolated from 75% of admitted burns (Colebrook et al, 1945) and was responsible for considerable morbidity and mortality. Now it can be readily controlled, but other bacterial species, especially *Ps. aeruginosa*, have replaced the streptococcus and the problem of wound colonization and sepsis has remained (Lowbury, 1979). Nevertheless, since 1950, the incidence of all bacterial species has declined (Lawrence, 1985; Figure 4). The introduction of silver compounds for topical prophylaxis in 1965 led to a decrease in the incidence of gram-negative bacilli which was associated with a significant decrease in mortality (Bull, 1971). The increase in *Ps. aeruginosa* from 1980 to 1983 correlated with the emergence of gentamicin-resistant strains (Fujita et al, 1982). Similarly the increase in *Staph. aureus* between 1976 and 1979 was associated with a virulent strain resistant to penicillin, erythromycin and tetracycline which caused an outbreak of boils among patients and staff (Lilly et al, 1979).

A comparison of the incidence of bacteria isolated from wound swabs and their incidence in patients during 1985 and 1986 is shown in Table 2 together with the mean acquisition time. Swab analyses have the merit of providing a rapid means of assessing the overall pattern but analysis by patient provides a more accurate pattern and is more relevant to infection control. The incidence of bacteria in 'shock cases', i.e. burns exceeding 15% body surface area in adults or 10% in children, is much higher than that in other patients but the acquisition time is often longer. This may be due, in part, to the fact that such cases are usually isolated at least during the early part of their hospital stay and more staff are allocated to their care.

The low incidence of *Strep. pyogenes* of Lancefield Group A in exten-

**Table 2.** The incidence of bacteria in burn wound swabs and patients admitted during 1985 and 1986.

| Species | Percentage incidence of bacterial species in: | | | | | |
|---|---|---|---|---|---|---|
| | Wound swabs | | | Patients | | |
| | All cases | Extensive burns | Non-extensive burns | All cases | Extensive burns | Non-extensive burns |
| *Pseudomonas aeruginosa* | 14.5 | 15.3 | 12.8 | 15.3 (10.9) | 31.2 (12.0) | 9.1 (9.9) |
| *Staphylococcus aureus* | 19.5 | 18.7 | 21.2 | 41.6 (6.0) | 53.5 (7.6) | 36.9 (5.2) |
| 'coliform' bacilli | 3.5 | 3.7 | 3.1 | 15.9 (6.8) | 28.6 (2.4) | 9.6 (7.0) |
| *Proteus* spp. | 2.5 | 1.5 | 4.4 | 8.3 (13.3) | 13.0 (17.9) | 6.5 (9.7) |
| *Klebsiella* spp. | 1.6 | 1.5 | 1.2 | 8.5 (15.0) | 18.2 (17.0) | 4.8 (12.0) |
| *Acinetobacter anitratus* | 7.7 | 9.2 | 4.4 | 16.0 (8.7) | 33.5 (8.6) | 9.3 (10.5) |
| *Streptococcus pyogenes* | | | | | | |
|   Group A | 0.2 | <0.1 | 0.4 | 1.9 (5.3) | 1.9 (12.4) | 2.6 (2.6) |
|   Group C | 0.1 | 0 | 0.4 | 0.8 (4.0) | 0 | 1.7 (4.0) |
|   Group D | 0.3 | 0.3 | 0.3 | 2.2 (9.3) | 4.5 (12.2) | 1.3 (5.4) |
|   Group G | 0.1 | 0.1 | 0.2 | 1.4 (9.2) | 1.9 (14.0) | 1.2 (6.2) |
|   None of the above groups | <0.1 | 0 | <0.1 | 0.1 (2.0) | 0 | 0.1 (2.0) |
| *Streptococcus faecalis* | 0.7 | 0.8 | 0.5 | 6.1 (11.0) | 15.2 (12.1) | 2.6 (9.2) |
| *Streptococcus viridans* | 0.3 | 0.2 | 0.5 | 5.0 (6.4) | 8.6 (7.8) | 3.6 (4.7) |
| Micrococci | 19.0 | 18.7 | 19.7 | 61.6 (3.1) | 78.1 (2.1) | 55.1 (3.7) |
| Skin diphtheroid bacilli | 6.4 | 6.9 | 7.7 | 35.2 (4.5) | 57.2 (4.4) | 26.6 (4.7) |
| Aerobic sporing bacilli | 1.1 | 0.8 | 1.5 | 13.1 (5.4) | 25.7 (5.9) | 8.2 (4.8) |
| No bacteria detected | 22.4 | 22.8 | 21.6 | 26.4 | 20.8 | 28.5 |
| Total swabs/patients | 18 793 | 12 619 | 6174 | 960 | 269 | 691 |

Acquisition time (days) in parentheses.

**Table 3.** The incidence of bacteria in extensive and non-extensive burned patients admitted during 1985 and 1986.

| Species | All patients | Patients admitted promptly | Delayed admissions | Extensive burns — Admitted promptly | Extensive burns — Delayed admissions | Non-extensive burns — Admitted promptly | Non-extensive burns — Delayed admissions |
|---|---|---|---|---|---|---|---|
| *Pseudomonas aeruginosa* | 15.3 (11.0) | 17.2 (11.4) | 14.0 (10.7) | 31.6 (6.8) | 30.9 (5.2) | 11.3 (11.0) | 7.6 (8.9) |
| *Staphylococcus aureus* | 41.6 (6.0) | 38.4 (7.1) | 43.8 (5.4) | 49.5 (6.4) | 56.6 (7.0) | 33.8 (6.2) | 39.1 (5.4) |
| 'coliform' bacilli | 14.8 (6.8) | 15.7 (8.7) | 14.3 (5.7) | 31.6 (7.5) | 26.3 (5.8) | 9.2 (10.4) | 9.8 (4.8) |
| *Proteus* spp. | 8.3 (13.3) | 9.5 (11.7) | 7.5 (14.8) | 12.0 (15.9) | 13.8 (19.2) | 8.5 (9.4) | 5.2 (10.2) |
| *Klebsiella* spp. | 8.5 (15.0) | 8.5 (13.3) | 8.6 (16.1) | 16.2 (14.4) | 19.7 (18.6) | 5.3 (11.9) | 4.4 (12.0) |
| *Acinetobacter anitratus* | 16.0 (8.7) | 18.0 (9.0) | 14.7 (8.4) | 34.2 (8.2) | 32.9 (7.1) | 11.3 (10.1) | 7.9 (10.9) |
| *Streptococcus pyogenes* | | | | | | | |
| Group A | 1.9 (5.3) | 2.0 (4.9) | 1.8 (6.2) | 0.9 (2.0) | 2.6 (11.2) | 2.5 (3.3) | 1.5 (1.7) |
| Group C | 0.8 (4.0) | 1.5 (4.1) | 1.1 (3.8) | 0 | 0 | 2.1 (4.1) | 1.5 (3.8) |
| Group D | 2.2 (9.3) | 2.7 (9.4) | 1.8 (9.2) | 6.0 (8.6) | 3.3 (14.0) | 1.4 (6.8) | 1.2 (4.4) |
| Group G | 1.4 (9.2) | 1.7 (9.4) | 1.1 (9.0) | 2.6 (12.0) | 1.3 (17.0) | 1.4 (7.5) | 1.0 (4.0) |
| None of the above groups | 0.1 (2.0) | 0 | 0.2 (2.0) | 0 | 0 | 0 | 0.2 (2.0) |
| *Streptococcus faecalis* | 6.1 (11.0) | 6.0 (14.8) | 6.3 (8.4) | 13.7 (17.7) | 16.4 (8.5) | 2.8 (11.1) | 2.5 (7.7) |
| *Streptococcus viridans* | 5.0 (6.4) | 6.5 (7.7) | 3.9 (4.9) | 9.4 (11.6) | 7.9 (4.2) | 5.3 (4.5) | 2.5 (5.7) |
| Micrococci | 61.6 (3.1) | 63.6 (3.3) | 60.1 (2.9) | 76.1 (2.2) | 79.6 (2.1) | 58.5 (4.0) | 52.8 (3.2) |
| Skin diphtheroid bacilli | 35.2 (4.5) | 36.2 (3.6) | 34.5 (5.2) | 56.4 (3.2) | 57.9 (5.3) | 27.8 (4.1) | 25.8 (5.3) |
| Aerobic sporing bacilli | 13.1 (5.4) | 13.5 (6.4) | 12.9 (4.7) | 22.2 (8.1) | 28.3 (4.6) | 9.9 (4.9) | 7.1 (4.8) |
| No bacteria detected | 26.4 (–) | 24.4 (–) | 27.7 (–) | 22.2 (–) | 19.7 (–) | 25.4 (–) | 30.7 (–) |
| Number of patients | 960 | 401 | 559 | 117 | 152 | 284 | 407 |

Acquisition time (days) in parentheses.

sively burned patients is probably due to the use of either penicillin or erythromycin by reason of tetanus prophylaxis during the week following burning. The incidence of other β-haemolytic streptococci is also low.

The high incidence of 'no growth' can be attributed to the fact that about 25% of all wound swabs are taken during the first week of a patient's hospital stay; the acquisition time of many bacteria is about 6 days. Short term cases (i.e. patients kept in hospital for less than a week), patients whose wounds are grafted early, and patients who die, also contribute to what, at first sight, might appear to be a remarkably high incidence of bacteria-free wounds. The term 'other coliform bacilli' in Tables 2 and 3 encompasses a variety of species which are listed in Table 4. Over 97% of *Proteus* spp. were *Proteus morganii*, the remainder *Prot. vulgaris*. *Providencia* spp., were only isolated once but Curreri et al (1973) reported a high incidence of *Providencia stuartii* in burns which was difficult to eradicate.

The incidence of *Acinetobacter* spp. has steadily increased in recent years and now is as commonly isolated as *Ps. aeruginosa*; Shereretz and Sullivan (1985) report a similar observation.

Rather more than half of the patients are not admitted direct but some come via other hospitals, and others are delayed for a variety of reasons.

**Table 4.** The distribution of bacterial species initially classified as 'coliform bacilli' during 1985 and 1986.

| Species | Number of strains | Percentage |
|---|---|---|
| *Escherichia coli* | 164 | 47.7 |
| *Enterobacter* spp. | 105 | 30.5 |
| *Citrobacter* spp. | 18 | 5.2 |
| *Serratia* spp. | 5 | 1.5 |
| *Aeromonas* spp. | 2 | 0.6 |
| Non typeable | 12 | 14.2 |
| Total typed | 155 | 100 |

**Table 5.** Potentially pathogenic bacteria detected in minor burns on presentation.

| | Burns first seen | | |
|---|---|---|---|
| | All cases | Within 24 h of injury | 24 h or longer after injury |
| No. of patients | 624 | 435 | 189 |
| No. of burn sites | 661 | 459 | 202 |
| Mean area burned (%) | 1.2 | 1.2 | 1.2 |
| Organisms isolated (%) | | | |
| None | 19 | 21 | 14 |
| *Staphylococcus aureus* | 22 | 11 | 50 |
| *Streptococcus pyogenes* Group A | 1 | 1 | 2 |
| *Streptococcus faecalis* | 3 | 2 | 6 |
| *Clostridium welchii* | 0.5 | 0.6 | 0 |
| *Pseudomonas aeruginosa* | 0.3 | 0 | 1 |
| *Proteus* spp. | 1 | 1 | 0 |
| 'coliform' bacilli | 8 | 3 | 18 |

Based on specimens taken over 10 week periods during 1982, 1983, 1984 and 1986.

There are bacteriological differences between such cases—an analysis is shown in Table 3. In delayed patients the incidence of pathogenic bacteria tends to be higher with a reduced acquisition time. The ease with which burns acquire bacteria has been demonstrated by sampling outpatients. Cases that present within 24 h of injury yield comparatively few pathogens, but patients who delay seeking advice beyond this time yield significantly higher numbers (Lawrence, 1977; Table 5).

It is likely that most other British burns units experience similar bacteriological patterns, though there is a paucity of comparative data. A comparison between the Birmingham and Billericay units (Lawrence, 1985) suggested that the incidence of wound colonization by a variety of potentially pathogenic bacteria did not appear to differ.

## MEANS OF MINIMIZING THE BACTERIAL PROBLEM

Despite the current low incidence of *Strep. pyogenes* of Lancefield Group A the high pathogenicity of this organism makes it desirable regularly to monitor patient's noses and throats (and those of the attending staff or visitors if they have sore throats). If *Strep. pyogenes* is isolated penicillin V is the antibiotic of choice with erythromycin as the alternative for persons who are penicillin-sensitive (Lawrence and Groves, 1983). If *Strep. pyogenes* is isolated from wounds flucloxacillin should be the first choice, since a substantial proportion of the wounds will also be colonized with *Staph. aureus*, thus rendering benzyl penicillins ineffective. Undetected pyogenic streptococci, even in relatively small wounds, can sometimes cause death (Cruickshank et al, 1981). It is unwise to make erythromycin the first choice, since its widespread use can result in the emergence of resistant staphylococci which may become endemic within the unit (Lilly et al, 1979). This disadvantage may well not apply to outpatients.

The general principle of bacteriological control in this and many other centres relies on topical antibacterial prophylaxis. Although a variety of products have been evaluated over the last 35 years most have some disadvantages. Three particular difficulties are:

1. The bacterial problem tends to change following introduction of any particular topical therapy. In part this can be attributed to the fact that most antibacterial agents tend to be less active against some species than against others (Lowbury, 1979).
2. The commercial availability of reasonably effective preparations is limited such that only silver sulphadiazine or mafenide creams are available at present in the UK. With hospital pharmacy co-operation the range can be extended (Lawrence et al, 1982).
3. Some topical preparations cause undesirable side effects. Mafenide is painful and can cause acidosis (Gillett, 1985). Silver nitrate stains all material it contacts and can cause electrolyte imbalance by removal of chloride ions which are precipitated as silver chloride (Gillett, 1985); moreover, maintenance of silver nitrate compresses requires intensive

nursing care. Silver sulphadiazine can result in an increased proportion of gram-negative bacilli other than *Ps. aeruginosa* becoming sulphadiazine-resistant. This negates the use of other antibacterials containing sulphonamides, and the resistance is linked such that strains are also resistant to antibiotics such as tetracycline, cephaloridine, chloramphenicol, ampicillin and carbenicillin (Bridges and Lowbury, 1977). If silver sulphadiazine is withdrawn the resistance problem declines to low levels within a few weeks.

Phenoxetol/chlorhexidine cream has proved a satisfactory alternative for non-extensive burns (Lawrence et al, 1982) and preliminary results suggest that it is also suitable for extensive burns.

Topical antibiotics, particularly gentamicin, have enjoyed some success (MacMillan, 1975) but emergence of resistant strains render such use undesirable especially as it is often deployed systemically; moreover, it has a significant renal and ototoxicity (Gillett, 1985). Resistance problems are associated with other antibiotics used topically and it is becoming increasingly accepted that they are best avoided. As far as burns are concerned, topical antibiotics should never be used for prophylactic purposes and only rarely for therapy.

It is our practice to dress burns whenever it is practical to do so; awkward sites such as the face, neck and perineal region are more conveniently left exposed. However, exposure of all burns is practised in some units, its success depends on achieving drying of the burn surface to create an unfavourable environment for bacterial growth. The merits of exposure and occlusion were discussed by Lowbury (1978); success depends on rapid drying. A warm, dry environment created artificially (Davies et al, 1977) or climates such as that of the Middle East achieve this but the UK environment usually does not (Groves, 1985). If exposure is used, application of topical antibacterial agents will reduce the incidence of pathogenic bacteria (Lowbury, 1978). Use of aqueous solutions of either povidone-iodine (10% containing 1% available iodine) or 0.5% silver nitrate is recommended. These are applied 3–4 times a day until the eschar is reasonably dry, usually within 6–8 days.

Despite the ever increasing range of innovative wound dressings (Lawrence, 1982, 1983b), modern technology has not produced a satisfactory material for covering extensive burns (Lawrence, 1987). Absorbent cotton wool and gauze essentially similar to those described by Gamgee over one hundred years ago are still in universal use. Tulle gras dressings, either medicated or plain, are also of value especially for covering minor burns or skin graft donor sites but those impregnated with antibiotics should be avoided (Lawrence, 1977).

A strict discipline of asepsis and hygiene must be observed by all persons involved with the management of burns. It is not always appreciated that non-injured sites may harbour pathogens (Lawrence, 1985)—assuming that a freshly dressed patient presents no bacteriological hazard is unwarranted. Patients' hands may become contaminated (Fujita et al, 1982) and so attention must be paid to adequate disinfection of all equipment that a patient may contact.

Problems of airborne infection were mentioned previously and discussed by Ayliffe and Lilly (1985). Sophisticated equipment such as 'life islands' with plastic curtains and downward laminar flow can virtually eliminate cross infection (Burke et al, 1977), but whether the cost of such systems can be justified is debatable. It is pertinent to note that bacterial comparison of a modern air conditioned unit with the Birmingham unit yielded essentially similar results (Lawrence, 1985). Given the choice, it is likely that extra space is preferable to sophisticated air conditioning other than in certain specialized areas.

Ayliffe and Lilly (1985) consider that contact spread, mainly by the hands of staff, is the principal route of bacterial transfer thus proper hand hygiene is a high priority. Normal washing can be inadequate as critical areas such as the finger tips and thumb web can be missed and a systematic hand disinfection scheme is desirable (Lawrence, 1985). Alcoholic chlorhexidine is a convenient material to have available in dispensers at various strategic points within the unit.

Although the dry environment is not normally a reservoir or route of spread of gram-negative bacilli, regular thorough cleaning is necessary since Ps. aeruginosa and other bacteria will survive for long periods in sloughs on floors (Ayliffe and Lilly, 1985). All equipment used must be regarded as a possible reservoir or vector of infection. Inadequately cleaned sinks and baths are obvious hazards but taps, trolleys, straps etc. can also become contaminated. Salads and other uncooked foods may also be sources of infection (Kominos et al, 1972).

## INFECTION

The classical signs of infection—cellulitis, lymphangitis and lymphadenitis—are relatively unusual in burns during the earlier stages of treatment but cellulitis can often be discerned in chronic unhealed areas. Despite the frequent lack of clinical evidence of infection, burns often yield bacterial numbers greater than $10^5$ per g tissue—the value quoted as the threshold for infection. It is to be remembered that most pathogenic bacteria produce toxins and toxic metabolic products (Lawrence, 1983a); for example the pigment pyocyanin produced by Ps. aeruginosa is more toxic than mercuric chloride.

Although infection in burns is usually silent, septicaemic episodes can occur at any time during treatment of the burned patient (Cason, 1981). The criteria for suspected septicaemia include a temperature exceeding 39.5°C or a lowered blood pressure and an enhanced pulse rate. Septicaemia should also be suspected if the patient is disorientated or the urinary sodium–potassium ion ratio is reversed. Development of petechial emboli (Figure 5) is also suggestive of septicaemia though nowadays such appearances are relatively rare. Ileus of the small bowel may also herald developing septicaemia. It is pertinent to make blood cultures from such cases but the incidence of positive cultures is low, currently between 6 and 8%, so antibacterial therapy often has to be guided by the wound flora. Since this is

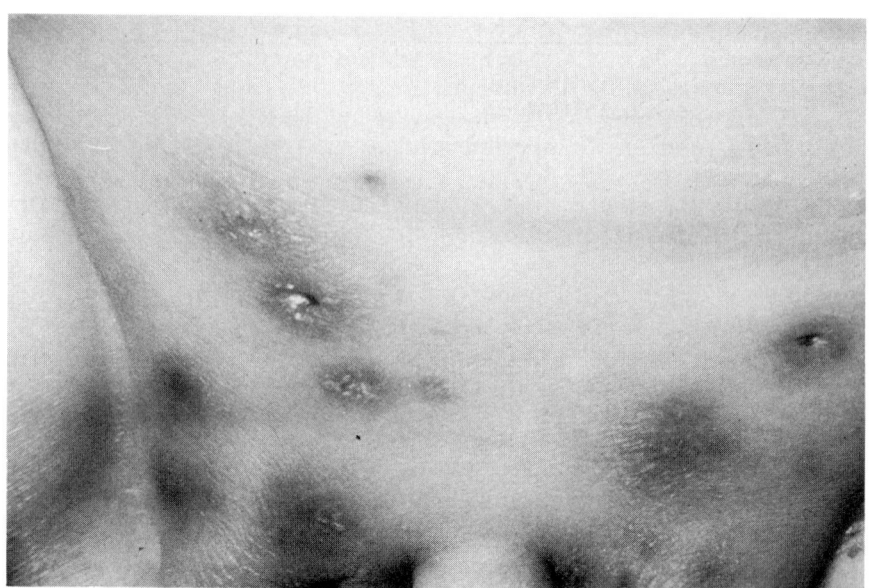

**Figure 5.** Petechial emboli seen in a young child who developed septicaemia caused by *Ps. aeruginosa*.

usually mixed, recourse to broad-spectrum antibiotics, usually aminoglycosides, is almost inevitable. Recently netilmicin has been our first choice, with amikacin as a reserve should gentamicin/netilmicin-resistant organisms occur. Combinations of aminoglycosides with either azlocillin, ticarcillin or mezlocillin may be more appropriate in some circumstances. However, the ultimate choice must depend on knowledge of local epidemiology and bacterial resistance patterns (Gillett, 1985). Results can be disappointing. None of the newer antibiotics have been evaluated clinically in burned patients, but our own laboratory studies suggest that ciprofloxacin, ceftazidime and timentin might be reasonable alternatives. Others, such as cefaclor, moxalactam and cefotaxime, appear to offer little advantage.

Burn patients are often given sub-therapeutic concentrations of aminoglycosides due to altered antibiotic pharmacokinetics in such cases. It is recommended that an adult with normal renal function is given a loading dose that is double the normal maintenance dose and subsequent doses 1½ times normal (Gillett, 1985). Serum concentrations should be monitored on the second day and dosage adjusted according to results.

Until recently the most common organisms isolated from blood cultures were *Staph. aureus* and *Ps. aeruginosa*. Confirmed staphylococcal septicaemia can be treated with flucloxacillin or fusidic acid plus erythromycin. In recent years other gram-negative bacilli, especially *Acinetobacter anitratus*, have become increasingly implicated in septicaemia.

Usually strains of *Staph. aureus* isolated from burn patients appear to be relatively avirulent and their appearance normally does not merit antibiotic therapy. However, virulent strains can appear at times and may become endemic within a unit (Lilly et al, 1979). Other units have reported outbreaks of staphylococcal scalded skin syndrome (Dowsett et al, 1984) and this particular problem has been reviewed by Dowsett (1984). Similarly methicillin-resistant *Staph. aureus* can occur in burns (Lacey et al, 1986); the problems associated with this organism and its control have been reviewed (Sanderson, 1986). Mupirocin, which can only be used topically, appears to be an efficient means of eradicating *Staph. aureus* (Casewell, 1986).

The only immunization available for burns is that employed to achieve prophylaxis against *Cl. tetani* (Lawrence and Groves, 1983). Trials of an anti-pseudomonas vaccine yielded promising results (Jones et al, 1980) but supplies of such vaccines are not available. Non-specific commercial immunoglobulins are available but their value in treating burns has yet to be determined.

## SUMMARY

Estimates concerning the current annual number and extent of injury of burn victims in the UK are given together with a brief review of burn epidemiology in other countries.

The need for thorough bacteriological monitoring of burns is stressed. Since this generates a large workload a modified standard bacteriological scheme is described enabling specimens to be processed efficiently from the clinician's point of view. The incidence of bacteria in burns in recent years is reported with comments on the significance of particular organisms, the nature of infection in burns and means for minimizing the infective problem.

Even small burns tend to rapidly acquire a variety of pathogenic bacteria thus presenting a cross-infection hazard. This problem increases with the extent of injury. The role of topical antibacterial prophylaxis in delaying bacterial acquisition is emphasized and the available range of materials for this purpose described. Guidance is given concerning the diagnosis and treatment of infection.

The need for rigorous hygiene in the management of burns is stressed and information given concerning the common routes of infection and cross-infection. Methods are described to help minimize these particular problems with especial emphasis on the need for careful attention to hand disinfection by all attending personnel.

## REFERENCES

Agha RB & Benhamia A (1978) Epidemiology of burns in Algeria. *Burns* **5:** 204–205.
Akhtar M & Gang RK (1980) Epidemiology of burns in Benghazi, Libya. *Burns* **7:** 351–356.
Artz CP & Reiss ER (1957) *The Treatment of Burns.* Philadelphia: WB Saunders & Co.
Ayliffe GAJ & Lilly HA (1985) Cross infection and its prevention. *Journal of Hospital Infection* **6**(supplement B): 47–57.

Bornside GH & Bornside BB (1979) Comparison between moist swab and tissue biopsy methods for quantitation of bacteria in experimental incisional wounds. *Journal of Trauma* **19:** 103–105.

Bridges K & Lowbury EJL (1977) Drug resistance in relation to the use of silver sulphadiazine cream in a burns unit. *Journal of Clinical Pathology* **30:** 160–164.

Bull JP (1971) Revised analysis of mortality due to burns. *Lancet* **ii:** 1133–1134.

Burke JF, Quinby WC, Bondoc CL, Sheehy EM & Moreno HC (1977) The contribution of a bacterially-isolated environment in the prevention of seriously burned patients. *Annals of Surgery* **186:** 377–387.

Casewell MW (1986) Epidemiology and control of the 'modern' methicillin-resistant *Staphylococcus aureus*. *Journal of Hospital Infection* **7**(supplement A): 1–11.

Cason JS (1981) *Treatment of Burns*. London: Chapman & Hall.

Colebrook L, Gibson T & Todd JP (1945) *Studies of Burns and Scalds*. Special Report Series, Medical Research Council No. 249. London: HMSO.

Cruickshank JG, Hart RJC, George M & Feest TG (1981) Fatal streptococcal septicaemia. *British Medical Journal* **i:** 1944–1945.

Curreri PW, Bruck HM, Lindberg RB, Mason AD & Pruitt BA (1973) *Providencia stuartii* sepsis: a new challenge in the treatment of thermal injury. *Annals of Surgery* **177:** 133–138.

Davies JWL, Lamke L-O & Liljedahl L-O (1977) Metabolic studies during the successful treatment of three adult patients with burns covering 80–85% of the body surface. *Acta Chirurgica Scandinavica* **468**(supplement): 25–60.

de Kock M (1978) The Cape Town Burn Profile. *Burns* **5:** 210–211.

Domestic Thermal Injuries (1983) A study of 1000 accidents admitted to specialised treatment centres. London: The Consumer Safety Unit, Department of Trade, Millbank.

Dowsett EG (1984) The staphylococcal scalded skin syndrome. *Journal of Hospital Infection* **5:** 347–354.

Dowsett EG, Petts DN, Baker SL et al (1984) Analysis of an outbreak of staphylococcal scalded skin syndrome: strategies for typing non-typable strains. *Journal of Hospital Infection* **5:** 391–397.

Fujita K, Lilly HA & Ayliffe GAJ (1982) Spread of gram-negative bacilli in a burns unit. *Journal of Hospital Infection* **3:** 29–37.

Gillett AP (1985) Antibiotic prophylaxis and therapy in burns. *Journal of Hospital Infection* **6**(supplement B): 59–66.

Groves AR (1985) Open and closed treatment of burns. *Journal of Hospital Infection* **6**(supplement B): 43–46.

Groves AR, Lawrence JC & Lilly HA (1981) Elimination of pseudomonas from burned bone. *Lancet* **i:** 676.

Home Office Accident Surveillance System (1986) Ninth Annual Report—1985 data. London: Consumer Safety Unit, Department of Trade.

Jones RJ, Roe EA & Gupta JL (1980) Controlled trials of pseudomonas immunoglobulin and vaccine in burned patients. *Lancet* **ii:** 1263–1265.

Keswani MH (1986) The prevention of burning injury. *Burns* **12:** 533–539.

Kidson A & Lowbury EJL (1979) Candida infection of burns. *Burns* **6:** 228–230.

Kominos SD, Copeland CE, Grosiak B & Postic B (1972) Introduction of *Pseudomonas aeruginosa* into hospital via vegetables. *Applied Environmental Microbiology* **24:** 567–570.

Lacey RW, Barr KW, Barr VE & Inglis TJ (1986) Properties of methicillin-resistant *Staphylococcus aureus* colonising patients in a burns unit. *Journal of Hospital Infection* **7:** 137–148.

Lawrence JC (1977) The treatment of small burns with a chlorhexidine medicated tulle gras. *Burns* **3:** 239–244.

Lawrence JC (1982) What materials for dressings? *Injury* **13:** 500–512.

Lawrence JC (1983a) Bacteriology and wound healing. In Fox JA & Fischer H (eds) *Cadexomer Iodine*, pp 19–31. Stuttgart: Schattauer.

Lawrence JC (1983b) Laboratory studies of dressings. In Lawrence JC (ed.) *Wound Healing Symposium*, pp 115–128. Oxford: The Medicine Publishing Foundation.

Lawrence JC (1985) The bacteriology of burns. *Journal of Hospital Infection* **6**(supplement B): 3–17.

Lawrence JC (1987) A century after Gamgee. *Burns* **13:** 77–79.

Lawrence JC & Groves AR (1983) Are systemic prophylactic antibiotics necessary for burns? *Annals of the Royal College of Surgeons of England* **65:** 279.

Lawrence JC & Lilly HA (1972) A quantitative method for investigating the bacteriology of skin: its application to burns. *British Journal of Experimental Pathology* **53:** 550–557.

Lawrence JC & Wilkins MD (1987) The epidemiology of burns. In Lawrence JC (ed.) *Burncare*, pp 13–26. Hull: British Burn Association/Smith & Nephew Ltd.

Lawrence JC, Lilly HA & Wilkins MD (1981) Evaluation of a portable air purifier. *Journal of Hygiene, Cambridge* **86:** 203–208.

Lawrence JC, Cason JS & Kidson A (1982) Evaluation of phenoxetol-chlorhexidine cream as a prophylactic antibacterial agent in burns. *Lancet* **i:** 1037–1040.

Lilly HA & Lowbury EJL (1972) Cetrimide nalidixic acid agar as a selective medium for *Pseudomonas aeruginosa. Journal of Medical Microbiology* **5:** 151–153.

Lilly HA, Lowbury EJL, Wilkins MD & Cason JS (1979) Staphylococcal sepsis in a burns unit. *Journal of Hygiene, Cambridge* **83:** 429–435.

Lilly HA, Kidson A & Fujita K (1982) Investigation of hospital infection from a damaged mattress and the demonstration of its mechanism. *Burns* **8:** 408–413.

Lowbury EJL (1960) Infection in burns. *British Medical Journal* **i:** 994–1001.

Lowbury EJL (1978) Fact or fashion? The rationale of exposure method, vaccination and other anti-infective measures. *Burns* **5:** 149–159.

Lowbury EJL (1979) Wits versus genes: the continuing battle against infection. *Journal of Trauma* **19:** 33–45.

Lowbury EJL (1985) Introduction from the Chairman. *Journal of Hospital Infection* **6**(supplement B): 1.

Lowbury EJL, Crockett DJ & Jackson DM (1954) Bacteriology of burns treated by exposure. *Lancet* **ii:** 1151–1153.

Lowbury EJL, Ayliffe GAJ, Geddes AM & Williams JD (1981) *Control of Hospital Infection*, 2nd edn. London: Chapman & Hall.

Lund T, Goodwin CW, McManus WF et al (1985) Upper airway sequelae in burn patients requiring endotrachial intubation of tracheostomy. *Annals of Surgery* **201:** 374–382.

Lyngdorf P, Sørensen B & Thomsen M (1986) The total number of burn injuries in a Scandinavian population—a prospective analysis. *Burns* **12:** 567–571.

MacKay A, Halpern J, McLoughlin E et al (1979) A comparison of age specific burn injury rates in five Massachusetts communities. *American Journal of Public Health* **69:** 1146–1157.

MacMillan BG (1975) Burn wound sepsis—a 10 year experience. *Burns* **2:** 1–13.

MacMillan BG, Law EJ & Holder IA (1972) Experience with candida infections in the burned patient. *Archives of Surgery* **104:** 509–513.

Nathan P, Law EJ, Murphy DF & MacMillan B (1978) A laboratory method for selection of topical antimicrobial agents to treat infected burns wounds. *Burns* **4:** 177–187.

Neal GD, Lindholm GR, Lee MJ, Marvin JA & Heimbach DM (1981) Burn wound histologic culture—a new technique for predicting burn wound sepsis. *Journal of Burncare and Rehabilitation* **2:** 35–39.

Pegg SP, Gregory JJ, Hogan PG, Mottarelly IW & Walker LF (1979) Epidemiological pattern of adult burn injuries. *Burns* **5:** 326–334.

Phillips W, Mahairas E, Hunt D & Pegg SP (1986) The epidemiology of childhood scalds in Brisbane. *Burns* **12:** 343–350.

Pruitt BA (1984) The diagnosis and treatment of infection in the burned patient. *Burns* **11:** 79–81.

Pruitt BA & Foley FD (1973) The use of biopsies in burn patient care. *Surgery* **73:** 887–897.

Report on The Hospital In-Patient Enquiry (1981) Part I Tables (published annually). London: HMSO.

Röding H (1978) The epidemiology of burn injuries in the German Democratic Republic. *Burns* **5:** 208–209.

Selwyn S & Ellis H (1972) Skin bacteria and skin disinfection reconsidered. *British Medical Journal* **i:** 136–140.

Settle JAD (1986) Severe burns: a continuing challenge. *Care of the Critically Ill* **2:** 184.

Shereretz RJ & Sullivan ML (1985) An outbreak of infections with *Acinetobacter calioaceticus* in burn patients: contamination of patients' mattresses. *Journal of Infectious Diseases* **151:** 252–258.

Sleigh JD & Timbury MC (1986) *Notes on Medical Bacteriology*, 2nd edn. Edinburgh: Churchill Livingstone.

Spebar MJ & Lindberg RB (1979) Fungal infection of the burn wound. *American Journal of Surgery* **138**: 879–882.
Thomas CH (1987) Early respiratory problems after burn injury. In Lawrence JC (ed.) *Burncare*, pp 35–41. Hull: British Burn Association/Smith & Nephew Ltd.
Wang de Wang, Li Ngao, Xiao Guang-Zia & Zhan Ya-Pin (1985) Anaerobic infection in burns. *Burns* **11**: 192–196.

# Plastic and Maxillofacial Surgery

# 9

# The anaesthetist's contribution to good patient care

## D. J. F. MACDONALD

'Plastic surgery was founded on the work of Magill and his tube: it would not have been possible without it.' Sir Harold Gillies.

Anaesthesia was developed in order to make it possible for lifesaving operations to be carried out with less pain for the patient. A byproduct of this was that the surgeon had better operating conditions and consequently was able to do a better job and consider procedures which would previously have been impossible. The various techniques of modern anaesthesia with the associated development of sophisticated monitoring have made possible ever more ambitious and aggressive surgery. With all this technological development, we do well to remind ourselves that the basic aims of anaesthesia and the duties of the anaesthetist remain unchanged:

1.  To ensure maximum safety and comfort for the patient.
2.  To provide the surgeon with the best possible operating conditions.

### THE CHALLENGE

Conditions which come under the care of plastic surgeons can be broadly classified into five groups—neoplastic, congenital, traumatic, burns (early and late) and cosmetic. Within each of these groups a proportion of the patients will present the anaesthetist with a specific challenge.

With so many of the operations involving the head and neck, control of the airway, difficulty with intubation and access to the patient during the operation can all cause problems. Tumours in the mouth, for example, with the frequent concomitant induration of the tongue, can make visualization of the larynx impossible.

Some of the severe congenital malformations can also cause extreme difficulty with intubation. Many present during the neonatal period: the child may be premature and one always has to be aware of the possible coexistence of other congenital anomalies.

Traumatic cases may present in a collapsed state, they may have swallowed large quantities of blood, and the possibility of other injuries must be borne in mind. One particularly challenging situation is the emergency intubation of a patient in whom there is reason to suspect a fracture of the cervical spine. Later, the anaesthetist may be involved in the longer term care of pulmonary or hepatorenal failure.

Anaesthesia in burned patients has justified a separate section in this book. The late scarring may require multiple corrective procedures, often at short time intervals. Scars around the face and neck may cause difficulty—occasionally it may be necessary for the surgeon to divide the contractures before the patient can be intubated.

Even operations with a large cosmetic component, such as mandibular osteotomies, present their peculiar challenge. As one of the aims of the operation is to improve the patient's appearance, there is a reluctance to perform a routine prophylactic tracheostomy with the possibility of leaving an unsightly scar. In addition, the patient may be left at the end of the operation with his jaws wired together: while this may ensure that the tongue does not fall back, it makes emergency intubation difficult! These patients require intense nursing attention and the immediate availability of skilled medical personnel.

Many of the extensive dissections and reconstructions may involve considerable blood loss. For this reason and also to make the surgery easier and safer, controlled hypotension is frequently employed and many surgeons infiltrate large amounts of adrenaline.

Many plastic surgical procedures require repeated anaesthetics at short intervals. The anaesthetic management of these patients should be planned from the beginning.

## RELATIONSHIP WITH THE SURGEON

In the interests of the patient it is important for a good relationship to exist between the surgeon and anaesthetist (and indeed through the entire team). The surgeon will perform best when he has confidence that the patient is being optimally cared for. The anaesthetist, as the most senior unscrubbed person in the theatre, has an important influence on the atmosphere in the operating room. Even such non-anaesthetic activities as adjustment of the operating light and choice of background music can influence the smooth running of the theatre and ultimately benefit the patient. And on the rare occasion when the anaesthetist has to intervene in the interests of safety, he should command the attention of everyone in theatre.

The mutual respect between surgeon and anaesthetist should work itself out in the practical management of the patient. There should be adequate preoperative discussion of the patient so that anaesthesia can be planned in good time: position of the patient, desirable level of induced hypotension, performance of an elective tracheostomy, bladder catheterization, ordering of blood and blood products, and the need for postoperative intensive care should all be anticipated in most cases. The better informed the anaesthetist is, the better the operating conditions he can provide for the surgeon. Conversely, when there is any doubt about the patient's fitness to withstand or benefit from the operation, the anaesthetist's opinion may influence the surgeon's plans regarding either the timing or the extent of surgery.

## THE PREOPERATIVE VISIT

It would be a great benefit if patients scheduled for surgery were seen by their own anaesthetist a week or two before their admission to hospital. This way they could be better informed of what will happen to them, problems could be anticipated and any necessary measures could be instituted to improve their condition. Unfortunately, in the UK at least, the workload of anaesthetic departments does not usually allow for the setting up of such an outpatient service. As things stand, most patients are only seen after publication of the theatre list on the afternoon prior to surgery. Thus if patients prove to be in a less than optimal state of physical health, the choice is limited to cancellation or postponement of the operation, or proceeding at increased risk of morbidity or mortality. The subtle psychological pressure on the anaesthetist not to cancel an operation for which the patient is 'all keyed up' makes it difficult to arrive at the right decision.

The preoperative visit has several important purposes.

### Assessment of fitness for operation

Only the anaesthetist can assess the patient's fitness for operation, as he alone can anticipate the physical, physiological and pharmacological effects of the proposed operation and anaesthetic. Other specialists, such as a cardiologist, may be consulted where appropriate, but their role is limited to making an assessment of the patient's physical status and advising on how to improve it. They may on occasion give valuable advice on the management of the patient during the operation (e.g. in diabetes), but it is the anaesthetist who will be taking responsibility for the patient and it is he who should make the final decision as to whether the risks are justified.

### Explanation of the planned procedure

While it is the surgeon's duty to explain to the patient both the need for and the nature of the planned operative procedure, it is surprising how often the anaesthetist, as the last professional visitor before the operation, finds himself having to answer some very basic questions about the operation. It is important to ensure that the patient knows what to expect postoperatively, as it can be a very alarming experience to wake up in an intensive care environment. Even an intravenous infusion is regarded by many patients with considerable awe. Where continued intubation or a tracheostomy is anticipated, the patient should have this explained and where appropriate should be reassured that the inability to speak will be only temporary.

In this age of increasing litigation, more and more emphasis is being placed on the need for full explanation of any planned procedure, including the spelling out of any risks involved (Forrest, 1984). Again, this is mainly the responsibility of the surgeon, but where there are specific anaesthetic problems or risks these must be faced honestly. For most patients, however, the greater need is to inspire them with confidence and allay any unfounded fears. An operation considered routine by the medical and nursing staff is still a major crisis in any patient's life. Many, presented with detailed explanation of the procedure, appear to 'switch off' mentally and one could question whether it is ever possible to obtain truly 'informed consent', no matter what detailed information has been imparted to the patient. At the end of the day it is still a matter of 'their life in your hands'.

### Rapport with the patient

During the course of the foregoing assessment and explanation, a rapport should be built up with the patient so that he has confidence in his anaesthetist based on the knowledge that the latter has a thorough understanding both of the patient and of the operation proposed, that if risks are involved these are recognized and prepared for and that he will have his anaesthetist's undivided attention throughout the operation. It is surprising how many patients think that the 'anaesthetic' consists of the initial injection and that if the dose is miscalculated they will either wake up before the end of the operation or fail to wake at all!

### Premedication

The fourth and perhaps least important reason for the preoperative visit is to prescribe suitable medication. This includes the adjustment of any regular medication which the patient is receiving, the provision of sedation if necessary in the period preceding surgery, including the night before operation, and the traditional 'premedication' given 1–2 h before the scheduled time of operation.

## INDUCTION

The anaesthetic room should be a haven of peace and tranquillity. In spite of all the necessary preparations when he is first brought into the anaesthetic room, from the moment the patient is wheeled in he should be conscious that everything is under control. As much preparation as possible should have been done before the patient is sent for. There should be no unnecessary persons present and no conversations taking place on the side. There is a place for initial light-hearted conversations between the patient and theatre staff, but from the moment that the anaesthetist prepares to commence, all other conversation should cease and the anaesthetist should have the patient's undivided attention. This is particularly important when dealing with children. Where for reasons of hospital design anaesthesia is induced in the operating room, these conditions are more difficult to achieve but are all the more necessary. Difficult airway and intubation problems will be dealt with in detail in a subsequent chapter: suffice it to say here that the emphasis must be on maintaining control of the situation at all times. The anaesthetist must have as much time as necessary to secure a safe airway, adequate venous access and all necessary monitoring.


## CONDUCT OF ANAESTHESIA

Anaesthesia involves the care of the whole patient for the whole of the perioperative period. The conduct of long operations such as free tissue transfer or replantation surgery is as akin to intensive care as it is to other forms of anaesthesia. In all reconstructive surgery involving skin or muscle flaps an understanding of circulatory physiology is essential if the anaesthetist is to provide optimal conditions not only for the surgery but for flap survival. The interplay of the various cardiovascular reflexes can be manipulated to maximize blood flow to the flap (Macdonald, 1985). Unfortunately, some of the measures taken in theatre to produce local vasodilatation or general hypotension can result in vasoconstriction on emergence from anaesthesia. (The author recalls having to re-anaesthetize a patient in order to relieve the strangulation of a deltopectoral flap caused by intense shivering.) Attention to heat conservation, fluid and blood balance, and analgesia from the commencement of the operation pays dividends in the postoperative period.


## POSTOPERATIVE CARE

Measures instituted in the theatre with their associated monitoring should be continued into the immediate postoperative period. True intensive care is no different from good anaesthetic practice. For this reason anaesthetists have been very involved in the development of intensive care units throughout the world, and although there is much disagreement about the way the specialty of 'intensivism' should be organized there is much to be said for the continued involvement of clinical anaesthetists (Stoddart, 1986). Ideally, major reconstructive surgery should be performed in specialized units where one anaesthetist—or a small manageable team—is involved with the patient throughout the entire perioperative period. This unit should, however, preferably be sited within a larger hospital complex where the assistance of other disciplines and laboratory services is conveniently available.


## PAIN RELIEF

Pain causes reflex vasoconstriction. Therefore, the adequate relief of pain intraoperatively and postoperatively is not only a moral and humane service to the patient but could influence the success or failure of the operation. The routine prescription of morphine or papaveretum intramuscularly 'prn' leaves much to be desired. Better methods of producing analgesia are available, but analgesia is always achieved at a price—frequently the risk of respiratory depression. Therefore, in the current state of knowledge many of the newer techniques should only be employed in an intensive care or high-dependency set-up.

So much of plastic and reconstructive surgery is performed on the surface of the body that regional analgesia is an appropriate technique in many cases. For the longer operations this should be combined with adequate basal sedation or light general anaesthesia, as it is unfair to ask the patient to lie on a hard narrow table for many hours. Regional blocks are attractive because they give good operating conditions and pain relief which continues into the postoperative period; in addition, the sympathetic block produced may improve the circulation to the operated area. There is some evidence that a concomitant general anaesthetic allows the administration of larger doses of local anaesthetics without toxic effects (Neill and Watson, 1984).

Intrathecal or extradural opiates have become popular for postoperative pain relief. However, the anaesthesia is insufficient to ablate the sharp pain of surgery and the technique is inappropriate for head and neck surgery as it cannot be used to produce analgesia in the area supplied by the cranial nerves. Even lumbar injection may produce profound respiratory depression several hours after the injection, necessitating close observation of the patient for 24 h (Morgan, 1982). Techniques of continuous infusion of opiates with or without patient-controlled bolus injection give good control of postoperative pain (Owen et al, 1986). The development of the necessary equipment and the advent of newer drugs with a short therapeutic half-life make continuous intravenous infusion a popular technique in the intensive care unit. Just as anaesthetic skills were adapted for use in intensive care so now these techniques developed in intensive care are finding their way back into the operating theatre. In the long term it seems that total intravenous anaesthesia with or without controlled ventilation is the logical development.

As the boundary between anaesthesia and intensive postoperative care has become blurred, so the distinction between general and local anaesthesia for all but the most minor cases is less clearly defined. It is a strange contradiction that while there is a growing concern about patients claiming to have been aware during a general anaesthetic (Jones and Konieczko, 1986; Hargrove, 1987) many major operative procedures are performed under some form of regional block with varying degrees of sedation. Surely the emphasis must be not on the state of consciousness of the patient but on his comfort throughout the operative experience.

## SUMMARY

A high standard of conscientious anaesthesia can mean the difference between failure and success of plastic and reconstructive surgery. Good operating conditions brought about by smooth anaesthetic management and controlled manipulation of the blood pressure can make for better surgery and a better final result. Poor anaesthetic control may lead to inadequate excision of tumours, excessive blood loss and non-survival of flaps.

Consideration of the patient as an individual and adequate consultation with the surgeon are essential for the optimal conduct of the anaesthetic. The high standard of monitoring and rapid correction of any deleterious changes which characterize good anaesthetic management in theatre should be continued in the postoperative period. The whole perioperative period should be viewed as an integrated process and planned accordingly.

## REFERENCES

Forrest JB (1984) Editorial. Defensive medicine: anaesthetic practice in the 80's. *Anaesthesia* **39:** 1165–1167.

Hargrove RL (1987) Awareness under anaesthesia. *Journal of the Medical Defence Union* **3:** 9–11.

Jones JG & Konieczko K (1986) Hearing and memory in anaesthetised patients. *British Medical Journal* **292:** 1291–1293.

Macdonald DJF (1985) Anaesthesia for microvascular surgery: a physiological approach. *British Journal of Anaesthesia* **57:** 904–912.

Morgan M (1982) Editorial. Epidural and intrathecal opiates for post-operative pain relief. *Anaesthesia* **37:** 527–529.

Neill RS & Watson R (1984) Plasma bupivacaine concentrations during combined regional and general anaesthesia for resection and reconstruction of head and neck carcinomata. *British Journal of Anaesthesia* **56:** 485–492.

Owen H, Glavin RJ, Reekie RM & Trew AS (1986) Patient-controlled analgesia: experience of two new machines. *Anaesthesia* **41:** 1230–1235.

Stoddart JC (1986) Editorial. A career post—with intensive therapy? *Anaesthesia* **41:** 1181–1183.

# 10

Special considerations in children

FRANK J. M. WALTERS

Children require plastic surgery for the treatment of disfiguring pathology which may be either congenital or acquired, burns being the most common acquired cause. Anaesthesia in children undergoing plastic surgery procedures, which are often multiple and involve repeat anaesthesia, grafts and delicate suture lines, has important and interesting implications for the anaesthetist. Finally, there are sometimes specific problems associated with coexisting congenital abnormalities; in particular, the airway, which may be compromised in children with cleft lip and palate defects and cystic hygromas. The airway may also be seriously at risk following burns to the face or neck when contractures develop. The treatment of an acute burn is considered elsewhere in this issue. Later, reconstructive surgery demands similar anaesthetic considerations as are generally described later.

## GENERAL PREPARATION

Patients requiring plastic surgery can present at all ages, although it is uncommon to have to deal with neonates. The newborn have specific problems as a result of their immaturity, making them unable to maintain body temperature and blood sugar, and more sensitive to anaesthetic drugs, neuromuscular blocking drugs in particular, although this point has been disputed (Goudsouzain, 1975). There is also a risk of causing the onset of retrolental fibroplasia in infants of less than 45 weeks gestational age during anaesthesia because of the raised arterial oxygen tension. Thus, it is preferable to postpone elective surgery for patients in this age group until later, so reducing the risk of anaesthesia and surgery.

It is not uncommon to find children and their parents under considerable psychological stress as many of these patients present with a disfiguring abnormality. The surgical procedure is often one of a series and, therefore, handling of the patient is particularly important, as any emotionally traumatic event may have effects on future anaesthesia and surgery. Children are often sensible and able to co-operate once a good rapport has been established. It is essential to be honest about the impending procedure, as deceit will ultimately be recognized and will totally destroy the child's confidence in both medical and nursing staff and, possibly, his parents. The combination of firm parental support and a simple honest explanation of the plan of events to the patient is far more effective than any pharmaceutical preparation.

Many congenital abnormalities are associated with other defects and may form part of a particular syndrome, such as Apert's, which includes facial abnormality, making intubation difficult, congenital heart disease and raised intracranial pressure (Figure 1). There are many eponymous syndromes, some of which have particular significance for the unwary anaesthetist (Jones and Pelton, 1976) as they may affect the heart, requiring evaluation and pretreatment with antibiotics, and the airway. The severity of the coexistent condition, particularly congenital heart disease with the associated risk of anaesthesia, may alter the significance and need for surgery. With good communication, consultation with others involved in the management of the child can take place in good time, thereby allowing adequate preparation before surgery and perhaps avoiding unnecessary admission.

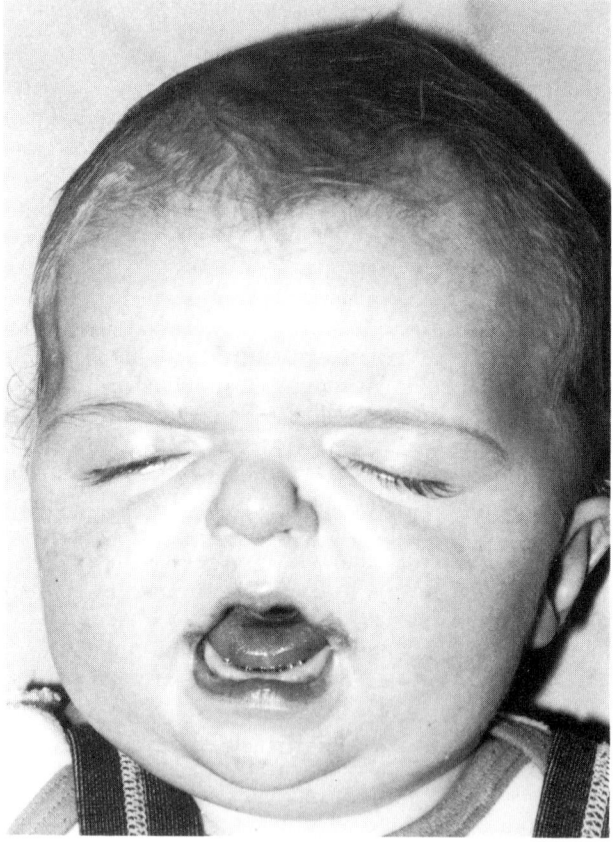

**Figure 1.** A child with Apert's Syndrome who presented for repair of a cleft palate.

Infants with a history of prematurity or respiratory distress need particular consideration. Minor surgical procedures should be performed on an inpatient basis if they are carried out in the first few months of life. Steward (1982) reviewed two groups of patients; the first consisted of 33 preterm babies where operation was carried out at between 3 and 28 weeks postnatally. The second contained 38 term infants where surgery was performed between 1 and 36 weeks of age. Eleven preterm infants had complications, the most common being apnoea occurring either operatively or after up to 12 h in the postoperative period, whereas only one of the term babies had a problem, an episode of breath-holding which occurred peroperatively. The incidence of complications is significantly higher in the premature group and is particularly alarming, as the complications can occur up to 24 h after surgery.

Urgent surgery is rarely indicated, and thus patients should be in an optimal condition prior to surgery. A common problem is the snuffly child. It is difficult to differentiate, sometimes, between an active cold and chronic rhinitis which is commonly seen in children, especially those presenting for cleft lip and palate surgery. Children in both instances will present with a runny nose and mouth breathing. Symptoms which would indicate a viral upper respiratory tract infection include malaise, loss of appetite and fever. If a viral infection is suspected then surgery should be postponed, as pneumonia or encephalitis may develop in the postoperative period.

## ANAESTHESIA

### Premedication

There is considerable variation in the use of premedication, from none at all to heavy sedation. There are no absolute rules but a number of factors will affect the type or degree of sedation required. Sedative premedication is unnecessary in babies who are less than 12–15 months, as they are too young to become anxious. In children who are over 3 years, a sedative premedication is omitted in some units, as it is believed that the child is often able to cope with their anxiety, especially if a good rapport has been established. The hospital theatre layout provides an anteroom which is set out as a play room where the children romp about, supervised by a tireless team of adults. The secret for success is the complete absence of waiting in the anaesthetic room or theatre, rapid induction and the consistent management of all children by the anaesthetic team.

When premedication is used, it is particularly important to avoid injections in children over 18 months, as they may make anyone in a white coat an instant enemy. This is not a problem for infants under 18 months of age, who should receive atropine, 0.02 mg/kg intramuscularly 30 min preoperatively. Older children receive oral premedication, trimeprazine 2–4 mg/kg or diazepam syrup 0.2 mg/kg 2 h preoperatively. The long-acting sedatives have a particular advantage, as they result in a sleepy child in the immediate postoperative period, and this reduces the likelihood of damage to delicate suture lines or bleeding under new skin grafts or tissue anastomoses.

Hypoglycaemia is a problem in infants, especially those who are less than 6 months, when normal feeding will be prevented for more than 5 h. In children less than 2 years, the stomach empties in 3 h, and therefore, if there is no pathology which might delay stomach emptying, a milk feed can be given electively 4 h preoperatively to reduce the period of starvation to a minimum. If there is any delay in the start of the operation, clear fluids can be given orally to ensure that hydration and blood sugar are maintained.

**Table 1.** Normal pulmonary function in infants (mean values). Adapted from Scarpelli (1979).

| Variable | Newborn | Adult |
|---|---|---|
| Body weight (kg) | 3 | 70 |
| Tidal volume (ml/kg) | 6 | 6 |
| Respiratory rate (breaths/min) | 35 | 15 |
| Volume expired (ml/kg/min) | 210 | 90 |
| Alveolar gas volume (ml/kg/min) | 130 | 60 |
| Anatomical dead space (ml/kg) | 2.5 | 2.0 |
| Physiological dead space/tidal volume ratio | 0.30 | 0.33 |
| Tracheal length (mm) | 57 | 120 |
| Tracheal diameter (mm) | 4 | 16 |

**Induction**

Careful handling is all-important. A recent report and subsequent correspondence in the literature have highlighted one of the difficulties, the presence of parents in the anaesthetic room during induction (While, 1985; Leader, 1986). Over the last few years, greater parental involvement has occurred generally. Ideally, the child should not be separated immediately from their parents before a stressful event, as they should be the best people to support and control their child, but there is a variation in parents' ability to cope with the situation. Good supportive parents are a positive asset in the anaesthetic room and should be encouraged but, unfortunately, nervous, distressed parents will only make worse the stress of the unfortunate child. Thus, there are no rules and each situation should be assessed separately, with the anaesthetist and nursing team being as flexible as possible.

There are three methods which can be used for induction. The first is heavy sedation followed by a gaseous induction, which is a popular technique in the UK. However, it has been argued that this apparently trauma-free method can cause psychological problems later, as the child may become afraid that each time he goes to sleep in his bed he may wake up having had another operation. Alternatively, following the establishment of an intravenous route, anaesthesia is induced intravenously. The recent introduction of EMLA cream has resulted in a significant decrease in painful reactions to venipuncture (Hannington-Kiff, 1986; Maunukesela, 1986). This is a 5% local anaesthetic cream, a eutectic mixture with equal weights of lignocaine and prilocaine, which is rubbed on to the injection site 1–2 h before operation. The author's personal experience is limited but very successful. Thirdly, thiopentone 25–30 mg or methohexitone 25 mg/kg may be given rectally in or just outside the anaesthetic room, but *never in the ward*. This method is a 'middle ground' approach which is employed in the USA but rarely in the UK. Finally, if there is difficulty with the airway, then it should be emphasized that the only acceptable method of induction is a gaseous one.

### Airway maintenance

The majority of patients undergoing plastic surgery are intubated, the exception being those having short surgical procedures performed peripherally, and who are both supine and have a good airway. Care must be taken during intubation and with the selection of the size of tube, as any oedema following intubation is particularly hazardous, because the tracheal diameter is as little as 4 mm in the neonate; any further decrease is very significant, as the resistance to gas flow increases by the 4th power of any decrease in radius. The cricoid is the narrowest part of the airway in children up to 10 years, and thus a small air leak is the only guarantee that the tube is not too large. Intubation is carried out following paralysis with suxamethonium 1 mg/kg or a non-depolarizing neuromuscular blocker (e.g. alcuronium 0.3 mg/kg) provided that the airway can be maintained.

Endotracheal tubes most commonly used are the RAE (Ring et al, 1975) tube, the anatomical tube (Morgan and Steward, 1982) and the Oxford tube (Alsop, 1955). All are preformed tubes made of polyvinyl chloride, except the Oxford, which is manufactured from rubber (Figure 2). The RAE has been criticized for being too long, but if the black ring is fixed at the lips, endobronchial intubation is less likely. The anatomical tube has been

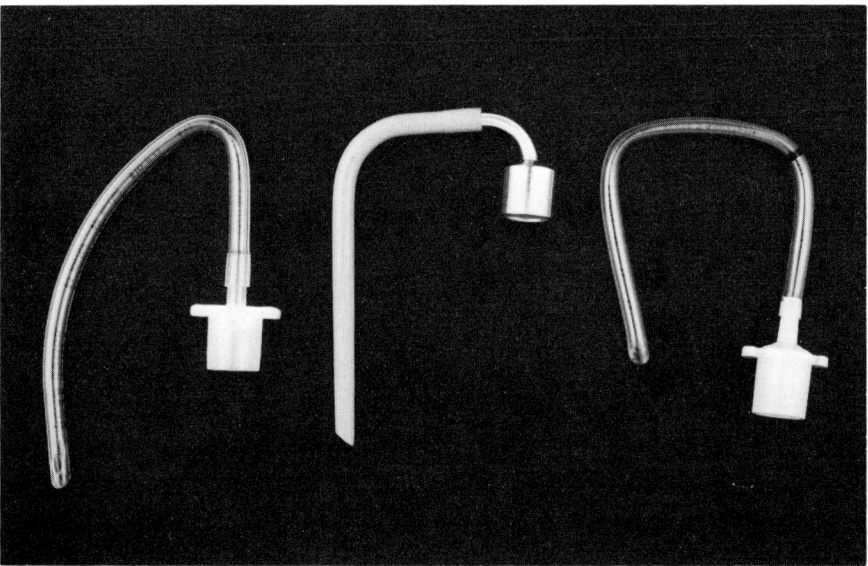

**Figure 2.** Three endotracheal tubes commonly used in paediatric plastic practice. From left to right, the tubes are: RAE™, Oxford, Anatomical.

designed from radiographic measurements of the children's airways. The Oxford tube, in contrast, is conical with a constant internal diameter but a gradually increasing external diameter. All these endotracheal tubes have 15 mm connectors which can fit directly into the ISO standard circuit. A modified Ayre's T-piece is used for small children, the Bain circuit (a coaxial modified Mapleson D circuit) being used for older children.

After ensuring air entry into both sides of the chest, the tube is firmly fixed by taping it to an airway or bite block which in turn is strapped to the face. This gives support to the endotracheal tube and is especially useful for small tubes, where often the weight of the breathing attachment can dislodge or kink the tube. Flexion and extension of the neck in an intubated patient with a tube fixed at the mouth makes the tip of the endotracheal tube move down and up the trachea respectively. In a postmortem study of infants, it has been shown that flexion shortens the distance between the carina and the tip of an orotracheal tube, while extension lengthens the distance, the implication being that with extension there is a risk of extubation and with flexion of endobronchial intubation (Bosman and Foster, 1977). The problems of difficult intubation are dealt with elsewhere in this issue. Suffice it to say here that one can always resort to using a flexible bronchoscope technique, especially as it is now possible to anaesthetize the child first, maintaining ventilation and anaesthesia with a transtracheal catheter (Ravussin and Freeman, 1985).

## Maintenance

Plastic surgery demands a good surgical field to allow accurate surgery to take place, followed by calm emergence from anaesthesia. Timing of the length of surgery is difficult as it can never be assumed that all is finished until the surgeon has left the theatre! Depending on the surgery involved, the anaesthetic technique may range from spontaneous breathing with a face mask to a full muscle relaxant technique with IPPV and a volatile agent with or without the addition of a narcotic. Factors to consider include the use of vasoconstrictor agents by the surgeons and repeat anaesthesia, which will be discussed later. The author's personal preference for the maintenance of anaesthesia is papaveretum, 0.1–0.3 mg/kg IM, given after induction with the addition of a volatile agent. Where the patients are ventilated, in older children 40% of the papaveretum dose may be given IV.

When a spontaneous breathing technique is used, the patient is connected to either a T-piece or Bain circuit with a fresh gas flow 2½ times the predicted minute volume. When the patients are ventilated, a simple system consists of connecting a ventilator to the expiratory limb of the T-piece or manual port of the Bain circuit with the valve closed (Figure 3). When minute ventilation is twice fresh gas flow, $PaCO_2$ becomes dependent on the fresh gas flow and the effect of minute ventilation is minimized. The Nuffield Anaesthesia Ventilator series 200 (Penlon Limited, Abingdon, Oxford) is a suitable machine, being a time-cycled ventilator, able to deliver flows of 0.2–1.0 litre/s at a rate of 10–85 breaths/min. When used with the Newton Valve (Penlon Limited) the system can ventilate all children. A suitable

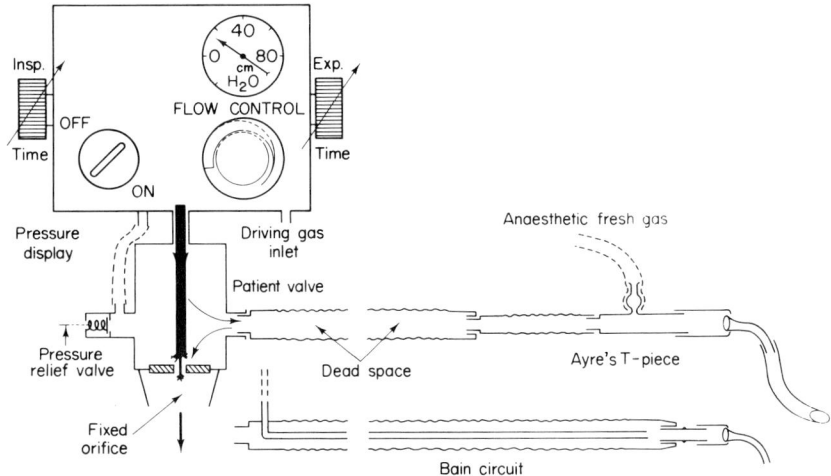

**Figure 3.** Diagrammatic representation of the arrangement, showing connection of the Nuffield series 200 ventilator to the T-piece or Bain circuit; from Newton et al (1981).

formula to calculate fresh gas flow has been derived from clinical practice by Rose and Froese (1979) (Table 2).

Temperature maintenance in infants and neonates is difficult because of the considerable heat losses from the relatively large surface area and underdeveloped temperature-regulating mechanisms. Methods to reduce the loss have been described in detail (Steward, 1979), and each technique depends on the surgery involved. Intravenous fluids are given to supply basal maintenance needs; 3–4 ml/kg/h in patients up to 20 kg, 2 ml/kg/h for 20–40 kg, and for those over 40 kg, 1 ml/kg/h. Other losses are made up with the relevant solutions. A difficult loss to assess is the steady ooze over a long period of time from large raw areas. The anaesthetist has to rely on other signs of hypovolaemia and to be prepared to transfuse despite an apparent absence of bleeding. Routine monitoring includes the use of precordial stethoscope and ECG. Blood pressure can be measured with a conventional sphygmomanometer using a flat Doppler flow probe placed over the radial artery as a pulse detection monitor. Temperature should be monitored routinely, the most accurate core temperature being measured two-thirds down the oesophagus. Central venous pressure is rarely required, but can be measured using a basilic, internal jugular or subclavian vein cannulation.

**Table 2.** Fresh gas flow requirement (controlled ventilation). $V_E$ (on the ventilator) must be twice this FGF. From Rose and Froese (1979).

| Weight | Predicted | Predicted |
|---|---|---|
| | $P_aCO_2$ 4.9 kPa (37 mm Hg) | $P_aCO_2$ 4.0 kPa (30 mm Hg) |
| 10–30 kg | 1000 ml + 100 ml/kg | 1600 ml + 100 ml/kg |
| > 30 kg | 2000 ml + 50 ml/kg | 3200 ml + 50 ml/kg |

The subclavian route has the highest risk of pneumothorax, and it has been suggested that a chest x-ray should be taken following cannulation.

## REPEAT ANAESTHESIA

For many years there has been a controversy over the use of halothane repeated at short intervals and the risk of postoperative jaundice. This has persisted because of the numerous causes of postoperative jaundice, which include viral hepatitis, sepsis, hypoxia and hypovolaemia, making it difficult to assess the evidence and perform clinical studies. The issue has been further clouded by the fact that millions of patients have been safely anaesthetized with this agent, which when it was introduced revolutionized anaesthetic practice. Despite this, there has been established a number of cases of jaundice which have followed repeat halothane anaesthetics, with an incidence which varies between 1 in 7000 and 1 in 30 000 (Bunker et al, 1969; Inman and Mushin, 1969; Fee et al, 1979). Neuberger and Williams (1984) suggested that there are two forms of halothane jaundice. The first is mild and is characterized by malaise, low-grade pyrexia and raised serum aminotransferase levels; it affects 25% of patients exposed to halothane. The second form occurs more rarely in patients following a repeat exposure to halothane and is characterized by fulminant hepatic failure with a high incidence of severe encephalitis and associated mortality.

Halothane is metabolized by either an oxidative or reductive pathway, the latter occurring under hypoxic conditions induced by either arterial desaturation or hepatic ischaemia following hypotension. Human cytochrome P-450 can convert halothane to free radicals which will combine with tissue macromolecules which initiate the events which result in hepatocellular death (Leader, 1986). Patients who develop fulminant hepatic failure have a history of previous halothane exposure with a reaction of postoperative pyrexia or jaundice, and antibodies to halothane-altered liver-cell membrane are present. Finally, Hoft et al (1981) and Farrell et al (1985) reported evidence which indicated that in humans susceptibility to halothane hepatitis was genetically determined. Lymphocytes from patients who suffered from halothane jaundice were susceptible to electrophilic attack by drug metabolites. Thus, it appears that a percentage of the population are susceptible to halothane jaundice following repeat exposure, the only sign of this susceptibility being perhaps a mild reaction which may only be a low-grade postoperative pyrexia.

Wark (1983) argued that this syndrome rarely affects children, following a retrospective study of patients at Great Ormond Street and, more recently, a prospective study conducted in Sydney, Australia (Wark et al, 1986). However, Whitburn and Sumner recently reported (1986) a case of halothane jaundice in an 11-month old baby who had the diagnostic evidence already described for adults. Furthermore, in a discussion of two other series of patients, children do not appear to be immune (Leader, 1986).

Should halothane be used as a volatile agent, particularly in patients who are highly likely to be undergoing repeat procedures? Firstly, the alternative volatile agents, isoflurane and enflurane, do not appear to produce free radicals and have a limited degree of metabolism when compared to halothane: enflurane 2%, isoflurane 0.2% and halothane 20% (Watson, 1986). Secondly, in a busy clinical practice, if the patient has a history of a previous anaesthetic, it may be relatively simple to establish the agent used, but very difficult to be certain that there was no evidence of pyrexia in the postoperative period. Finally, despite some reported difficulties in the use of the alternative agents (Pandit et al, 1985) and their considerable cost, it is difficult to justify the use of halothane routinely in the more affluent parts of the world. Equally, when there is a particular clinical or economic indication to use halothane, then there is no justification for increasing the risk to the patient by not using halothane. If halothane does have to be repeated, then the interval should be not less than 3 months, unless clinical considerations dictate otherwise (CSM, 1986).

## TECHNIQUE FOR BLOODLESS FIELD

Blood loss during cleft lip and palate surgery ranges between 2 and 280 ml blood (Tempest, 1958; Jennings et al, 1980; Black et al, 1969). It is rarely significant from a cardiovascular point of view, as the loss is slow and can easily be replaced, but blood transfusion has many hazards and therefore it is better if it can be avoided. A persistently flooded field will make surgery difficult and prolonged, thereby increasing morbidity because there is more diathermied tissue and less accurate and prolonged surgery. A common technique used to reduce blood loss includes infiltration with an adrenaline solution. Gordon-Jones (1962) established that there was a significant reduction in blood loss when using 2% lignocaine solution with 1 in 80000 adrenaline. Halothane sensitizes the heart to adrenaline, which has resulted in numerous studies to establish the safe dose. Wallbank (1970) and Karl et al (1981) most recently reported respectively the safe use of 1.5–5.5 µg/kg in spontaneously breathing children and 0.4–15.7 µg/kg in hyperventilated children, confirming the author's opinion that tolerance is reduced in the presence of hypercapnoea.

Much of this is academic, since the advent of the newer volatile agents, enflurane and isoflurane, which do not appear to sensitize the heart to adrenaline. Johnston et al (1976) established an $ED_{50}$ of adrenaline which would produce three extra systoles in patients who are ventilated and anaesthetized with either halothane, enflurane or isoflurane. The $ED_{50}$ were 2.1 µg/kg (halothane), 3.7 µg/kg (halothane + lignocaine), 10.9 µg/kg (enflurane) and 6.7 µg/kg (isoflurane). The maximum recommended amount is 50% of the $ED_{50}$ dose. In our own practice, Moffett's solution (3% cocaine and 1 in 4000 adrenaline) 0.1 ml/kg, is applied topically on gauze producing blanching of the tissues (Figure 4). In a small double-blind study, a significant reduction in blood loss from 25.2 ml to 14.4 ml during cleft palate surgery was observed in those babies treated with topical Moffett's solution. The patients were in two groups, with the palates of the control group (12 patients) being infiltrated with lignocaine and adrenaline,

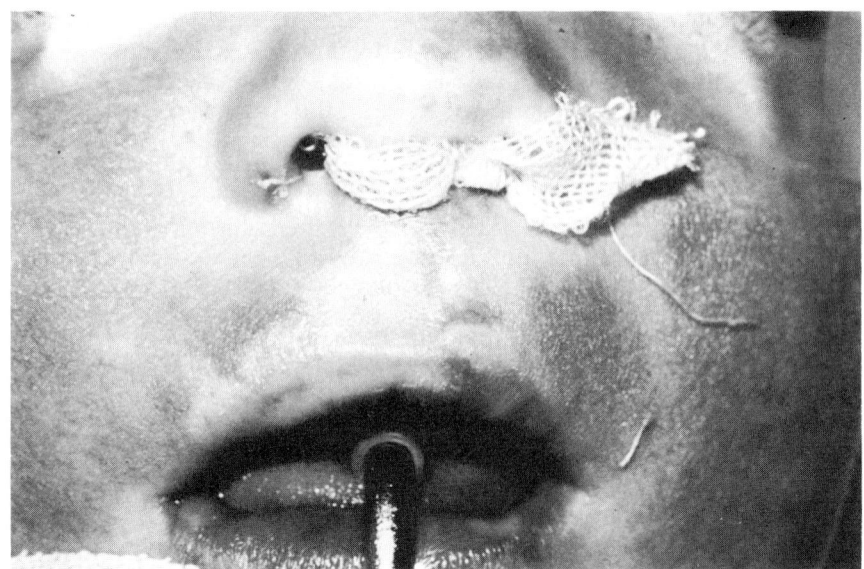

**Figure 4.** Nasal pack soaked in Moffett's solution. Note blanching of the upper lip and cupid's bow.

and those of the test group (11 patients) receiving the topical Moffett's solution in addition (Walters, unpublished data).

Finally, the trial introduction of POR-8, a synthetic derivative of the natural neurohypophyseal hormone, should be followed closely, as, provided it is equally effective and has no cardiac effect, it should prove safer than adrenaline as significant amounts of the infiltrated dose of adrenaline, 21.8%, may appear in the intravascular compartment (Low et al, 1984).

## CLEFT LIP AND PALATE SURGERY

### Classification

The overall incidence of this defect is 1 in 600. Cleft lip occurs alone, right or left, with an incidence of 25%, unilateral cleft lip and palate with a 40% incidence, bilateral cleft lip and palate with a 10% incidence, and cleft palate alone with a 25% incidence (Hathorn, 1986). Other congenital abnormalities occur in 3–13% of patients with an isolated cleft lip, in between 2 and 11% of those with both lip and palate defects, and in 13–15% of patients with a single cleft palate.

Important conditions associated with cleft lip and palate defects include Pierre–Robin syndrome with macroglossia and micrognathia. This has important implications for the anaesthetist, as in these patients it is difficult to intubate the airway, which may easily become obstructed, depending on the size of the tongue. Other syndromes include Treacher Collins with micrognathia, down-slanting palpebral fissures, absent zygoma and low-set ears. Finally, cleft defects may be associated with hemifacial microsomia (Goldenhar's syndrome) which also includes cardiac defects and renal and vertebral abnormalities.

## Primary surgery

Primary surgery for cleft lip repair can take up to 2 h and is performed at 3 months of age. Definitive surgery for cleft palate repair is performed at 6–12 months, and takes approximately 1 h. The preoperative visit must include an assessment of the airway, which often presents no problem, but if associated with one of the syndromes already listed may cause marked difficulty with intubation and with airway maintenance once anaesthesia has been induced. Potential airway obstruction can be assessed by asking about sleeping, snoring and the position of the patient during sleep. Enquiries about feeding will give a general impression of the patient and more information about the airway.

## Anaesthesia

Preoperative preparation, premedication and induction have already been described. All patients are intubated and a throat pack inserted to prevent blood reaching the oesophagus. Rarely, intubation of a patient with a cleft lip defect may be difficult because the laryngoscope slips into the cleft. This can be prevented by packing the cleft with gauze. It is important to fix the orotracheal tube centrally without distorting the lips and to protect the eyes with ointment if they have to be exposed. Topical vasoconstriction can be obtained by packing a gauze soaked in Moffett's solution into the nose and over the cleft.

Cleft plate surgery requires the insertion of a gag with a split tongue blade which acts as a slot for the endotracheal tube. While the gag is being positioned and opened it is possible for the tube to become crushed between the blade and the alveolus (Figure 5). Moffett's solution can be applied topically with a gauze draped over the soft and hard palate.

## Postoperative period

Ideally, the patient should be tranquil and pain-free in the postoperative period, as crying and struggling will almost invariably start some oozing. Analgesia can be given in the postoperative period, codeine phosphate 1.0–1.5 mg/kg IM, in addition to the residual analgesia from the pre-operative narcotic. Sometimes these babies cry because they are hungry. Therefore, all fluids should be started as soon as possible postoperatively (2–5 h), working up to a full feed as quickly as the baby can manage.

In the meantime, intravenous fluids should be continued until oral nourishment has been established. Special sleeves should be put on the baby's arms to prevent the fingers from being sucked, which may damage the repair.

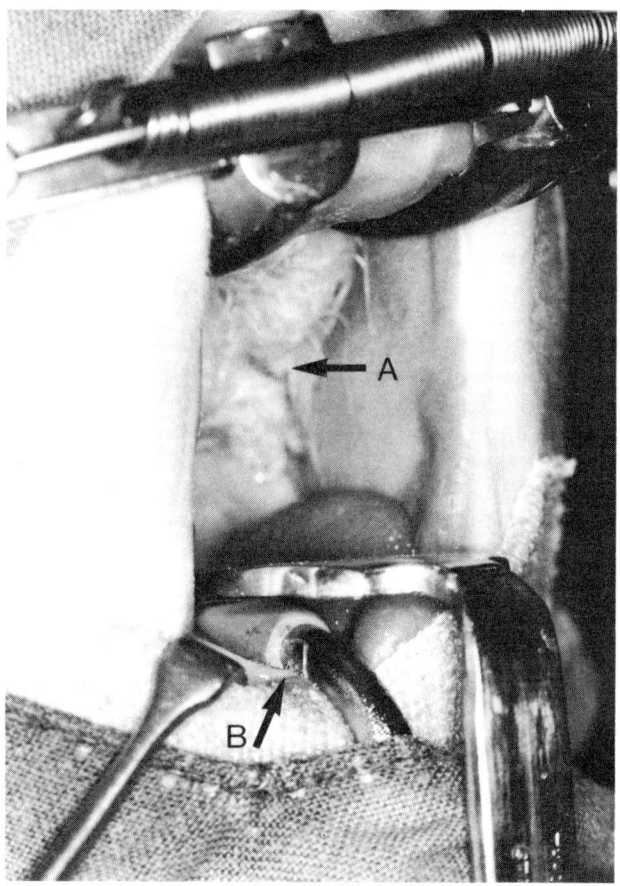

**Figure 5.** Boyle–Davies gag in position prior to repair of cleft palate. A indicates gauze soaked in Moffett's Solution placed on the palate. B indicates the ET tube crossing the alveolus beneath the tongue gag where it can be crushed.

A major postoperative complication is airway obstruction. The large preoperative cavernous airway is reduced by surgery, particularly following a cleft lip repair. Generally, this presents no problem for the child in the postoperative period as he learns very quickly to adapt to the new airway, but occasionally a tongue suture may be needed to pull the tongue forward. If this method fails to keep the airway clear, an oral airway may be inserted to establish the airway. It can then be taped in position for a few hours while the baby learns to adapt to mouth breathing. Rarely, nasotracheal intubation is required, but this should only be performed after consultation with the surgeon to avoid damage to the repair.

**Secondary surgery**

Secondary surgery is performed on children between 5 and 15 years.

Revisions to the lip include columella lengthening and the Abbé flap, which is performed when the upper lip is short of tissue and the lower lip is protuberant. A wedge of tissue is swung up to the upper lip, which means that when the child wakes up the lips are joined by a tissue pedicle. Between 10 and 14 days later, after the tissue has picked up a new blood supply, the bridge is divided under anaesthetic following intubation which can be quite 'sporting'. The airway is not difficult to maintain, so following an intravenous induction intubation is performed by passing the laryngoscope and tube down opposite sides of the bridge. Other secondary surgery includes nose revisions and surgery to the hard palate and alveolus.

Secondary speech surgery is performed for hypernasality resulting from nasal escape when the gap between the soft palate and the posterior pharyngeal wall is too large. At operation, pharyngoplasty, the posterior pharyngeal wall may be brought forward, thereby reducing the airway. The anaesthetic considerations are similar to those for cleft palate surgery. Occasionally, chronic obstruction occurs if the gap has been made too small and may result in a failure to thrive, cor pulmonale and possibly sleep apnoea. These systemic complications must be borne in mind if these patients are anaesthetized to have their obstruction reduced. Finally, nasal intubation is contraindicated for any procedure in these patients.

## REFERENCES

Alsop AF (1955) Non-kinking endotracheal tubes. *Anaesthesia* **10**: 401–403.
Black GW, Coppel DL, Hughes NC et al (1969) Anaesthesia for cleft palate surgery: a comparative study of anaesthetic methods. *British Journal of Plastic Surgery* **22**: 343–350.
Bosman YK & Foster PA (1977) Endotracheal intubation and head posture in infants. *South African Medical Journal* **52**: 71–73.
Bunker JP, Forrest WH, Mosteller F & Vandam DJ (1969) *The National Halothane Study*. Washington DC: US Government Printing Office.
Committee on Safety of Medicines (1986) *Halothane hepatotoxicity* pp 18.
Farrell G, Prendergast D & Murray M (1985) Halothane hepatitis. Detection of a constitutional susceptibility factor. *New England Journal of Medicine* **313**: 1310–1314.
Fee JPH, Black GW, Dundee JW et al (1979) A prospective of liver enzyme and other changes following repeat administration of halothane and enflurane. *British Journal of Anaesthesia* **51**: 1133–1141.
Gordon-Jones RG (1962) The reduction of bleeding in hare-lip and cleft-palate surgery. *British Journal of Anaesthesia* **34**: 481–488.
Goudsouzian NG, Donlon JV, Savarese JJ et al (1975) Re-evaluation of dosage and duration of action of D-tubocurarine in the pediatric age group. *Anesthesiology* **43**: 416–425.
Hannington-Kiff JC (1986) Anaesthesia for children. *Lancet* **ii**: 1031.
Hathorn IS (1986) Classification. In Alberry EH, Hathorn IS & Pigott RW (eds) *Cleft Lip and Palate: a Team Approach*, pp 17–19. Bristol: Wright.
Hoft RH, Bienker JP, Goodman HI & Gregory PB (1981) Halothane hepatitis in three pairs of closely related women. *New England Journal of Medicine* **304**: 1023–1024.
Inman WHW & Mushin WW (1969) Jaundice after repeat exposure to halothane: an analysis of reports to the Committee on Safety of Medicines. *British Medical Journal* **i**: 5–10.
Jennings FO, Delaney EJ & Prendiville JB (1980) Ether—cyclopropane anaesthesia for the primary repair of cleft lip and palate. *British Journal of Plastic Surgery* **33**: 301–304.
Johnston RR, Eger EI II & Wilsin C (1976) A comparative interaction of epinephrine with enflurane, isoflurane and halothane in man. *Anesthesia and Analgesia* **55**: 709–712.

Jones AEP & Pelton DA (1976) An index of syndromes and their anaesthetic implications. *Canadian Anaesthetists' Society Journal* **23:** 207–226.

Karl HW, Swedlow DB, Lee KW & Downes JJ (1981) Epinephrine–halothane interactions in children. *Anesthesiology* **55:** A336.

Leader (1986) Parents in the anaesthetic room. *Lancet* **ii:** 903.

Leader (1986) Halothane-associated liver damage. *Lancet* **i:** 1251–1252.

Low JM, Harvey JT, Cooper GM et al (1984) Plasma concentrations of catecholamines following adrenaline infiltration during gynaecological surgery. *British Journal of Anaesthesia* **56:** 849–853.

Maunuksela E-L & Korpela R (1986) Double-blind evaluation of a lignocaine–prilocaine cream (EMLA) in children. *British Journal of Anaesthesia* **58:** 1242–1245.

Morgan GAR & Steward DJ (1982) A pre-formed paediatric orotracheal tube design based on anatomical measurements. *Canadian Anaesthetists' Society Journal* **29:** 9–11.

Neuberger J & Williams R (1984) Halothane anaesthesia and liver damage. *British Medical Journal* **289:** 1136–1139.

Newton NI, Hillman KM & Varley JG (1981) Automatic ventilation with the Ayres T-piece: a modification of the Nuffield Series 200 ventilatory for neonatal and paediatric use. *Anaesthesia* **36:** 22–36.

Pandit UA, Steude GM & Leach AB (1985) Induction and recovery characteristics of isoflurane and halothane anaesthesia for short outpatient operations in children. *Anaesthesia* **40:** 1226–1230.

Ravussin P & Freeman J (1985) A new transtracheal catheter for ventilation and resuscitation. *Canadian Anaesthetists' Society Journal* **32:** 60–64.

Ring WH, Adair JC & Elwyn RA (1975) New paediatric endotracheal tube. *Anaesthesia and Analgesia* **54:** 273–274.

Rose DK & Froese AB (1979) The regulation of $PaCO_2$ during controlled ventilation of children with a T-Piece. *Canadian Anaesthetist's Society Journal* **26:** 104–113.

Scarpelli EM (ed.) (1979) *Pulmonary Physiology in the Fetus, Newborn, and Child*, pp 168. Philadelphia: Lea and Febiger.

Steward DJ (1979) *Manual of Pediatric Anesthesia*, 1st edn. New York: Churchill Livingstone.

Steward DJ (1982) Preterm infants are more prone to complications following minor surgery than are term infants. *Anesthesiology* **56:** 304–306.

Tempest MN (1958) Some observations on blood loss in hare-lip and cleft palate surgery. *British Journal of Plastic Surgery* **11:** 34–44.

Vergani D, Mieli-Vergani G, Alberti A et al (1980) Antibodies to the surface of halothane altered rabbit hepatocytes in patients with fulminant hepatic failure. *New England Journal of Medicine* **303:** 66–71.

Wallbank WA (1970) Cardiac effects of halothane and adrenaline in hare-lip and cleft-palate surgery. *British Journal of Anaesthesia* **42:** 548–552.

Walton B (1986) Halothane hepatitis in children. *Anaesthesia* **41:** 575–578.

Wark HJ (1983) Postoperative jaundice in children. The influence of halothane. *Anaesthesia* **38:** 237–242.

Wark H, O'Halloran M & Overton J (1986) Prospective study of liver function in children following multiple halothane anaesthetics at short intervals. *British Journal of Anaesthesia* **58:** 1224–1228.

While A (1985) Personal view. *British Medical Journal* **291:** 343.

Whitburn RH & Sumner E (1986) Halothane hepatitis in an 11-month-old child. *Anaesthesia* **41:** 611–613.

# 11

Local and regional anaesthesia

DEREK J. DYE

Plastic surgery provides an unsurpassed opportunity to employ local anaesthetic techniques for a variety of operations over a wide age range. Used alone or with sedation, local anaesthesia can provide excellent operating conditions and postoperative analgesia, along with useful sympathetic blockade. If used in combination with general anaesthesia, e.g. in children or anxious adults, local anaesthesia reduces anaesthetic requirements, attenuates the stress response to surgery, and can ensure a pain-free recovery period. In addition, local anaesthetic techniques may improve red cell deformability (thus reducing blood viscosity) and are associated with a lower incidence of thrombotic complications when used for orthopaedic surgery (McKenzie and Loach, 1986).

The recommended doses of local anaesthetics for some nerve blocks are in excess of the maxima quoted in drug data sheets. It is therefore sensible to consider briefly the toxicity and pharmacokinetics of local anaesthetics and the management of their toxic manifestations. A detailed account of the pharmacokinetics of local anaesthetics is given by Tucker (1986).

## LOCAL ANAESTHETIC TOXICITY

Toxicity developing immediately after injection is indicative of intravascular injection. Signs of toxicity appearing 10 min or more after injection are suggestive of rapid absorption, and progress relatively slowly, allowing time for appropriate action to minimize toxic effects.

Intravenous access and resuscitation facilities must be available if local anaesthetic techniques are to be used safely. As with most unwanted drug effects, local anaesthetic toxicity is more easily prevented than treated and is rare if scrupulous care is taken to avoid intravascular injection and if injections are made slowly. It is important to watch for early signs of toxicity and, particularly, to ask the patient to report any untoward symptoms.

### Central nervous system toxicity

The pattern of symptoms and signs of CNS toxicity ranges from patients complaining of feeling 'odd', 'vague' or anxious, sometimes with numbness of the tongue, through tinnitus, nausea and visual disturbance, and the more serious signs of slurred speech, inco-ordination and muscle twitching, to unconsciousness and convulsions. Convulsions may occur without warning after inadvertent intravascular injection and are likely if arterial plasma levels exceed 4 μg/ml for bupivacaine (Moore et al, 1979) and 10 μg/ml for lignocaine (Tucker, 1986). The quantity of local anaesthetic reaching the brain after intravascular injection will be greatly increased if the cardiac output is low.

Sedation or general anaesthesia may mask the symptoms and signs of CNS toxicity and, to some extent, protect against the worst manifestations. It is most unlikely that premedicant doses of benzodiazepines would protect against the CNS effects of an accidental IV bolus, but in borderline cases where the rise in plasma levels is gradual and peak levels are lower, convulsions may sometimes be averted by intravenous diazepam up to 0.35 mg/kg (Moore et al, 1979). If frank convulsions occur, thiopentone (with respiratory support if necessary) is a more appropriate anticonvulsant. CNS toxicity of local anaesthetics is well reviewed by Scott (1986).

**Cardiovascular toxicity**

The cardiovascular effects of local anaesthetic agents are potentially far more serious than the CNS effects and are responsible for most local anaesthetic-related deaths. Leaving aside arterial hypotension caused by central blocks, the untoward effects of local anaesthetics on the CVS include myocardial depression, ventricular arrhythmias (particularly from bupivacaine), conduction defects and cardiac arrest (Reiz and Nath, 1986). Most reports of cardiac arrest have concerned the use of 0.75% bupivacaine in labour (an unnecessarily high concentration which has now been withdrawn from obstetric use) or the use of bupivacaine in i.v. regional anaesthesia. There have also been cardiac arrests after caudal block, and after interscalene block. Bupivacaine remains in the myocardium longer than lignocaine, and when cardiac arrest follows administration of the former it is likely to be particularly refractory, requiring prolonged cardiac massage (Reiz and Nath, 1986). Animal studies indicate that bupivacaine in equianalgesic doses may be as much as 2.5 times as cardiotoxic as lignocaine (Tanz et al, 1984; Moller and Covino, 1985). The margin between the plasma level likely to cause convulsions and that associated with cardiac effects may be smaller for bupivacaine than for lignocaine (Tanz et al, 1984).

## LOCAL ANAESTHETIC DOSAGE

The maximum safe dose of local anaesthetic agents administered at one time will depend upon drug concentration, the use of vasoconstrictors, the characteristics of the chosen drug and, perhaps most importantly, the route of administration. The latter factor has received little attention in published tables of 'maximum' doses. Although the 1986/7 Data Sheet Compendium (UK) states that the maximum dose will depend upon the size and physical status of the patient and the rate of absorption from particular injection sites, the maximum dose for peripheral nerve block is quoted as 30 ml of 0.5% bupivacaine. This is unnecessarily restrictive for some blocks, in which clinical studies have demonstrated the safety of much greater volumes (Tucker, 1986).

In adults, body weight is a poor guide to dose requirements, stature being better. In children of normal body build, weight is an acceptable indicator of dose requirement and is a readily available parameter in most hospitals.

## CENTRAL BLOCKS

### Spinal subarachnoid block

The reliability of subarachnoid block and its speed of onset make this technique highly suitable for operations below the waist, although if there is likely to be prolonged or severe postoperative pain, an epidural block with a catheter for postoperative analgesia may be a better option. Many plastic surgical procedures involve the taking of split skin grafts from the legs, and spinal subarachnoid anaesthesia is often very useful for this purpose, combined, if necessary, with other forms of local anaesthesia, e.g. axillary block, for the primary procedure. Heavy 0.5% bupivacaine is a very satis-factory agent, having a long duration of action (3–4 h) and predictable spread. Isobaric 0.5% bupivacaine, although useful if the side to be operated upon is painful (e.g. in burns of the leg), is less predictable in its spread (Logan et al, 1986).

### Lumbar epidural block

Lumbar epidural block may be used for anaesthesia and, if a catheter is inserted, to provide excellent postoperative analgesia. Epidural anaesthesia markedly improves blood flow in pedicle flaps, mainly because of the sympathetic block produced.

For postoperative analgesia, an epidural infusion of 0.25% bupivacaine at the rate of 3–10 ml/h is usually satisfactory in adults, but if a large number of segments are to be blocked or if motor blockade is a problem, then a larger volume of more dilute solution may be preferable. A lower concentration may also be safer in the event of dural penetration by the catheter tip and may give early warning without high spinal motor block (Ewen et al, 1986). Plasma levels of bupivacaine may be quite high during continuous infusion (up to 4 μg/ml in one study: Ross et al, 1980) but have not been associated with clinical problems. The technique considerably improves patient com-fort after such operations as cross leg flaps, but the patient is deprived of protective sensation, so great care must be taken to avoid pressure necrosis and other positional injuries. 0.125% bupivacine may not remove all sensation and may be safer in this respect, as may epidural opiates. If epidural block is to be used after free flap surgery it is essential to avoid arterial hypotension; this is less likely to occur if analgesia is maintained by infusion rather than bolus injections. Epidural opiates are free of sympathetic effects but have not been shown to have any beneficial effects on fibrinolysis or blood viscosity.

### Caudal block

Caudal epidural block, although little used in adults, is particularly suited to small children in whom it may be used to provide analgesia of skin donor sites and after hypospadias correction. In the latter case it is better than penile nerve block since the latter does not anaesthetize the whole of the ventral surface of the penis. Caudal block in children is most easily performed after the induction of general anaesthesia with the child in the lateral position.

Age correlates well with dose requirements (Schulte-Steinberg and Rahlfs, 1977) but so does weight. The latter measurement is readily available, and gives a better guide to dosage in children who are unusually small or large for their age. A lumbosacral block requires 0.5 ml/kg body weight. 0.25% plain bupivacaine is usually sufficient to provide good postoperative analgesia (Armitage, 1985) and allows the simultaneous administration of axillary blocks (using 0.25% bupivacaine) for hand operations. 0.25% bupivacaine also has the advantage that it does not usually cause urinary retention or motor block. Children find the latter distressing, which may be a factor in the restlessness often reported after caudal blocks with 0.5% bupivacaine.

Although full aseptic precautions are vital, it is not necessary to use a special pack; a standard 23 SWG (standard wire gauge) 2.5 cm needle is quite satisfactory. If this is only inserted far enough to encounter a loss of resistance to injection and care is taken to aspirate before injection and after every 2 or 3 ml, there is very little risk of subarachnoid or significant intravascular injection. Arterial hypotension, often seen in adults after epidural blocks, does not seem to be a problem in children, in whom caudal block is a safe and reliable procedure (Armitage, 1985).

## BRACHIAL PLEXUS BLOCKS

Brachial plexus blocks are useful for procedures ranging from carpal tunnel release to reimplantation of severed digits. It is possible to use them for prolonged operations on adults without heavy sedation or general anaesthesia, but unless great care is taken to position the patient comfortably on the operating table and to ensure that the bladder is empty before surgery commences, patients are likely to become restless. This can be a great hindrance to the surgeon, particularly if microsurgery is being undertaken. If the patient is not heavily sedated (and heavy sedation can lead to the patient becoming restless and unco-operative) it is helpful to provide some distraction in the form of taped music or quiet conversation.

Uptake of local anaesthetic after brachial plexus blocks is relatively slow, and peak plasma levels are lower than those seen after other blocks, increasing in the order: axillary–supraclavicular–interscalene (Vester-Andersen et al, 1981).

For a number of reasons, the axillary route is the only safe option for brachial plexus block in small children (Arthur and McNicol, 1986), and although it is sometimes feasible to use axillary blocks in awake children it is generally preferable to insert the block after induction of general anaesthesia, with the aim of providing good postoperative analgesia. There is a theoretical risk of unrecognized intraneural injection, and if there is any resistance to injection the needle must be withdrawn slightly before injecting more local anaesthetic. The use of a lower concentration of drug (e.g. 0.25% bupivacaine) allows the simultaneous employment of another block, e.g. a second axillary block or a caudal block to cover skin donor sites.

## Axillary block

Axillary block has major advantages; there is no risk of inadvertent subarachnoid or epidural injection, or of pneumothorax, or of phrenic or recurrent laryngeal nerve block. Its main disadvantage is that, even in experienced hands, there is an appreciable failure rate (as high as 20% in some reported series). A less serious disadvantage is that the block can take an hour or more to develop and this may complicate theatre logistics. The block is less likely to be successful in obese patients, partly because it is often more difficult to identify the axillary sheath but probably also because fat within the sheath takes up part of the dose of local anaesthetic; also, the block which develops, although widespread, is sometimes insufficiently dense to permit surgery without supplementary anaesthesia.

### Practical details

For a detailed consideration of the technique of axillary block the reader is referred to Eriksson (1979), but the local anaesthetic doses recommended in this publication are rather meagre and likely to be rewarded with a very low success rate. It has been shown that in adults the use of 50 ml of local anaesthetic solution results in a higher success rate than 40 ml, but that further increase in volume makes no difference (Vester-Andersen et al, 1984). For supraclavicular block, where uptake is more rapid, doses as high as 60 ml of 0.5% bupivacaine with 1:240 000 adrenaline have been shown to produce peak arterial plasma bupivacaine levels of less than 2.5 µg/ml in patients weighing as little as 53 kg (Moore et al, 1976), while for axillary block 40 ml of bupivacaine 0.5% without a vasoconstrictor was shown by Tuominen et al (1983) to produce blood levels well below the toxicity threshold.

The author's preference is to use either 0.5% plain bupivacaine or a mixture of plain bupivacaine 0.5% and lignocaine 1%, which seems to give a faster onset (see Table 1). This gives a success rate of about 90% overall without supplementary measures. A light tourniquet or digital pressure below the point of injection prevents downward spread of local anaesthetic. The use of an immobile needle technique (using a plastic extension tube) makes the block technically easier, and deposition of 5 ml of local anaesthetic superficial to the sheath usually ensures blockade of the musculo-

Table 1. Local anaesthetic dosages—brachial plexus blocks.

| Axillary | Adults | Children* |
|---|---|---|
| Bupivacaine 0.5% plain | 45–50 ml | 0.7 ml/kg |
| Bupivacaine 0.5%/lignocaine 1% mixture 2:1 | 45–50 ml | 0.7 ml/kg |
| Supraclavicular and interscalene | | |
| Bupivacaine 0.5% plain | 40 ml | N/A |

* For children 0.25% bupivacaine will provide postoperative analgesia.

cutaneous nerve after it has left the axillary sheath and before it enters the coracobrachialis muscle. Although analgesia is usually not dense in the tourniquet areas, it is generally sufficient to prevent patient discomfort. Adduction of the arm as soon as the injection is complete removes the restrictive effect of the head of the humerus on the axillary sheath and favours the upward spread of the injected agent. It is not necessary to seek paraesthesia, and indeed there is evidence that deliberately doing so may lead to a higher incidence of nerve damage (Selander, 1979).

Short bevelled needles cause less nerve damage than standard intravenous needles (Selander et al, 1977), but the latter may be used without clinical problems provided that the operator is gentle and careful to avoid intraneural injection and that small-gauge needles are used. If paraesthesiae are evoked, if there is resistance to injection or if the patient complains of pain on injection, the point of the needle should be slightly withdrawn before injecting more local anaesthetic. Arterial puncture should be avoided; blood in the sheath may reduce the effectiveness of the block and a haematoma may cause pain and paraesthesia when the block wears off.

The duration of anaesthesia with 0.5% bupivacaine is usually at least 6 h, even without the use of a vasoconstrictor. Catheter techniques (Selander, 1977) are rarely called for, although they may be of use for multiple finger replantation. It is not necessary to use epidural needles and cannulae for this purpose; simple i.v. cannulae inserted obliquely are suitable and much easier to insert. The 23 SWG Y-can (Wallace) with its short length of flexible tubing is very useful in this respect. Even with a single injection of plain 0.5% bupivacaine, analgesia often persists for up to 12 h, after which simple oral analgesics will usually suffice.

## Supraclavicular block

The reader is again referred to Eriksson (1979) for details of this block. Unlike axillary block, this technique anaesthetizes the shoulder, but this is rarely an advantage in plastic surgery, and the risk of pneumothorax (which may be slow to develop) is a major disadvantage if the block is used in patients with chest disease or in small children; in the latter the risk of recurrent laryngeal nerve block is also a problem (Arthur, 1983). This block does, however, provide good analgesia in the tourniquet area.

Although supraclavicular block is generally less useful than axillary block in plastic surgery, it can be so if patients are unable to abduct their arm (e.g. in rheumatoid arthritis or following trauma) and it is more likely than interscalene block to produce good anaesthesia of the hand. A major disadvantage of this and of interscalene block is that both require a high degree of patient co-operation.

### Interscalene block

Interscalene block, first described by Winnie in 1970, has the advantage of a very high success rate in experienced hands (98% is quoted by Vester-Andersen et al, 1981) and gives excellent anaesthesia of the shoulder and upper arm. Unfortunately, block of the hand is less reliable because the ulnar nerve is often missed. This is less likely if paraesthesia is sought down the arm rather than over the shoulder, and digital pressure is applied above the point of injection. Pneumothorax is rare, but recurrent laryngeal and phrenic nerve blocks are common and pose a serious threat to patients with restrictive ventilatory defects or respiratory failure. For the same reason the block is unsuitable for use in children, the more so because it requires an awake and co-operative patient. Inadvertent subarachnoid or epidural injection is also a risk, although both can be avoided by care in the positioning of the needle. Like supraclavicular block, this technique may be helpful in patients who are unable to abduct their arms. The uptake of local anaesthetic is more rapid than that after axillary or supraclavicular blocks.

## SIMPLE INFILTRATION

Infiltration is widely used in plastic surgery. The recommended doses of local anaesthetics used in this way are given in Table 2. As is true of other routes of administration, the safe doses of bupivacaine, especially if used with a vasoconstrictor, are in excess of the data sheet recommendations, which allow only 60 ml of 0.25% bupivacaine for a 70 kg man, or 120 ml of 0.125%. Colley and Haevner (1981) showed that, using doses around this level, even without a vasoconstrictor, for scalp infiltration, peak blood levels did not exceed 1.23 and 0.77 µg/ml respectively. If the solutions contained 1:400 000 adrenaline, the levels were 1.01 and 0.12 µg/ml respectively. If a vasoconstrictor is used with bupivacaine, it is probably safe to allow 100 ml of 0.25% bupivacaine or 200 ml of 0.125%. It is important to reduce the concentration of vasoconstrictor in the latter solution or toxic doses may be exceeded (see Table 2).

**Table 2.** Anaesthetic dosages—infiltration.

|                                                                      | Adults | Children |
|----------------------------------------------------------------------|--------|----------|
| Bupivacaine 0.25% plain                                              | 60 ml  | 1 ml/kg  |
| Bupivacaine 0.25% (+ adrenaline 1:200 000)                          | 100 ml | 1.5 ml/kg |
| Bupivacaine 0.125%—double the above quantities.                     |        |          |
| Lignocaine 0.5% plain                                               | 25 ml  | 0.4 ml/kg |
| Lignocaine 0.5% (+ adrenaline 1:200 000)                           | 60 ml  | 1 ml/kg  |
| Prilocaine 3% (+ felypressin 0.03 units/ml) (in dental cartridges)  | 20 ml  | 0.33 ml/kg |
| Prilocaine 1% plain                                                 | 40 ml  | 0.5 ml/kg |

Besides reducing the uptake of local anaesthetic and permitting the use of a greater volume, vasoconstrictors produce a relatively bloodless field; while this is often an advantage, it may be counterproductive if local rotation flaps are utilized to fill skin defects, and in these circumstances nerve blocks are to be preferred.

Many minor procedures on the head and neck are performed with simple infiltration, which may be used for quite extensive superficial operations such as facelifts.

## PERIPHERAL NERVE BLOCKS

Peripheral nerve blocks are useful where only a small area of anaesthesia is required. They avoid the motor blockade and haemodynamic effects associated with more central blocks.

### Head and neck

Procedures in the head and neck involving deeper structures or rotation flaps are usually better conducted with the aid of specific nerve blocks, rather than simple infiltration. In the past, particularly during World War II, local anaesthesia was used extensively for major operations on facial soft tissue and skeleton. To some extent this was because local anaesthesia offered a more satisfactory alternative to the general anaesthetic techniques then available. With the advent of more modern general anaesthesia, the art of local anaesthesia to the face has fallen into disuse in the UK, but it is possible to conduct major operations on the head and neck using nerve blocks with either sedation or light general anaesthesia. For eyelid surgery, Neill (1983) has demonstrated that local anaesthesia with sedation provides operating conditions which are at least as good as those obtained with induced hypotension. The underutilization of local anaesthesia for surgery of the head and neck in the UK is largely due to lack of patient acceptability: in general, the closer the operation site is to the eyes, the less acceptable is local anaesthesia.

### Gasserian ganglion block

The Gasserian or trigeminal ganglion may be blocked by inserting a fine spinal needle through the foramen ovale into Meckel's cave. This block, which anaesthetizes the face above the line of the mandible, provides excellent anaesthesia for operations in this area. Patients often find the experience disagreeable and it is difficult to justify in awake patients unless there are good reasons to avoid general anaesthesia. Inadvertent intrathecal injection is the most serious potential complication, and haematoma along the needle track may be a problem (Eriksson, 1979). Bilateral Gasserian ganglion block combined with bilateral cervical plexus block, although it leads to high plasma bupivacaine levels, will provide satisfactory operating conditions for major cancer resections in the head and neck if combined with light general anaesthesia (Neill and Watson, 1984).

## Trigeminal nerve—branches

Blocks of the branches of the trigeminal nerve can be useful if only a small area of anaesthesia is required. For a detailed account of the anatomy and blocks of the trigeminal nerve and its branches, the reader is again referred to Eriksson (1979). Particularly useful in plastic surgery are blocks of the frontal, supratrochlear and infraorbital nerves, all of which may be blocked as they emerge from foramina above and below the orbit. In elderly patients presenting with minor skin tumours, a combination of these nerve blocks with local infiltration and sedation is often the preferred anaesthetic technique.

## Local anaesthesia of the pinna

This may be achieved by subcutaneous infiltration in the form of a V around the pinna commencing at a wheal of local anaesthetic just below the lower pole of the ear. This will block the great auricular nerve posteriorly and the auriculotemporal nerve anteriorly and is less painful for the awake patient than direct infiltration of the pinna for 'bat ear' correction. Used in conjunction with general anaesthesia in children, the technique considerably improves postoperative patient comfort, for up to 6 h if a vasoconstrictor is used.

## Cervical plexus block

This will be required in addition to Gasserian ganglion block if operations extend below the line of the mandible. There is a risk of subarachnoid or epidural injection and a substantial risk of phrenic and recurrent laryngeal nerve block. Intravascular injection is also a hazard. Because high blood levels of local anaesthetic will result from the combination of Gasserian ganglion and cervical plexus block, it is prudent to use a vasoconstrictor in the local anaesthetic.

## Arm

Peripheral nerve blocks in the arm have to compete with brachial plexus blocks and are rarely used as a primary measure, being of more use as an adjunct to partially successful or patchy brachial plexus blocks. The nerve blocks most useful in this respect are described below.

## Ulnar nerve block

The ulnar nerve is sometimes missed by axillary block and, more frequently, when the interscalene route is used. If may be easily blocked with 2–5 ml 0.5% bupivacaine 2 cm proximal to its sulcus behind the medial epicondyle of the humerus. If paraesthesia is elicited, it is wise to withdraw the tip of the needle 2 or 3 mm before injecting, to reduce the likelihood of neuritis; for the same reason, injection should not be made into the ulnar nerve sulcus itself. Unless the injection is made very close to the nerve, the block usually requires some 15 min to become effective if bupivacaine is used; lignocaine works more quickly.

It is also possible to block the palmar and dorsal branches of the ulnar nerve at the wrist (Eriksson, 1979).

### Median and radial nerves

These nerves are less commonly missed by brachial plexus blocks. In patients in whom it is important to avoid general anaesthesia, otherwise lost brachial plexus blocks may sometimes be salvaged by blockade of the median or radial nerves at the elbow.

The median nerve may be blocked at the elbow where it lies superficially, about 0.5 cm medial to the brachial artery in the epicondylar plane. Paraesthesia should be sought with a short 25 SWG needle inserted 0.5 cm medial to the artery at right angles to the skin. Care should be taken to avoid intraneural injection; 5 ml of local anaesthetic solution will suffice to block the nerve but further subcutaneous infiltration is required to block the more proximal cutaneous branches.

### Lateral cutaneous nerve of the forearm

This nerve, which is the sensory branch of the musculocutaneous nerve, is often missed when the brachial plexus is blocked by the axillary route. It may be blocked at the level of the lateral epicondyle with the elbow extended. The needle should be inserted lateral to the biceps tendon and paraesthesia sought some 0.5 cm superficial to the bone. Although the block is more likely to be effective if paraesthesia is obtained, it is important to avoid intraneural injection. 3–5 ml of local anaesthetic solution will suffice if paraesthesia has been elicited, but in its absence a fanwise injection of 10–15 ml of 0.25% bupivacaine lateral to the biceps tendon in the epicondylar plane, starting 0.5 cm superficial to bone and ending in subcutaneous tissue, will block the nerve and also the radial nerve.

## Leg

Peripheral nerve blocks in the leg are less useful because central blocks are so easy and reliable. They are rarely required to bolster up failed central blocks but can be useful when only a small area of anaesthesia is required or central blocks are contraindicated. Femoral nerve block combined with block of the lateral cutaneous nerve of the thigh is sometimes very convenient as a means of anaesthetizing split skin donor sites on the anterolateral aspect of the thigh.

## Intercostal nerve block

Intercostal nerve block may be useful if rib grafts are taken, and may be inserted under direct vision by the surgeon; this will considerably improve patient comfort for several hours after operation and the blocks may be repeated as required. An alternative is to use intercostal catheters for repeat injections, or to use a thoracic epidural, although this may cause unacceptable arterial hypotension which can endanger the perfusion of free flaps. This may be avoided if epidural opiates are used rather than local anaesthetic. Uptake of local anaesthetic agents from the intercostal spaces is very rapid (Moore et al, 1976) and, although doses as high as 600 mg of bupivacaine have been used without any reported problems, it is prudent to use a vasoconstrictor if more than 20 ml of 0.5% bupivacaine or its equivalent is used.

## INTRAVENOUS REGIONAL ANAESTHESIA

Intravenous regional anaesthesia (IVRA) is of limited utility in plastic surgery because analgesia is short-lived after cuff deflation, and the need to work within safe tourniquet time is a serious limitation. If local anaesthesia for hand or arm surgery is essential and brachial plexus block is impossible, IVRA may offer a satisfactory alternative for short operations. There have been a number of reports of fatalities in patients undergoing IVRA with bupivacaine, so bupivacaine must not be used for this purpose. There have also been reports of cardiovascular disturbance following the use of lignocaine. Prilocaine 0.5%, which is broken down in the bloodstream, is by far the safest agent in the event of premature cuff deflation (McKeown et al, 1984). Provided that dosage is less than 600 mg, methaemoglobinaemia is unlikely to occur.

## SYMPATHETIC NERVE BLOCKS

Sympathetic nerve blocks may be useful to improve the circulation in skin flaps but usually this function is better served by the use of appropriate somatic nerve blocks. Specific sympathetic nerve blocks are of more use in the treatment of patients in whom chronic circulatory insufficiency is compromising healing (e.g. of leg ulcers) or in whom there is sympathetic dysfunction following injury, particularly in the hand. Patients with painful neuromata or general hyperaesthesia following nerve injuries are particularly likely to be helped by block of the sympathetic nerve supply to the affected part. This may be done either with specific nerve blocks (i.e. stellate ganglion or lumbar sympathetic chain) or by the use of regional intravenous guanethidine (Hannington-Kiff, 1979). The latter seems to be less effective for cases where the sympathetic dysfunction affects the leg, and in these cases a lumbar sympathetic block with local anaesthetic, followed if necessary by phenol, is a better solution to the problem.

When an i.v. guanethidine block is performed for sympathetic dysfunction, the pain may initially be exacerbated by the injection of guanethidine and it is kind to perform IVRA with prilocaine 3 min before the guanethidine injection (Driessen et al, 1983). Intravenous guanethidine block lasts up to three days, while stellate ganglion block with bupivacaine lasts only some

10 h, so the former may be the preferred technique in the arm (Eriksen, 1981).

No matter which technique is used, it will generally be necessary to perform repeat blocks at intervals of a few days to two or three weeks before the symptoms totally abate, each successive block producing a longer period of relief. In patients with sympathetic dystrophy after hand injuries, it is helpful to synchronize sympathetic blocks with attendance at the physiotherapy department in order to capitalize on any improvement in mobility.

## TOPICAL APPLICATION

### Fibreoptic bronchoscopy and laryngoscopy

The fibreoptic laryngoscope has revolutionized the management of patients in whom conventional laryngoscopy is impossible, while the fibreoptic bronchoscope is increasingly being employed in the assessment of respiratory burn injury. Fibreoptic endoscopy in an awake patient, with or without sedation, requires satisfactory local anaesthesia of the mouth, pharynx, larynx and sometimes the nose. The latter may be anaesthetized with a 10% cocaine solution (5 ml sprayed into the chosen nostril) which has the useful effect of causing vasoconstriction and shrinking of the nasal mucosa. The mouth and pharynx are best anaesthetized with a 4% lignocaine spray. If the cricoid ring is palpable, local anaesthetic may be injected through the cricothyroid membrane direct into the airway, but if, as is often the case in plastic surgical patients, this is not possible, then modern fibreoptic laryngoscopes will allow 4% lignocaine solution to be administered via the suction channel. The total dose of lignocaine should not exceed 300 mg.

### Split skin donor sites

Lignocaine gel 2% applied to split skin donor sites before they are dressed is an effective analgesia for what is often the most painful part of skin grafting procedures. The technique is obviously only applicable to small donor areas and is of no use where excision and grafting has been extensive, but on small donor sites it is safe and effective, often avoiding the use of postoperative opiates. Using 2% lignocaine gel, Read and Bach (1980) reported plasma levels well below the toxic threshold, as did Bulmer and Duckett (1985), who used 1% lignocaine gel, which may be equally efficacious. The latter authors used approximately 20 ml of 1% gel and reported venous plasma levels of less than 0.51 μg/ml. On this basis, for adults it is safe to use 50 ml of 1% or 25 ml of 2% lignocaine.

## SUMMARY

Local anaesthetic techniques are widely applicable in plastic surgery and can bring considerable benefits to patients. The effective utilization of local anaesthesia often requires careful timing and many a block has been declared a failure because time was not allowed for it to become effective. The successful employment of many techniques requires dosages of local anaesthetics which are in excess of data sheet recommendations and close to toxic levels. Although toxic effects are uncommon in practice, it is essential that practitioners have the facilities and ability to cope with adverse reactions.

## REFERENCES

Armitage EN (1985) Regional anaesthesia in paediatrics. *Clinics in Anaesthesiology* **3:** 553–568.

Arthur DS (1983) Local anaesthesia for paediatric surgery. In *Practical Local Anaesthesia*, 1st edn. Edinburgh: Blackwell Scientific Publications.

Arthur DS & McNicol LR (1986) Local anaesthetic techniques in paediatric surgery. *British Journal of Anaesthesia* **58:** 760–768.

Bulmer JN & Duckett AC (1985) Absorption of lignocaine through split-skin donor sites. *Anaesthesia* **40:** 808–809.

Colley PS & Haevner JE (1981) Blood levels of bupivacaine after injection into the scalp with and without epinephrine. *Anesthesiology* **54:** 81–84.

Driessen JJ, Van Der Werken Chr, Nicolai JPA & Crul JF (1983) Clinical effects of regional intravenous guanethidine (ismelin R) in reflex sympathetic dystrophy. *Acta Anaesthesiologica Scandinavica* **27:** 505–509.

Eriksen S (1981) Duration of sympathetic blockade. *Anaesthesia* **36:** 768–771.

Eriksson E (1979) *Illustrated Handbook in Local Anaesthesia*, 2nd edn. London: Lloyd-Luke.

Ewen A, McLeod DD, McLeod DM et al (1986) Continuous infusion epidural analgesia in obstetrics. A comparison of 0.08% and 0.25% bupivacaine. *Anaesthesia* **41:** 143–147.

Hain WR (1978) Anaesthetic doses for extradural anaesthesia in children. *British Journal of Anaesthesia* **50:** 303.

Hannington-Kiff JG (1979) Relief of causalgia in limbs by regional intravenous guanethidine. *British Medical Journal* **2:** 367.

Logan MR, McClure JH & Wildsmith JAW (1986) Plain bupivacaine: an unpredictable spinal anaesthetic agent. *British Journal of Anaesthesia* **58:** 292–296.

McKenzie PJ & Loach AB (1986) Local anaesthesia for orthopaedic surgery. *British Journal of Anaesthesia* **58:** 779–789.

McKeown DW, Meiklejohn B & Scott DB (1984) Bupivacaine and prilocaine in intravenous regional anaesthesia. *Anaesthesia* **39:** 150–154.

Moller RA & Covino BG (1985) Toxic cardiac electrophysiologic effects of bupivacaine and lidocaine at high concentrations. *Anesthesiology* **63:** A223.

Moore DC, Mather LE, Bridenbaugh LD, Balfour RI et al (1976) Arterial and venous plasma levels of bupivacaine following peripheral nerve blocks. *Anesthesia and Analgesia* **55:** 763–768.

Moore DC, Balfour RI & Fitzgibbons D (1979) Convulsive arterial plasma levels of bupivacaine and the response to diazepam therapy. *Anesthesiology* **50:** 454–456.

Neill RS (1983) Regional analgesia combined with iv sedation in major eyelid surgery: an alternative to induced hypotension. *British Journal of Plastic Surgery* **36:** 29–35.

Neill RS & Watson R (1984) Plasma bupivacaine concentrations during combined regional and general anaesthesia for resection and reconstruction of major head and neck carcinomata. *British Journal of Anaesthesia* **56:** 485–492.

Read JM & Bach PH (1980) Sterile topical lignocaine jelly in plastic surgery. *South African Medical Journal* **57:** 704–706.

Reiz S & Nath S (1986) Cardiotoxicity of local anaesthetic agents. *British Journal of Anaesthesia* **58:** 736–746.

Ross RA, Clarke JE & Armitage EN (1980) Postoperative pain prevention by continuous epidural infusion. A study of the clinical effects and the plasma concentrations obtained. *Anaesthesia* **35:** 663–668.

Schulte-Steinberg O & Rahlfs VW (1977) Spread of extradural analgesia following caudal injection in children. *British Journal of Anaesthesia* **49**: 1027–1034.

Scott DB (1986) Toxic effects of local anaesthetic agents on the central nervous system. *British Journal of Anaesthesia* **58**: 732–735.

Selander D (1977) Catheter technique in axillary plexus block. *Acta Anaesthesiologica Scandinavica* **21**: 324–329.

Selander D (1979) Paraesthesia or no paraesthesia? *Acta Anaesthesiologica Scandinavica* **23**: 27–33.

Selander D, Dhuner KG & Lundborg G (1977) Peripheral nerve injury due to injection needles used for regional anesthesia. *Acta Anaesthesiologica Scandinavica* **21**: 182–188.

Tanz RD, Heskett T, Loehning RW & Fairfax CA (1984) Comparative cardiotoxicity of bupivacaine and lidocaine in the isolated, perfused mammalian heart. *Anesthesia and Analgesia* **63**: 549–556.

Tucker GT (1986) Pharmacokinetics of local anaesthetics. *British Journal of Anaesthesia* **58**: 717–731.

Tuominen M, Rosenberg PH & Kalso E (1983) Blood levels of bupivacaine after single dose supplementary dose and during continuous infusion in axillary plexus block. *Acta Anaesthesiologica Scandinavica* **27**: 303–306.

Vester-Anderson T, Christiansen C, Hansen M et al (1981) Interscalene brachial plexus block: area of analgesia, complications and blood concentrations of local aesthetics. *Acta Anaesthesiologica Scandinavica* **25**: 81–84.

Vester-Andersen T, Husum B, Lindeborg T, Borits L & Gothgen I (1984) Perivascular block IV: blockade following 40, 50, 60 ml of mepivicaine 1% with adrenaline. *Acta Anaesthesiologica Scandinavica* **28**: 99–105.

Wildsmith JAW, Tucker GT, Cooper S, Scott DB & Covino BG (1977) Plasma concentrations of local anaesthetics after interscalene brachial plexus block. *British Journal of Anaesthesia* **49**: 461–466.

Winnie AP (1970) Interscalene brachial plexus block. *Anesthesia and Analgesia Current Researches* **49**: 455–466.

# 12

Hypotensive anaesthesia

H. P. PATEL

Deliberate hypotension has been one of the most controversial subjects in anaesthesia in the last 35 years. This technique has attracted ardent protagonists and doggedly severe critics and opponents. The debate usually hinges around the subject of mortality and morbidity as weighed against the advantages to the patient in terms of speed of operation and reduction of blood loss. Other anaesthetic techniques invite similar controversy, e.g. epidural analgesia in obstetrics, hyperventilation in neurosurgical anaesthesia, induced hypothermia, halothane and hepatitis and many more. It might be pointed out by their protagonists that all these latter techniques, in spite of a certain morbidity, bring definite advantages to the patient without which the outcome might be more detrimental to the patient. The case for deliberate hypotension has unfortunately not been argued passionately, though in many ways it resembles these techniques as far as the advantage to the patient and reduction in surgical morbidity is concerned. Indeed, the late Sir Archibald McIndoe described the benefit of induced hypotension as constituting 'a major surgical advance'. In only one surgical procedure, the clipping of cerebral aneurysm, did hypotension ever become an accepted practice because it allowed the 'impossible to become possible'! Like many trends in medicine it looks as if deliberate hypotension might become re-established in the armamentarium of the anaesthetist in the near future as transfusions of blood and its allied products are increasingly incriminated in disseminating alarming and new diseases.

## INDICATIONS

### Reduction of blood loss

One of the main reasons for deliberate hypotension is to reduce blood loss during surgery, thus avoiding blood transfusions totally or minimizing the amount transfused to the patient. The transfusion of blood into a patient is a matched homograft as well as a potential means of transmitting disease and is therefore not without its risks and complications.

### Provision of a clear and dry surgical field

In the majority of plastic surgical cases, deliberate hypotension is used to provide a clear and relatively bloodless surgical field so that delicate, intricate and definitive procedures can be carried out with ease and rapidity (McIndoe, 1956). It is this indication which prompts many practitioners to question its justification in view of the potential mortality and morbidity of the technique. However, it has many real advantages to the patient and these have been succinctly pointed out by a plastic surgeon intimately involved with the technique for the last 30 years (Beare, 1985).

1. *Duration of operation* is curtailed as less time is required for haemostasis.
2. *Accuracy of operation* is enhanced and there is less likelihood of accidental damage to vital and easily identifiable structures.
3. *Pathological tissues* are more easily identified and thus excised with greater precision.
4. *There is no distortion of tissues* as would occur with local infiltration with a vasoconstrictor drug.
5. *Relative absence of tissue oedema* resulting from low pressure allows better healing with fewer complications and reduced wound infection.
6. *Reactionary haemorrhage*, postoperative bleeding and haematoma are less common.

Operations which fall in this group are those on the eyelids, nose, face, neck dissection, parotid gland surgery, facial nerve anastomosis, etc.

**When to use hypotension?**

Apart from the obvious contraindications on medical grounds, the decision whether or not to induce hypotension must always be a matter of discussion between surgeon and anaesthetist. Obviously, if the surgeon is of the opinion that a particular operation can be done without the help of hypotension then it should not be provided by the anaesthetist.

There are three absolute requirements which must be met before the use of hypotensive anaesthesia is considered (Beare, 1985). These requirements are:

1. That the patient will derive positive benefit from application of the technique to that particular operation.
2. That the anaesthetist has been properly trained and is competent to carry out the technique safely and effectively.
3. That the surgeon is sufficiently skilled and experienced to take positive advantage of the improved conditions so that he may carry out the operation more swiftly, more accurately or with reduced blood loss.

If any of the three individuals concerned, patient, anaesthetist or surgeon, does not meet these criteria, then hypotensive anaesthesia should not be used.

On the other hand, if these criteria are present, the ultimate responsibility of deciding whether hypotension can be induced safely in that particular patient should rest with the anaesthetist.

The anaesthetist, however skilled, should never persuade an unwilling and unversed surgeon to operate on a patient under induced hypotension. Conversely, it is equally unwise and more dangerous for an enthusiastic surgeon to persuade an unwilling and unpractised anaesthetist into using it against his wishes (Enderby, 1975).

It is clear that a successful and satisfactory use of the technique, which, one must re-emphasize, is for the benefit of the patient alone, is impossible unless the anaesthetist and surgeon have a genuine rapport with one another (Beare, 1985).

## CONTRAINDICATIONS

Some of the absolute and relative contraindications to deliberate hypotension are listed below.

1. History of cerebrovascular disease.
2. History of cardiovascular disease.
3. History of severe respiratory disease.
4. Haemoglobin level of less than 11 g/100 ml.
5. Diabetic and asthmatic patients.

### Diabetes

The diabetic patient is sensitive to ganglion-blocking and beta-adrenergic blocking drugs and these should be avoided. In the insulin-dependent diabetic patient there is evidence that cerebral blood flow (CBF) is unstable (Dandona et al, 1979). High blood glucose concentrations have a deleterious effect during partial brain ischaemia and recovery, and this is believed to be due to increased brain lactoacidosis (Siesjö and Wieloch, 1985; Lanier et al, 1985).

It is interesting to note that the preoperative starvation regime used clinically may have been more advantageous than was realized. It can be inferred that infusions of glucose should not be given to any patient before or during deliberate hypotension and that anaesthetics which increase blood glucose should be avoided (McDowall, 1985).

### Asthma

Should bronchospasm occur in the presence of ganglion-blocking agents in the asthmatic patients, a severe and dangerous hypotension will ensue. Sodium nitroprusside (SNP) is the preferred alternative if induced hypotension is indicated.

### High blood pressure

A symptomless benign hypertension is not a contraindication to induction of hypotension. However, great care should be taken in the level and rate of reduction of arterial pressure. Synergism between medication for raised blood pressure and hypotensive drugs should be borne in mind and the ECG should be continuously monitored.

## TECHNIQUES

There are a number of techniques, using different drugs and controls, which have evolved over the last 36 years since the introduction of deliberate hypotension in clinical practice. They all have their enthusiasts and opponents, and are not without their advantages and disadvantages. It is obvious that no one technique is inherently better than the others. A technique which works well for a particular patient, operation, surgeon, and/or available postoperative recovery facility might be totally unsuitable for another. Again, given the same conditions, a technique which works well in the hands of one anaesthetist might not do so for another. Therefore, the comparison of different techniques in clinical situations becomes difficult. Comparisons as regards physiological changes produced in cerebral blood flow (CBF), cardiac output (CO), pulmonary blood flow etc. might be valid for different drugs and techniques when carried out in animal experiments under strict uniform conditions for each technique, but there still remains the difficulty of interpreting animal work for human application and establishing the superiority of any drug or technique over the others.

It is incontrovertible that smooth induction and maintenance of anaesthesia, a clear airway and unimpeded respiration—preferably controlled, with good oxygenation, proper elimination of carbon dioxide and adequate analgesia—are essential to make any technique work well. Meticulous attention to detail is more important than the use of a particular agent (MacRae, 1985).

In head and neck surgery, the posture of the patient on the operating table is of considerable importance. A head-up tilt of about 25°–30° provides good venous drainage, establishes a gradient of arterial pressure and provides a comparatively clear operating field in many instances, even without recourse to the use of hypotensive agents. For other situations, some sort of hypotensive technique will be essential in addition to tilt to provide optimum operating conditions.

The different techniques in clinical use are composed of three main components.

1. *Drugs*:
    (a) Ganglion blocking drugs, e.g. Pentolinium Tartrate (Ansolysen), Trimetaphan (Arfonad).
    (b) Direct acting vasodilators: (i) Sodium Nitroprusside (SNP); (ii) Glyceryltrinitrate (TNG); (iii) Adenosine Triphosphate (ATP).
2. *Adjuvants*:
    (a) Adrenergic blocking drugs: (i) Propranolol; (ii) Practolol; (iii) Labetalol.
    (b) Anaesthetic agents: (i) Halothane; (ii) Enflurane; (iii) Isoflurane.
    (c) Analgesic agents: (i) Fentanyl; (ii) Alfentanil.
3. *Physical controls*:
    (a) Posture.
    (b) IPPV.
    (c) PEEP.

Any one of the above components, or a combination, may be used to advantage to achieve hypotension in different types of patients, operations and available facilities.

A detailed account of various drugs and techniques as described by Enderby (1985) cannot be given in a short chapter of this nature. However, a short description of the main drugs and the technique used at the plastic surgery unit at East Grinstead follows.

## Drugs

### Ganglion blocking drugs

Historically, apart from high spinal anaesthesia these were the first drugs used to reduce blood pressure and to achieve a bloodless operating field. The two commonest drugs are a long-acting ganglion blocker, pentolinium, and a short-acting one, trimetaphan.

*Pentolinium tartarate (Ansolysen).* The long duration of action of 1–4 h has been considered by many to be a disadvantage of this drug, and a longer period of possible 'postural hypotension' in the recovery room has positively dissuaded many from using it. However, this long-acting effect has been exploited to advantage in the speciality of plastic surgery, as the return to normotension is slow over a period of 2–3 h. This reduces postoperative bleeding and helps prevent haematoma. Ansolysen only needs to be given in a single intravenous dose, obviating the need for sophisticated means of regulating i.v. infusion, and the hypotension is much smoother as opposed to the see-saw effect sometimes seen with other drugs. Among its disadvantages are pupillary cycloplegia, tachyphylaxis, and postural hypotension which requires the patients to be kept in bed for 12–24 h postoperatively.

The dose normally used is 0.1–0.15 mg/kg i.v. The recommended dose produces very little or no reduction of blood pressure by itself but does produce a fair amount of venodilatation. This, in combination with head-up tilt and IPPV, helps to pool the blood in lower extremities. Smaller doses are required in the elderly and the drug is not needed in very old and frail patients where the use of posture with other adjuvants usually suffices to pool the blood in the legs.

Pentolinium, unlike SNP and TNG, does not activate the renin–angiotensin–aldosterone axis which antagonizes hypotension. Instead, it reduces plasma renin activity (PRA) and inhibits catecholamine release (Jones et al, 1981) and thus makes hypotension easier to achieve. It also inhibits the hyperglycaemic response induced by surgical stress, thereby limiting the rise in blood glucose levels (Fahmy and Battit, 1975). Recently it has been shown that presence of relative hyperglycaemia contributes significantly to neurological damage in the event of cerebral ischaemia (Lanier et al, 1985).

*Trimetaphan (Arfonad).* The short action of trimetaphan is considered by many to be an advantage, as the return to normotension is fairly quick at the end of the operation and there is less chance of postural hypotension. It is usually diluted and administered by a continuous infusion which allows it to produce hypotension without a head-up tilt if so required. Here the drug itself is used as a sole or main agent to achieve low blood pressure as opposed to pooling the blood in extremities in a head-up tilt. The disadvantages of its use in plastic surgery are the chances of postoperative bleeding and haematoma due to a quick return to normotension; and a lack of smoothness of hypotension due to a see-saw effect on blood pressure.

Though the total maximum amount is not limited by toxicity as in the case of SNP, it has been recommended that not more than 1 g should be administered (Eckenhoff, 1955). Recently, McRae (1981) reported using a 10:1 mixture of trimetaphan and SNP with good results and found synergism between the two agents. This might be due to trimetaphan inhibiting the plasma renin activity, which is activated by SNP (Green, 1985a).

## Direct-acting vasodilators

*Sodium nitroprusside (SNP).* The rapid, transient and potent action of SNP accompanied by the return of blood pressure to normal at the end of operation has persuaded many anaesthetists to make this drug an agent of choice. Cardiac output is maintained at normal values. CBF is increased, leading to a rise in ICP in the early stages of hypotension, but it returns to normal once arterial pressure has fallen by 30% or more (Turner et al, 1977).

Its main disadvantage is the risk of cyanide poisoning, but this can be avoided if the administration of the drug is kept within the recommended dosage of 1.5 mg/kg (Vesey et al, 1976), and potentiation of SNP is achieved by adjuvants in resistant cases. There is also the possibility of a rebound hypertension in the postoperative period. This is thought to be due to activation of renin–angiotensin–aldosterone system. However, this can be abated by the beta-adrenergic blocker, propranolol (Khambatta et al, 1981).

For details of practical considerations, see Verner (1985).

*Glyceryltrinitrate (TNG).* This drug has been used by intravenous infusion in recent times to induce systemic hypotension or to avoid hypertension during cardiac surgery. Its action is more variable than SNP and the return to normotension is slower (Aveling and Verner, 1981). It might be useful where only moderate hypotension is required. However, it has to be administered in glass or polythene containers, as polyvinyl chloride bags absorb a large proportion (40%) of TNG within 1 h.

*Adenosine triphosphate (ATP).* ATP and its active metabolite, adenosine, are potent vasodilators and have been used to produce hypotension in animal experiments (Newberg et al, 1985) and in clinical practice. Absence of tachyphylaxis, tachycardia and rebound hypertension are some of the advantages claimed for the drug (Fakunaga et al, 1982; Sollevi et al, 1984). Pretreatment with Dipyridamole, an adenosine uptake inhibitor, potentiates the vasodilator effects of adenosine in dogs. Adenosine-induced hypotension in the dog also prevents elevation of circulating plasma renin activity (Lagerkranser et al, 1984).

ATP can increase CBF and impair cerebrovascular reactivity, so care should be taken in patients with intracranial pathology (Van Aken et al, 1984).

Recently, Laycock et al (1986) demonstrated that at low perfusion pressures there was impairment in cortical oxygen which was similar with both SNP and adenosine.

ATP has been introduced fairly recently and its place in clinical practice is still to be fully evaluated.

## Adjuvants

### Adrenergic blocking drugs

*Propranolol and practolol.* The early attempts to achieve profound hypotension using only ganglion-blocking drugs were thwarted in younger patients by a reflex tachycardia associated with these drugs. Their use was later made possible by the introduction of beta-blockers and halothane in anaesthetic practice (Hellewell and Potts, 1966; Hewitt et al, 1967).

The two agents used to depress tachycardia were propranolol and practolol, the latter being the drug of choice today because of the better selective action on the cardiovascular system. It must be remembered that only a mild depression of tachycardia is needed rather than a potent blocking agent which causes bradycardia. Practolol in a small dose, 0.14 mg/kg (Enderby, 1980), is better for this purpose than the potent new beta-blockers currently available. In young patients this should be administered slowly after induction of anaesthesia and prior to administering the hypotensive agents. Beta-blockers usually are not required in elderly patients as these are less prone to develop tachycardia with ganglion blockade. Propranolol is an alternative agent used in a dose of 0.035 mg/kg i.v. but its tendency to cause occasional bronchospasm has limited its use in this field. Beta-blockers prevent the rise of plasma renin activity (PRA) and subsequent release of angiotensin associated with use of head-up tilt in younger patients.

*Labetalol.* A combined alpha-1 and beta adrenoceptor antagonist agent has been advocated by many to achieve desired hypotension in young patients. In anaesthetized patients it reduces blood pressure by a large decrease in systemic vascular resistance (Scott et al, 1978) and a modest reduction in heart rate and cardiac output. Care should be exercised with simultaneous use of halothane, especially higher concentrations, as they have a synergistic action. Smaller doses are suggested when using IPPV instead of spontaneous respiration. Bradycardia is the commonest untoward effect seen which sometimes is persistent in the postoperative period. It can be treated with atropine 0.6 mg, though this may restore the blood pressure to normal (Cope and Crawford, 1979).

*Anaesthetic agents*

*Halothane*. A useful adjunct to hypotension was made available with the introduction of halothane. It can be used either with other hypotensive agents or on its own.

With ganglion-blocking agents, halothane is effective in low concentration of 0.5–1.0% to start with. Once the effects of drugs, tilt, and controlled respiration on blood pressure have been established, the concentration of halothane can be increased to 1.5–2.0% if further fall in blood pressure is required or if surgical stimuli tend to raise the level. Used in such a way it plays only a secondary role.

Halothane on its own can produce hypotension when used in old and frail patients. Here it plays a primary role and can produce satisfactory results even in low concentrations. High concentrations are not recommended as it is a potent myocardial depressant.

*Enflurane*. Enflurane is similar to halothane except that it causes less dysrhythmia when used with adrenaline infiltration. It can be used in a similar way to halothane.

*Isoflurane*. Lam and Gelb (1983), Fairbain et al (1986) and Newman et al (1986) produced satisfactory hypotension using isoflurane alone or as an adjunct.

Isoflurane decreases arterial pressure to approximately the same extent as enflurane or halothane, though by a different underlying mechanism. Isoflurane causes a dose-related hypotension by reducing systemic vascular resistance more than contractility, in contrast to halothane and enflurane, which reduce cardiac output. It also has the advantage that it reduces cerebral metabolic activity with only moderate cerebral vasodilatation and may provide some cerebral protection against hypoxia or ischaemia (Newberg and Michenfelder, 1983; Newberg et al, 1983).

In view of the peripheral synergistic action, great care should be exercised when using isoflurane with ganglion-blocking agents or direct-acting vasodilators.

*Analgesic agents*

Without adequate analgesia the level of blood pressure often tends to rise in response to strong surgical stimulus. This can be prevented by use of potent short-acting analgesics like fentanyl and alfentanil. These agents will provide intense analgesia during the intraoperative period and will be relatively free of side-effects later in the recovery period.

**Physical controls**

*Posture*

Elevation of the part to be operated upon to a maximum possible height is one of the most important factors in achieving a bloodless field. In operations on the head and neck this is easily achieved by tilting the operating table in a head-up position. Apart from enhancing venous drainage from the elevated site, this manoeuvre produces a gradient of blood pressure in the entire body due to gravity. The pressure falls by 2 mmHg for each 2.5 cm of vertical height achieved. Thus a rise of 25 cm from the heart level will reduce the pressure by about 20 mmHg at the elevated site. A foot-down tilt of 25°–30° is essential to produce a sizeable gradient of this level. When an overall reduction of systolic pressure at heart level is added to this 'postural ischaemia', the elevated parts will now have a much lower tissue pressure, empty capillaries and veins and a relatively bloodless field.

This head-up posture plays a particularly important and synergistic role in producing hypotension when the technique of ganglionic blockade as used at East Grinstead is employed. Pooling of blood in the dilated lower half of the body decreases venous return, leading to fall in cardiac output and reduction of systolic pressure. In the absence of a head-up tilt, this fall in systolic pressure would not be easily achieved without recourse to higher doses of hypotensive drugs to produce further dilatation of vessels.

Thus with the use of posture, two objectives are achieved simultaneously:

1.  Pooling of blood in the venodilated dependent parts leading to reduction in overall systolic pressure.
2.  A 'postural ischaemia' with relative vasoconstriction and therefore less bleeding at the site of operation.

Obviously the head-up tilt is most useful in operations on the head and neck which incidentally forms a major proportion of plastic and maxillo-facial surgical procedures needing deliberate hypotension.

The control for tilting the operating table should be near the anaesthetist, preferably by the foot-end of the patient. Adjustment to the tilt of the table can then be carried out instantly when needed. The initial head-up tilt should be very gradual and increased step by step to avoid precipitous and uncontrolled fall in blood pressure. A period of 10–15 min to achieve a 25° tilt is recommended. A slow reduction of blood pressure, not more than 10 mmHg/min, allows time for full cerebral autoregulation to take place with little effect on CBF or cerebral activity (Patel, 1981).

## IPPV and PEEP

IPPV produces reduction of blood pressure by an increase of intrathoracic pressure and decrease in venous return, leading to a fall in cardiac output. It can be varied quickly when hand ventilation is used and thus provides a breath to breath control of blood pressure, which is especially useful when surgical stimuli are changing frequently. Occasionally, IPPV might need to be augmented with PEEP for a short time to control a large rise in blood pressure. However, a prolonged use of large PEEP is not recommended, as it tends to cause venous congestion leading to increased bleeding and may also increase intracranial pressure. It also causes a rise in $V_d/V_t$ ratio (Eckenhoff et al, 1963).

## MONITORING HYPOTENSIVE ANAESTHESIA

### Blood pressure

Obviously, the most important parameter that should be monitored vigilantly and continuously during hypotensive anaesthesia is the blood pressure. Which method one uses to achieve this depends on factors like available equipment, experience of the user, national standards and patient expectation. Whatever method is chosen, it should be accurate, reliable, preferably simple and easy to use, and familiar to the user.

Direct intra-arterial monitoring is considered by many to be the only reliable and accurate method of measuring blood pressure. It has been our choice of method for long, extensive surgery where wide and rapid changes in blood pressure and/or significant haemorrhage are expected. For short routine operations we prefer the noninvasive indirect method of blood pressure measurement by an oscillometer. The systolic pressure measured with an oscillometer correlates well with direct intra-arterial readings (Hutton and Prys-Roberts, 1982). It is used in a 'modified' manner so as to give a continuous beat to beat measurement of blood pressure rather than a single reading at specified intervals. Until recently this was the only monitoring carried out in the majority of patients at East Grinstead and there seems to be no evidence that it was inadequate. The introduction of noninvasive automated devices has found favour with some practitioners in recent times. However, even in ideal conditions the maximum number of readings per minute that can be achieved with such devices is limited and hence care is needed in their use. Unlike the oscillometer they cannot give a continuous measurement of blood pressure.

### Technique of 'modified' continuous monitoring

The double cuff of an oscillometer is applied to the right arm at the level of the heart and protected from interference by a metal guard. The cuff is inflated to the required systolic level and the oscillations are observed. If the amplitude increases it indicates that the blood pressure is rising, and conversely if the amplitude decreases then the blood pressure is falling (Figure 1). On observing rising amplitude a larger tidal volume is applied at the next breath until the amplitude size decreases, indicating that the blood pressure has fallen to the chosen systolic level. The opposite is done when the amplitude is observed to be decreasing. The cuff is left inflated for 5 min, after which it is deflated to restore circulation for 1 min. In this manner, a near-continuous monitoring and control of blood pressure is achieved. To use the oscillometer in this manner it is necessary to remove the return spring from the control lever. The repeated inflation and deflation of cuff releases fibrinolysins from the arm and provides a possible protection against deep vein thrombosis.

### Monitoring other parameters

In modern anaesthetic practice, routine ECG monitoring is considered by most to be obligatory. In hypotensive anaesthesia it can be of further value in detection of early ischaemic changes by observation of the S–T segment. The most useful lead for this purpose is precordial lead V5. It can be used as true lead V5 if lead selection is available, or in a modified configuration— CC5 or CM5—where this facility is absent (Froelicher et al, 1976).

Monitoring $O_2$ and $CO_2$ levels, body temperature, central venous pressure, pulse wave and blood loss have been recommended and can be most useful during prolonged hypotension. They provide additional information which can be interpreted along with blood pressure and ECG to form a basis for safe practice.

## Monitoring the brain

Interest in monitoring adequacy of cerebral perfusion in hypotensive anaesthesia has been pursued for a long time. Various parameters and

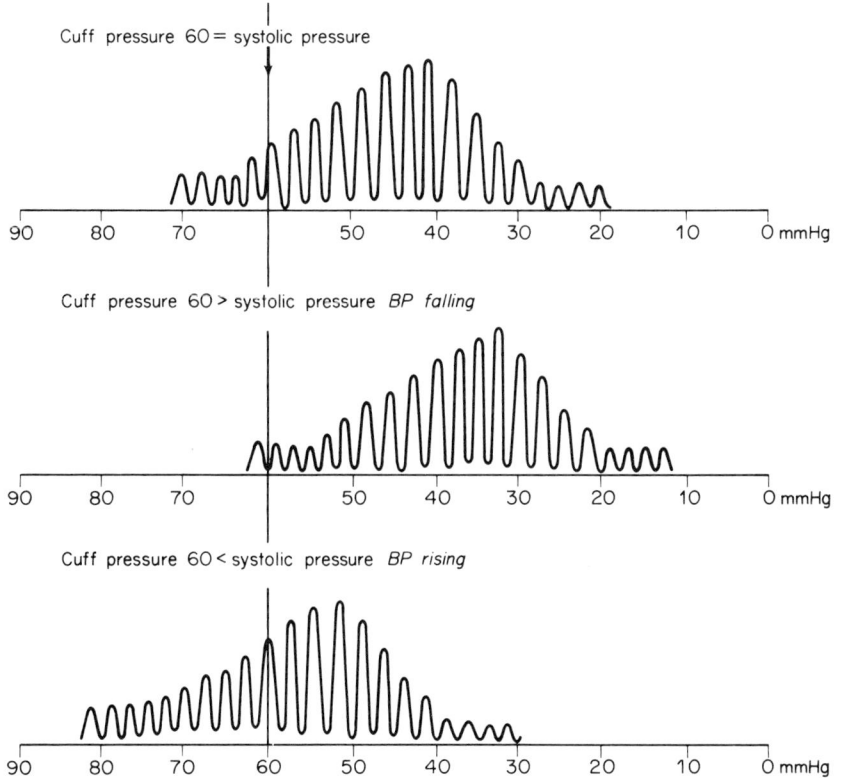

**Figure 1.** Illustrations of an oscillogram to explain how it can function as a continuous monitor of systolic blood pressure. (Cuff pressure constant at 60 mmHg in all traces.) Top trace indicates systolic end point of 60 mmHg. Middle trace indicates that the end point has moved to the right as blood pressure falls (oscillations decrease). Lower trace indicates that the end point has moved to the left as blood pressure rises (oscillations increase). From Enderby (1985), reproduced with permission of editor and publisher.

devices have been used intraoperatively to assess cerebral perfusion, each method having advantages and disadvantages of its own. At present it is unclear whether any of them are useful for routine monitoring.

There appears little evidence that major depression of CBF or electrical activity occurs at MAP greater than 60 mmHg in normotensive patients who are presumed capable of autoregulation (Prior, 1985). The EEG or somato-sensory evoked potential is abolished at cerebral blood flows of 15–20 ml/min/100 g (Symon, 1985). At this unit, using radioactive xenon-133 clearance technique, CBF was measured in patients hypotensive with ganglion blockade and head-up tilt. The lowest recorded MAP was 40 mmHg and the lowest CBF was 33 ml/min/100 g (unpublished data). There was no depression of activity as recorded by cerebral function monitor. Provided that the safe lower limit of blood pressure is never exceeded, it seems that a well-conducted hypotensive anaesthesia does not result in obvious postoperative brain dysfunction, except when it is associated with a catastrophe such as a cardiac arrest.

## POSTOPERATIVE MANAGEMENT

Of the reported deaths associated with deliberate hypotension in the years 1958–1963, 97% occurred during postoperative recovery (Larson, 1964). Therefore, the importance of providing a well-staffed and well-equipped recovery room, preferably in close proximity to the operating theatre, cannot be overstressed. The nursing staff should be specially trained to deal with airway problems, as maintenance of a clear airway, adequate venti-lation and administration of supplementary oxygen are of vital importance in this period of profound physiological change. Any respiratory obstruction in the presence of ganglion blockade is likely to lead to hypoxia and a fall in blood pressure and may eventually end in a cardiac arrest.

To avoid postural changes affecting arterial pressure, it is desirable to transfer the patient directly from the operating table to a bed, nursed preferably in lateral position. Arterial pressure, pulse rate and respiration should be monitored and recorded first at 5 min and then at 15 min intervals. Regular observations should be maintained until the patient is both con-scious and alert and arterial pressure is stable. Adequate analgesia and gradual head-up tilt may be employed to prevent quick rise of arterial pressure, thus helping to maintain haemostasis.

When conscious, the patient must remain in bed, preferably for 24 h, to prevent any postural hypotension in the presence of ganglion blockade. The first attempt by the patient to stand or walk should be supervised by a nurse or attendant.

## MORTALITY AND MORBIDITY

The ultimate question that remains to be answered is whether the use of hypotensive techniques increases the mortality and morbidity compared with anaesthesia where hypotension has not been used deliberately (so-called normotensive anaesthesia). Many studies have been carried out to record complications associated with the technique. Their results, on the whole, need careful interpretation and assessment with regard to increase in complications. It would be difficult to discuss these in detail here and the reader is referred to Green (1985b) for further information. Instead, it is proposed to report the results of 30 years of experience with hypotensive anaesthesia at Queen Victoria Hospital, East Grinstead.

20 558 hypotensive anaesthetics were carried out at the above unit during the years 1950–79. There were 10 deaths in this series (Enderby, 1985). Five of them were due to cardiac arrest caused by inadequate control of blood pressure during surgery (2 patients) and inadequate supervision of airway leading to respiratory obstruction in the recovery room (3 patients). The other 5 patients died as a result of other causes not directly attributable to hypotension, but are included here as they had all received ganglion-blocking drugs. The causes were air embolism, adrenal insufficiency, spon-taneous pneumothorax, viral hepatitis and more recently a case of malignant hyperpyrexia. Except for the last case all occurred during the early years between 1950 and 1961 (Enderby, 1985). If malignant hyperpyrexia is excluded, then since 1961 there has not been a single death in 15 853 hypotensive anaesthetics. This is the result of experience of the first 10 years, improvement in knowledge of the pharmacology and physiology of the technique, better monitoring and control of level of blood pressure, and lastly and most importantly provision of a recovery room open 24 hours a day situated in the vicinity of the operating theatre and staffed by trained and skilled nurses. Added to this is the improvement in the assessment and choice of patients who are fit to undergo the technique.

The morbidity of the technique is, however, more difficult to assess. Cerebral and myocardial complications occurred in 6 patients, all of them again during the early years (1950–60). Two patients had cerebral thrombosis, one of which occurred during recovery soon after a period of severe anoxia caused by a misplaced throat pack. Nominal aphasia, personality change, reduced learning capacity and myocardial infarct during surgery accounted for the remaining cases.

Enderby (1985) gives a very fine account and reports the occasional incidence of transient headache, depression, forgetfulness and lack of con-centration.

Thirty years of experience at East Grinstead therefore suggest that deliberate hypotension is a safe procedure provided strict guidelines are adhered to:

1. Careful preoperative assessment and choice of patients.
2. A clear and reliable airway with a non-kinking tube and good oxy-genation during hypotension (50% inspired $O_2$).
3. Continuous monitoring and precise control of blood pressure at the specific level chosen, ensuring that the lower limit of safety is never exceeded.
4. Meticulous attention to detail, with regard to (a) timing and sequence of

administration of drugs, (b) slow increase of head-up tilt, and (c) increased ventilation and/or introduction of higher concentrations of halothane or enflurane only after assessment of full effect of drugs and tilt.

5. Ensure a slow rate of reduction of blood pressure—not more than 10 mmHg/min.
6. Monitoring of ECG and ST segment changes in $V_5$, CC5 or CM5 lead.
7. Good and efficient postoperative recovery facilities with continuing care of the airway and oxygenation.

With diligent adherence to these guidelines, the technique has proved reliable, effective, simple and safe. Newer drugs and techniques are introduced in anaesthetic practice all the time, but the vast experience and unique safety record of achieving hypotension in the manner described here has made it very difficult for this author to contemplate changing over to other methods. It is suggested that, whatever techniques or drugs are used, the criteria and guidelines recommended above will provide a good foundation for the safe practice of hypotensive anaesthesia.

## FUTURE RESEARCH

There are two areas which are of current interest to investigators in the subject.

### New hypotensive agents

Apart from TNG and ATP, there has been a recent interest in the use of calcium blockers to produce hypotension. Diltiazem has been used clinically but the arterial pressure is difficult to control and the effect is unpredictable (Bernard et al, 1986).

Captopril, an angiotensin-converting enzyme (ACE) blocker, has recently been used to prevent rebound hypertension following SNP administration and to reduce the dosage of vasodilator required (Pasch et al, 1986; Woodside et al, 1984). Saralasin, an inhibitor of angiotensin II, has been used (Miller et al, 1981) for the same purpose with poor results.

### Cerebral protection from ischaemia

The possibility of reducing the threshold of cerebral blood flow where electrical or ionic failure occurs in brain ischaemia is of interest to many workers in the field (Symon, 1985; Siesjö and Wieloch, 1985). Anticonvulsants and drugs that depress cerebral metabolism, such as barbiturates, phenytoin, isoflurane and gammahydroxbutyrate, have been studied. Prostacyclin and indomethacin, calcium entry blockers, antioxidants and free radical scavengers have also been tried. As yet no accepted drug therapy has conclusively emerged, in spite of a great deal of experimental and clinical research. The only undisputed therapeutic principle is to improve the oxygen demand:supply ratio (Gisvold and Steen, 1985). This is best achieved by application of general measures to restore an adequate supply of oxygenated blood to the brain (Aitkenhead, 1986).

## SUMMARY

Deliberate hypotension performed skilfully by a competent anaesthetist brings great advantages to the patient undergoing plastic surgery. The obvious reduction of blood loss and avoidance of blood transfusion is easy to achieve but the requirements for producing a clear and dry surgical field are more exact and thus more difficult. Provided blood pressure is monitored continuously and reduced gradually to a safe level, there seems to be no more danger than with a normotensive anaesthetic. It does, however, require extra vigilance, proper assessment and choice of patients, special medical and nursing training, an equipped recovery room and more refined surgical techniques. Above all, it needs a good rapport among the operating theatre team to achieve the genuine advantages that it brings to the patient.

It has been suggested by opponents that deliberate hypotension is a physiological trespass. 'However it would appear that a well-considered and skilfully managed controlled hypotension is no more of a physiological trespass than anaesthesia, nor indeed the trespass of the surgeon's knife itself' (Leigh, 1975).

The value of the technique was recognized over 20 years ago: 'In the right hands controlled hypotension in anaesthesia is a major advance and should now be acceptable in properly judged circumstances' (McLaughlin, 1966). It was true then: it is true now.

## APPENDIX: HYPOTENSIVE ANAESTHETIC TECHNIQUE AT EAST GRINSTEAD

A safe, easy and reliable technique for inducing and maintaining hypotension has evolved over the last 30 years at East Grinstead. The chronological order and details of the technique, used in 23 200 hypotensive anaesthetics, is given below:

1. Anaesthesia is induced with a barbiturate (3–5 mg/kg of 2.5% thiopentone) as it provides limited protection to the brain in the event of ischaemia (Michenfelder et al, 1976).
2. Intubation is with a non-kinkable armoured tube to ensure a clear and reliable airway.
3. Intubation is assisted by a muscle relaxant whose action should persist until the patient is positioned on table, tilted and the full effect of ganglion and beta blockade assessed. To achieve this, without recourse to high concentration of inhalation agent, Decamethonium (C10) is the relaxant used. It lasts for 15–20 min, has few effects on pulse rate and blood pressure, and does not need reversal at the end.
4. ECG and intravenous infusion of Ringer's lactate.
5. Manual control of respiration is achieved using a circle system with a soda-lime absorber and avoiding hyperventilation. Administration of 50% inspired oxygen and minimal (0.5%) halothane or equivalent.
6. Ganglion blocker is preceded by a beta-blocker if indicated.
7. Patient is positioned on the table and the foot rest is secured.
8. Initial blood pressure reading while the table is flat.
9. Gradual head-up tilt in stages over a period of 10–15 min until maximum 20°–25° achieved. Assessment of its effect on blood pressure.

10. Further required fall in blood pressure is now achieved by increasing IPPV and/or the concentration of the volatile agent.
11. Beat to beat monitoring of arterial pressure by oscillometer used in a 'continuous' mode, as described in main body of chapter.
12. Short-acting analgesic if there is a reflex rise in blood pressure because of surgical stimuli.
13. At the end of the operation, there is a gradual reversal of tilt to allow autoregulation of CBF. Blood pressure returns to 80–90 mmHg on establishment of spontaneous respiration.

The advantages of this technique in maxillofacial and plastic surgery are:

(a) Wide fluctuations in blood pressure in response to surgical stimuli are easily and quickly controlled by increasing or decreasing IPPV. Thus breath to breath control of blood pressure and smooth hypotension is achieved.
(b) At the end of operation arterial pressure tends to return to a safe level of 80–90 mmHg and then gradually rises to its preoperative level over 1–3 h, thereby assuring haemostasis, and preventing cerebral hyperaemia.

## REFERENCES

Aitkenhead A (1986) Cerebral protection. *British Journal of Hospital Medicine* **35:** 290–298.
Aveling W & Verner IR (1981) Profound hypotension with intravenous nitroglycerin. In Robinson BF & Kaplan JA (eds) *The International Symposium on the Clinical Use of Tridil, Intravenous Nitroglycerin*, p 35. Oxford: The Medical Publishing Foundation Symposium Series.
Beare R (1985) Indications for hypotensive anaesthesia. In Enderby GEH (ed.) *Hypotensive Anaesthesia*, pp 99–108. London: Churchill Livingstone.
Bernard JM, Pinaud M, Carteau S, Hubert C & Sourou R (1986) Hypotensive action of diltiazem and nitroprusside compared during fentanyl anaesthesia for total hip arthroplasty. *Canadian Anaesthetists' Society Journal* **33:** 308–314.
Cope DHP & Crawford MC (1979) Labetalol in controlled hypotension. Administration of labetalol when adequate hypotension is difficult to achieve. *British Journal of Anaesthesia* **51:** 359–365.
Dandona P, James AM, Newburg ML & Becket AG (1979) Instability of cerebral blood flow in insulin-dependent diabetics. *Lancet* **ii:** 1203–1205.
Eckenhoff JE (1955) The use of controlled hypotension for surgical procedures. *Surgical Clinics of North America* **45:** 1579–1584.
Eckenhoff JE, Enderby GEH, Larson A, Edridge A & Judevin DE (1963) Pulmonary gas exchange during deliberate hypotension. *British Journal of Anaesthesia* **35:** 750–759.
Enderby GEH (1975) Some observations on the practice of deliberate hypotension. Guest Editorial. *British Journal of Anaesthesia* **47:** 743–744.
Enderby GEH (1980) Hypotensive anaesthesia. In Gray TC, Nunn JF & Utting JE (eds) *General Anaesthesia*, 4th edn, pp 1149–1168. London: Butterworths.
Enderby GEH (1985) *Hypotensive Anaesthesia*. London: Churchill Livingstone.
Fahmy NR & Battit GE (1975) Effects of pentolinium on blood sugar and serum potassium concentrations during anaesthesia and surgery. *British Journal of Anaesthesia* **47:** 1309–1313.
Fairbairn ML, Eltringham RJ, Young PN & Robinson JM (1986) Hypotensive anaesthesia for microsurgery of the middle ear. A comparison between isoflurane and halothane. *Anaesthesia* **41:** 637–640.
Fakunaga AF, Ikeda K & Matsuda I (1982) ATP-induced hypotensive anaesthesia during surgery. *Anesthesiology* **57:** A65.
Froelicher VF, Wolthins R & Keiser N (1976) A comparison of two Dipolar exercise ECG leads to lead V5. *Chest* **70:** 611–616.
Gisvold SE & Steen PA (1985) Drug therapy in brain ischaemia. *British Journal of Anaesthesia* **57:** 96–109.

Green D (1985a) Pharmacological blockade. In Enderby GEH (ed.) *Hypotensive Anaesthesia*, pp 109–137. London: Churchill Livingstone.

Green D (1985b) Cardiac and cerebral complications of deliberate hypotension. In Enderby GEH (ed.) *Hypotensive Anaesthesia*, pp 236–261. London: Churchill Livingstone.

Hellewell J & Potts MW (1966) Propranolol during controlled hypotension. *British Journal of Anaesthesia* 38: 794–801.

Hewitt PB, Lord PW & Thornton H (1967) Propranolol in hypotensive anaesthesia. *Anaesthesia* 22: 82–89.

Hutton P, Prys-Roberts C (1982) The oscillotonometer in theory and practice. *British Journal of Anaesthesia* 54: 581–591.

Jones RM, Hantler CB & Knight PR (1981) Use of pentolinium in post operative hypertension resistant to sodium nitroprusside. *British Journal of Anaesthesia* 53: 1151–1153.

Khambatta HJ, Stone JG & Khan E (1981) Propranolol alters renin release during nitroprusside induced hypotension and prevents hypertension on discontinuation of nitroprusside. *Anaesthesia and Analgesia Current Researches* 60: 569–573.

Lagerkranser M, Irestedt L, Sollevi A & Andreen M (1984) Central and splanchnic haemodynamics in the dog during controlled hypotension with adenosine. *Anesthesiology* 60: 547–552.

Lam AM & Gelb AW (1983) Cardio-vascular effect of isoflurane-induced hypotension for cerebral aneurysm surgery. *Anaesthesia Analgesia* 62: 742.

Lanier WL, Stangland KJ, Scheithauer BW, Milde JH & Michenfelder JD (1985) Effects of I.V. Dextrose and head position on neurologic outcome after complete cerebral ischaemia. *Anesthesiology* 63: A110.

Larson AG (1964) Deliberate hypotension. *Anesthesiology* 25: 682–706.

Laycock JRD, Coakham HB, Silver IA & Walters FJM (1986) Changes in brain surface oxygen tension during profound hypotension induced with Sodium Nitroprusside or adenosine in the sheep. *British Journal of Anaesthesia* 58: 1422–1426.

Leigh JM (1975) The history of controlled hypotension. *British Journal of Anaesthesia* 47: 745–749.

MacRae WR (1985) Induced hypotension. *British Journal of Hospital Medicine* 33: 341–343.

MacRae WR, Wildsmith JAW & Dale BA (1981) Induced hypotension with a mixture of sodium nitroprusside and trimetaphan camsylate. *Anaesthesia* 36: 312–315.

McDowell DG (1985) Editorial: Brain ischaemia—its prevention and treatment. *British Journal of Anaesthesia* 57: 1–2.

McIndoe A (1956) Hypotensive anaesthesia in surgery. *Plastic and Reconstructive Surgery* 17: 1–8.

McLaughlin CR (1966) Hypotensive anaesthesia: a surgeon's view. *Anesthesiology* 27: 239–241.

Michenfelder JD, Milde JH & Sundt TM Jr (1976) Cerebral protection by barbiturate anaesthesia. Use after middle cerebral occlusion in Java monkeys. *Archives of Neurology* 33: 345–350.

Miller ED, Delaney TJ & Beckman JJ (1981) Blood flow alteration induced by Saralasin or Sodium Nitroprusside in rats. *Anesthesiology* 54: 199–203.

Newberg LA & Michenfelder JD (1983) Cerebral protection by isoflurane during hypoxemia or ischaemia. *Anesthesiology* 59: 29–35.

Newberg LA, Milde JH & Michenfelder JD (1983) The cerebral metabolic effects of isoflurane at and above concentrations that suppress cortical arterial activity. *Anesthesiology* 59: 23–28.

Newberg LA, Milde JH & Michenfelder JD (1985) Cerebral and systemic effects of hypotension induced by adenosine or ATP in dogs. *Anesthesiology* 62: 429–436.

Newman G, Gelb AW & Lam AM (1986) The effect of isoflurane-induced hypotension on cerebral blood flow and cerebral metabolic rate for oxygen in humans. *Anesthesiology* 64: 307–310.

Pasch T, Kleierl-Lindner C, Gotz H & Pichl J (1986) Studies on rebound hypertension following controlled hypotension, and its prevention by captopril (Germ). *Anaesthetist* 35(2): 66–72.

Patel H (1981) Experience with the cerebral function monitor during deliberate hypotension. *British Journal of Anaesthesia* 53: 639–645.

Prior PF (1985) EEG monitoring and evoked potentials in brain ischaemia. *British Journal of Anaesthesia* **57:** 63–81.

Scott DB, Buckley FP, Littlewood DG, Macrae WR, Arthur GR & Drummond GB (1978) Circulatory effects of labetalol during halothane anaesthesia. *Anaesthesia* **33:** 145–156.

Siesjö BK & Wieloch T (1985) Cerebral metabolism in ischaemia: neurochemical basis for therapy. *British Journal of Anaesthesia* **57:** 47–62.

Sollevi A, Lagerkranser M, Irestedt L, Gordon E & Lindquist C (1984) Controlled hypotension and adenosine in cerebral aneurysm surgery *Anesthesiology* **61:** 400–405.

Symon L (1985) Flow thresholds in brain ischaemia and the effects of drugs. *British Journal of Anaesthesia* **57:** 34–43.

Turner JM, Powell D, Gibson RM & McDowall DG (1977) Intracranial pressure changes in neurosurgical patients during hypotension induced with sodium nitroprusside or trimetaphan. *British Journal of Anaesthesia* **49:** 419.

Van Aken H, Puchstein C, Fitch W & Graham DI (1984) Haemodynamic and cerebral effects of ATP-induced hypotension. *British Journal of Anaesthesia* **56:** 1409–1415.

Verner IR (1985) Direct-acting vasodilators. In Enderby GEH (ed.) *Hypotensive Anaesthesia*, pp 138–163. London: Churchill Livingstone.

Vesey CJ, Cole PV & Simpson PJ (1976) Cyanide and thiocyanate concentrations following sodium nitroprusside infusion in man. *British Journal of Anaesthesia* **48:** 651.

Woodside J, Garner L, Bedford RF et al (1984) Captopril reduces the dose requirement for Sodium Nitroprusside induced hypotension. *Anesthesiology* **60:** 413–417.

# 13

Anaesthesia for microvascular surgery

DAVID F. COCHRANE

The simultaneous development of the operating microscope, purpose-made instruments and microsutures in the 1960s enabled surgeons to anastomose blood vessels of 1.6–3 mm diameter in experimental animals, and still retain their patency. Successful replantation of amputated digits, scalps and other structures soon followed. In 1974, increasing confidence in these techniques led Taylor in Melbourne to successfully transfer a free skin flap, based on readily identifiable vessels, from the groin to the leg, and re-establish its blood flow through microvascular anastomoses to vessels at the recipient site.

This ability to transfer tissue from one part of the body to another in a single operation has led to the development of a variety of new procedures. The transfer of skin, bones, muscles, nerves and composite flaps of all these, including whole digits, is now commonplace in patients of all ages. It is therefore unlikely that anaesthetists in training will escape them.

The two main problems facing the anaesthetist are those of prolonged anaesthesia and the promotion of good tissue perfusion.

Table 1 shows the percentage of 88 operations lasting 7 h or more carried out in the plastic surgery theatres at Frenchay hospital over a four-year period. These are for the initial microvascular operation. Occasionally, a patient has to return for a 're-do' of the anastomosis and this can add several hours to these times.

**Table 1.** Operations lasting 7 h or more.

| | |
|---|---|
| 23% | 7–9 h |
| 24% | 9–11 h |
| 39% | 11–13 h |
| 13% | 13–16 h |
| 1% | 22 h (one case only) |

Prolonged operations are not the sole prerogative of the microsurgeon. A complicated neurosurgical operation, such as the removal of an acoustic neuroma, or a faciomaxillary reconstruction, can last most of the day. In the case of microvascular surgery, however, the anaesthetist is confronted not only with the problems of prolonged surgery, but also with the overriding need to maintain optimal perfusion to the graft. Failure in this respect can have catastrophic consequences. Not only is there the waste of many man-hours of operating time, but also the useless sacrifice of the donor graft, with the result that the patient is physically and in terms of morale worse off than before the operation.

There are several stages in a microvascular operation, each with different anaesthetic implications.

1.  Preparation of the recipient site.
2.  Preparation of the donor graft.
3.  Perfusion of graft on its isolated pedicle.
4.  Transfer of graft and microvascular anastomoses.
5.  Completion of operation, and transfer of patient to a high-dependency unit.

The recipient site can range from a relatively small skin defect in the leg, to that left after a major ablative procedure for cancer of the head and neck. The donor graft, likewise, could range from a small skin graft to a composite skin, muscle and bone flap. The problems of anaesthesia up to this point are no different from those for orthopaedic or major head and neck surgery, in any age group, although they might involve hypotensive anaesthesia. Where possible, the first two stages are carried out simultaneously, thus saving much time.

It is crucial that the final two stages follow on smoothly from each other. The surgeon must attach the graft in reasonable time and the anaesthetist ensure optimal perfusion, not only while in the operation theatre, but also during transfer to the ward or high-dependency unit.

It should be emphasized that it is primarily the surgeon who determines whether the graft will be successful or not. A well-chosen flap with relatively large vessels, anastomosed correctly, will survive, unless there is gross anaesthetic mismanagement. Nevertheless, there are many operations where the surgeon is obliged to use less than ideal sized vessels, e.g. in digital transplants, and here the anaesthetic management can determine success or failure.

## BLOOD FLOW TO THE GRAFT

Although free grafts are chosen with the largest possible blood vessels supporting them, their total blood supply will, with certain exceptions, be less than before they were raised. The edges of the graft will now be supplied by end arteries and be particularly susceptible to ischaemia.

The term 'microvascular' refers to the use of a microscope and not to the microcirculation. Both the arteries and veins of 1–4 mm size used in micro-vascular surgery still contain a large amount of smooth muscle, and although the blood vessels in a free graft are denervated, they still react to physical and chemical influences. Normally, the build-up of metabolites will ensure maximal dilatation, but cold and rough handling can send the vessels into spasm (Khashaba and McGregor, 1986). The vessels proximal to the anastomosis are, in addition, subject to the usual neural influences.

Two physical laws govern the flow of blood to the graft—the laws of Laplace and Poiseuille.

Laplace's law:

$$P = 2T/R$$

where $P$ is the intraluminal pressure, $T$ the wall tension and $R$ the radius of the vessel.

Poiseuille's law (simplified):

$$\text{Flow} = \frac{\text{Head of pressure} \times R^4}{\eta L}$$

*where* $\eta$ is the viscosity of the fluid and $L$ and $R$ the length and radius of the tube respectively.

Laplace's Law basically means that less pressure is needed to overcome wall tension to keep open a dilated vessel than a constricted one, as the pressure needed to do this is inversely proportional to its radius.

In Poiseuille's law, the flow through the vessels is proportional to the fourth power of the radius, for a given viscosity and pressure gradient. Thus with increasing dilatation the flow will increase substantially and the head of pressure needed to sustain the dilatation will decrease. On the other hand, if vasoconstriction is allowed to occur, there is a descent into a spiral of ever-decreasing flow and further vasoconstriction, culminating with sludging of the circulation and an ischaemic graft.

Poiseuille's law strictly applies to laminar flow in rigid tubes and not to a pulsatile, non-Newtonian fluid, such as blood, contained in elastic blood vessels. The influence of blood viscosity is therefore undervalued in comparison to that of the radius of the vascular bed ($\eta^1$ compared with $R^4$). Blood viscosity is not constant and can vary severalfold throughout the circulation. The factors involved in these changes are extremely complex. (For a comprehensive review, see Goslinga (1984).)

As blood progresses towards the microcirculation, its viscosity decreases as the vessels get smaller. This is because although its flow rate gradually *decreases* as vessels get progressively smaller, its flow, relative to the diameter of the vessels, *increases*. This increase in relative velocity results in an increased shear rate and lowered viscosity. At the level of the capillary, this high relative velocity of flow induces the erythrocytes to line up in single file, like a stack of saucers on their edges, to be carried along in a stream of plasma. The blood viscosity at this point can approach that of plasma.

In addition, because of their flexibility, the erythrocytes adopt a more streamlined shape. An increase in rigidity, such as occurs in acidosis or unusual shape (e.g. in sickle cell disease) will militate against this streamlining.

At the level of the postcapillary venule, the sudden fall in the rate of flow due to the rise in vessel size, allows the erythrocytes 'to break ranks' and hit the sides of the vessel wall, with a consequent sudden increase in viscosity and resistance, and a further decrease in flow. A similar retardant effect will be caused by platelet aggregation and rouleaux formation. At low shear rates the tendency of erythrocytes to clump is increased, although they will disengage if the shear rate rises above a critical level. There is thus a compounding effect, so that as blood flow improves, so do its rheological properties and vice versa.

The principal factors influencing blood viscosity are:

1.  Number of erythrocytes.
2.  Their tendency to aggregate, which is *increased* by substances of higher molecular weight, such as fibrinogen, macroglobulins and dextran 70 and 110, and *decreased* by dextran 40.
3.  Plasma viscosity, which is *increased* by fibrinogen, gelatin solutions and dextran 70, and *decreased* by albumin solutions.
4.  Velocity of flow.

The most important of these factors is the concentration of erythrocytes, although each has a 'knock-on' effect on the others. Haemodilution with plasma substitutes markedly improves its rheological properties, and although plasma substitutes such as gelatin solutions have viscosities almost twice that of plasma, their effects on diminishing the viscosity of whole blood by lowering the haematocrit predominate.

The experience of anaesthetists closely involved in this field has led them, often empirically, to the same conclusion, which is that in order to provide optimum perfusion for a graft, excellent total body perfusion should be the aim. The physiological basis of this is well reviewed by Macdonald (1985).

The player who has just come off the squash court, or a patient with thyrotoxicosis or anaemia, is a good example of a well-perfused person. This is typified by:

1.  Raised cardiac output.
2.  Vasodilatation and warmth.
3.  High pulse pressure.
4.  High velocity of flow.

The cardiac output can be raised by increasing the central venous pressure with a fluid load with consequent reflex vasodilatation, or the afterload can be decreased with vasodilators and fluids used to maintain the blood pressure. In practice, both methods are used simultaneously.

The aim is therefore to promote optimal blood flow by:

1.  High circulating volume with moderate haemodilution.
2.  Vasodilatation.
3.  Maintenance of peripheral and core temperatures.

The effect of lowering the haematocrit on viscosity and flow in small vessels has already been mentioned. There is abundant evidence, both experimental and clinical, of the benefits of haemodilution on the survival of tissues with borderline flow. The decrease in oxygen-carrying capacity from the loss of haemoglobin is more than compensated for by the increase in flow. Optimum oxygen transfer in the resting state is achieved at a haematocrit of 30%. Nevertheless, this presupposes that there will be a compensatory increase in cardiac output and that the patient is well-oxygenated.

It would therefore appear prudent, particularly in patients with poor cardiac reserve, to provide a safety margin and aim for a haematocrit of 35% (Macdonald, 1985).

In the operating theatre, the best indication we have of flow is the peripheral temperature, a fall of which precedes changes in the pulse rate and blood pressure.

## Blood loss

Blood loss in long microvascular cases can be grossly underestimated, as it is not easy to measure. A large donor and recipient site and a slow constant ooze, particularly from bone, can soon mount up, and there is always a sudden loss when tourniquets are released. In the transfer of a composite bone, muscle and skin flap from the iliac region to the leg a total (intra-operative + postoperative) transfusion of eight units of blood is not unusual.

The author's practice is therefore not to attempt to measure blood loss, but to maintain the central venous pressure at 1–2 cm $H_2O$ above the initial level. The initial level is taken as the level in the anaesthetized patient just prior to surgical stimulation. Blood is then given to maintain the haematocrit between 33 and 35%. Where SAG M blood is used, an equivalent volume of human albumin solutions is infused; otherwise the CVP is maintained with equal volumes of dextran 40 and Ringer lactate, up to a maximum volume of 1500 ml of the dextran per 24 h, when gelatin solutions are used. The maintenance of a good urine output is rarely a problem in these well-perfused patients. Their high circulatory volume and optimal perfusion, however, make them exquisitely sensitive to diuretics. The injudicious use of 10 mg of frusemide has been followed by a colossal output of urine with deleterious effects on the circulation. A test dose of 2 mg is recommended.

## Vasodilators

There appear to be very few vasodilators that have not been used at some time or another to overcome spasm and promote flow. Sympathetic denervation, adrenergic blockers, and direct-acting smooth muscle relaxants have all been tried. Their very number says much for their efficacy. In the author's view, their use lies in enabling a good cardiac output, vasodilatation and high velocity of flow to be attained, and not for their local effects.

Experience has shown that if good perfusion to a graft is obtained by regional block, volatile anaesthetic, or an agent such as sodium nitro-prusside, without also maintaining a high circulating fluid volume and general vasodilatation, then on withdrawal of the agent or block, peripheral constriction will occur. Isoflurane, unlike other volatile agents, has a direct vasodilator action without compromising the cardiac output and is therefore the volatile agent of choice.

Papaverine administered both topically or intravascularly has proved disappointing, but naftidrofuryl oxalate applied topically appears to be efficacious in treating local spasm. Adrenergic block of the isolated limb lasting up to 10 days by the use of 15–30 mg of guanethidine in a Biers block has been described by Holland et al (1977). Chlorpromazine in repeated doses of 2.5–5.0 mg i.v. has not only useful alpha-blocking effects, but also prevents postoperative shivering as well as having sedative and antiemetic properties.

## Vasoconstriction

This can be caused by cold, pain, hypocarbia and hypovolaemia, and must be avoided at all costs. The $PCO_2$ should be kept at near-normal levels. Generous doses of opiates (and relaxants) can be used during the first half of the operation, which is associated with the most surgical stimulation, in the knowledge that several hours still remain for their termination of action.

## Maintenance of body temperature

It cannot be stressed too strongly that a fall in body temperature should not be allowed to occur during and following the transfer of a free graft. Failure to maintain core temperature will result in a vasoconstricted and probably shivering patient. By the time rewarming has occurred, the sequence of vasoconstriction, poor flow, increased viscosity, further decrease in flow and clotting of the vessels to the graft may have occurred. The graft itself must be kept warm because, although denervated, its vessels constrict in response to cold.

Factors aggravating loss of heat during microvascular surgery include:

1. Prolonged surgery.
2. Vasodilatation.
3. Exposure of large areas of body with simultaneous surgery to donor and recipient sites.
4. Evaporation from wet drapes.
5. Good urine output.

Heat loss can be minimized by covering up as much of the body as possible with nonabsorbent drapes, the operative site(s) with sterile adhesive drapes, and the rest of the body with metallized plastic sheet. The latter may not have any advantage over simple polythene sheet in insulating the body (Marcus et al, 1977).

The head is an important source of heat loss in small children and should be covered. The legs, where possible, can be covered with antiembolic pneumatic cuffs which also serve to keep the heels off the table. In theory, one can diminish heat loss by raising the temperature of the operating theatre, but in practice this is not tolerated by the theatre staff for long periods. These measures alone have not been found to be adequate by themselves and active means of heating, such as a thermal mattress and heated anaesthetic gases, are required if large areas of the body are exposed. The need to warm infusion fluids is well recognized.

The contribution of the thermal mattress is overrated. Stone et al (1981) showed that there were no differences between the temperatures of exposed patients having major surgery whether the heating was turned on or not.

The problem is that only a relatively small area of the body is in contact with the mattress—about a third—when the patient is lying on his back, and rather less when he is on his side. Heat and fluid loss from the respiratory tract is substantial and can be minimized by the use of one of the many available condenser humidifiers. These are perfectly adequate for operations such as replants of fingers, or operations on the head and neck, but where a large proportion of the body is exposed, such as in a latissimus dorsi flap, the use of an efficient heated humidifier, able to warm and humidify the dry inspired gases to 37 °C, is essential if the temperature of the patient is not to fall.

There is a tendency for the temperature to rise towards the end of the operation. Once the donor site has been closed, the heat loss from this area will diminish. Measurements of the patient's steroid output in our unit showed that there was a continuing rise throughout the operation, except in those patients where a regional block was used. The rise in temperature was also less in the latter group, and it is assumed that the metabolic response to surgery resulting in the normal postoperative pyrexia is being seen during these lengthy operations. It is not unusual, therefore, to have to discontinue some of the heat-retaining appliances towards the end of the operation, particularly in children. Block (1986) has shown that in children the application of a tourniquet is associated with a rise in temperature, probably due to the exclusion of significant areas of the body from heat loss.

## CHOICE OF ANAESTHESIA

### Regional anaesthesia

Table 2. Advantages and disadvantages of regional anaesthesia.

| Advantages | Disadvantages |
|---|---|
| Sensory motor, and sympathetic block continued into postoperative period. | Not always applicable. |
| Minimal sedation or general anaesthesia. | Hypotension. |
| Stress-free anaesthesia. | False sense of security. |

Regional anaesthesia is attractive in theory, although few patients would be able to lie immobile for long periods, and supplementary sedation or a light general anaesthetic is required. The duration of action of even the longest-acting local anaesthetic will not be sufficient for these operations. In practice this limits their use to axillary and epidural blocks, where a catheter can be inserted and top-up doses given.

Operations below the waist, especially those involving bone work, are obvious indications for epidural anaesthesia, but in many cases the donor and recipient sites are situated widely apart. Hypotension can be a problem, especially if artificial ventilation using non-depolarizing relaxants with hypotensive effects are used. While hypotension may be desirable during the initial dissection, later on the blood pressure will be a compromise between the level needed to help the surgeon identify the blood supply to the graft, and the desire to minimize blood loss.

A systolic arterial pressure of 100 mmHg in the vasodilated fit patient is ideal (Macdonald, 1985). Once the anastomoses have been completed, the blood pressure must not be allowed to fall below this level. The author has in the past been lulled into a false sense of security when using a continuous epidural block for postoperative analgesia. The circulating fluid volume had not been kept at an adequate level and the vasodilatation in the lower half of the body had been compensated for by vasoconstriction in the upper half, thereby maintaining the blood pressure. When, however, the epidural wore off and for technical reasons could not be reinstituted, severe vasoconstriction occurred in the limb supporting the graft. As a result of this experience an intravenous continuous infusion of opiate is now used for postoperative pain, because not only is it applicable to all microvascular cases, but it is also effective in providing stable conditions and alleviating the general aches and pains that are caused by the prolonged immobility.

**General anaesthesia**

The 'unfavourable effects of prolonged anaesthesia', in so far as they relate to general anaesthetics, were enumerated by Vandam (1965). His view of many of the factors to be taken into consideration when choosing an anaesthetic agent are still applicable. They are:

1.  Direct toxicity.
2.  Toxicity of metabolites.
3.  Adverse cumulative effects.
4.  Ease of reversibility.

*Nitrous oxide*

The use of a nitrous oxide–oxygen-relaxant technique with supplementary analgesics appears at first glance to fulfil all of the above criteria. Recovery from nitrous oxide anaesthesia is extremely rapid, even after very long operations, due to its low solubility. Nevertheless, the well-known ability of nitrous oxide to cause bone marrow depression is a cause for concern. It used to be thought that several days of exposure were necessary for bone marrow depression to occur. The introduction of more sensitive tests has shown that abnormalities can occur following as little as 2–6 h of exposure in ill patients admitted to an intensive care unit (Amos et al, 1982). In healthy patients, these changes appear to be reversible, and balanced anaesthesia with nitrous oxide still remains the most common technique used for microvascular surgery. As more information comes to light concerning its long-term effects, the use of air as a carrier gas may replace it.

Nitrous oxide diffuses rapidly into air-filled cavities and can increase the pressure in an endotracheal cuff to well above capillary pressure within an hour. If this is allowed to occur for prolonged periods, tracheal mucosal damage will occur. There are three ways round the problem.

1.   Fill cuff with anaesthetic gases or water.
2.   Check pressure in cuff at periodic intervals.
3.   Use special tube with a pilot balloon made of a larger diameter than the tracheal cuff and made of thinner material, through which nitrous oxide can diffuse out.

### Volatile anaesthetics

In the present state of knowledge there must be many question marks against the use of volatile anaesthetics for prolonged anaesthesia. There is also the problem of repeated anaesthesia. The patients will quite often have had several general anaesthetics prior to the microsurgery, with the probability of more to come after it.

When volatile anaesthetics are used as the main anaesthetic for long periods, patients have a prolonged emergence with restlessness and agitation. This is the author's experience with halothane. In a case described by Caplan (1984), 26 MAC hours of enflurane were given over the course of a 47 h operation. Although the patient opened his eyes to command soon after reaching the intensive care unit, he could only be extubated on the second postoperative day, and even then was extremely agitated, thrashed about a great deal and did not properly wake up until the third postoperative day. This difference between partial and full recovery was predicted by Mapleson (1963), with an analogue model of uptake and elimination of halothane. In Mapleson's model, the time taken for the concentration of halothane in the brain to decrease to 75% and 10%, respectively, of the anaesthetic level, is illustrated for different lengths of administration.

*Partial recovery to 75% of anaesthetic level of halothane.*
4 min after 10 min  administration
6 min after 10 h   administration
7 min after 10 days administration

*'Complete' recovery to 10% of anaesthetic level.*
30 min after 10 min  administration
 9 h    after 10 h    administration
24 h    after 10 days administration

In other words, partial recovery is hardly affected by the length of administration, whereas 'full' recovery is markedly so. This disparity increases with the blood–gas solubility partition coefficient of the agent, and is thus minimal with nitrous oxide, but will increase respectively for isoflurane, enflurane and halothane.

The low blood–gas solubility and amount of metabolic degradation of isoflurane, in addition to its beneficial effects on the circulation, further enhance its position as the volatile anaesthetic of choice. The expense of the drug can be minimized by the use of low-flow closed-circuit anaesthesia, which because of its conservation of heat and moisture may render a heated humidifier unnecessary.

When volatile agents are withdrawn at the end of the operation, their vasodilator action also ceases. The ensuing vasoconstriction can result in a very sick-looking flap by the time the patient reaches the recovery area. If they are used, they should be turned off well before the end of the operation to check that the circulating volume is adequate and the flap is not agent-dependent.

## Total intravenous anaesthesia

Although eliminating many of the practical and theoretical disadvantages of inhalational agents, total intravenous anaesthesia brings problems of its own, and while the advent of new drugs may increase its use, at present it is not a valid alternative for most anaesthetists.

## Complications

Some of the complications particularly associated with microvascular surgery have already been referred to and relate mostly to the maintenance of the circulating volume, vasodilatation, core and peripheral temperatures. In addition the following have occurred during the use of anaesthetics given by the author:

1.  Failure of adequate ventilation due to
    (a) disconnection
    (b) dilatation of stomach
    (c) tension pneumothorax
    (d) atelectasis.
2.  Bladder distension (in patient) interfering with operative access.

These are immediately recognizable as the sort of complication that one sees more frequently in the intensive care unit than on the operating table. This is the key to managing these cases. They should be thought of as patients being ventilated on the ICU and should attract all the care associated with such patients. An implant-tested endotracheal tube, nasogastric tube and urinary catheter will be routine. Physiotherapy and skin care is limited to passive head and limb movements. As the patient cannot be turned, a ripple mattress is useful and particular care is taken with the positioning of the limbs and the protection of nerves, especially the ulnar. The use of a heated humidifier, with careful monitoring of the naso-pharyngeal and peripheral temperatures, has already been mentioned. An ICU type chart is more appropriate than the standard anaesthetic form with inflation pressure, CVP, regular blood gases and haematocrit being charted, as well as the temperatures(?), pulse, blood pressure and fluid balance.

## Monitoring

It is impossible to maintain constant vigilance for prolonged periods, particularly when there seems to be little happening. It is easy for gradual changes to go unnoticed until a major problem occurs.

The finger plethysmograph is the most useful of all the monitors available. Its output depends on peripheral flow to the finger and can be used to trigger an audible bleep, which if set at an appropriate level, will not be a source of irritation to the theatre staff, but whose sudden absence, or change of rate, would be immediately noticed.

There is a natural reluctance to cannulate arteries for surgery in which flaps based on a functioning radial artery are commonplace. An automatic noninvasive oscillometric blood pressure monitor is perfectly adequate for most cases. Capnographs obviate the need to puncture arteries, and many of them have useful alarm functions. A ventilator disconnection alarm is mandatory.

The function of the anaesthetist during these long cases has been likened to that of the pilot of an aircraft. The well-designed aircraft cockpit has all the relevant instruments set out in a regular pattern, and all controls to hand. So it should be with the anaesthetist. If he is not careful, he can find himself uncomfortably squeezed into a small space by two teams of surgeons and nurses, with all their impedimenta, to say nothing of the microscope. It is of the utmost importance that he marks out his territory and defends it against all comers. It helps to organize the operating table so that he can be near the door where he can be passed things without people falling over all the equipment. The abundance of electrical equipment requires extra electrical sockets.

The great majority of free flaps are elective procedures and can be carried out within an extended normal working day, and as such should not provide any logistical problems, although a short break from the theatre enhances the vigilance of the anaesthetist enormously. Emergencies and the occasional case that extends into the small hours are another matter altogether. It was expected that emergency microvascular surgery would cause major staffing problems by effectively removing an important member of the emergency anaesthetic team. The early enthusiasm for replantation of limbs and digits has, however, been tempered by a critical reassessment of the long-term results, and the emergency load has fallen substantially. Nevertheless, when emergencies do occur it is essential to draft in an additional member of the emergency team to relieve the emergency anaesthetist, who may have already worked a full day. During the day, the vigilance of the anaesthetist can be enhanced by giving practical instruction to junior anaesthetic or ancillary staff. The use of the nerve stimulator for monitoring relaxants and practical measurements in closed-circuit anaesthesia are obvious examples. At night, however, the relative absence of extraneous activity causes major problems in attentiveness.

## POSTOPERATIVE CARE

The circulation to the graft is particularly vulnerable for 48 h, after which the failure rate of free grafts falls off sharply. Transfer to a high-dependency area is therefore advisable in order to maintain an equivalent standard of care, particularly of temperature and circulatory control, to that of the operating theatre. Early detection of poor perfusion is essential if a surgically correctable complication is to be treated. The temperature of the graft is an unreliable guide to detection of early problems with flow. The graft itself may be kept warm by heat conducted from the surrounding tissues, especially in the case of small grafts. Various instruments have been described to monitor perfusion. These include laser reflective photometry and implanted electromagnetic flow meters, but until such time as their value has been established and they are widely available, the eye of an experienced observer, monitoring the colour of the flap and the capillary return in response to pressure, is as good a method as any. A trap for the unwary is that an 'instant' capillary return may be due to venous obstruction.

Some grafts, particularly composite ones containing bone and muscle, will continue to ooze postoperatively, and in some cases this will be a desirable way of relieving venous obstruction until such time as new venous channels are established. Close monitoring of the CVP and appropriate fluid balance is therefore imperative.

It is interesting that, in spite of the prolonged immobility of these patients, many suffering from serious injuries to the limbs and the major surgery involved, deep vein thrombosis and pulmonary embolism do not appear to be a problem. It may be that the obsession with the promotion of blood flow plays a contributory part.

Microvascular surgery highlights many shortcomings in anaesthetic technique that would perhaps go unnoticed in routine anaesthesia. The experience gained in managing these cases is relevant to providing better care for others.

## SUMMARY

The number and scope of operations involving microvascular surgery is rapidly increasing. The anaesthetic management involves not only the problem of very prolonged surgery, but also the need to optimize the circulation to the graft during the operation and the early postoperative period. This requires a sound knowledge of the factors influencing blood rheology. A hyperdynamic circulation with high velocity of flow and an adequate arterial pressure is ideal, and is obtained by hypervolaemic haemodilution in a vasodilated warm patient.

Heat loss is a problem due to exposure of large areas of the body for prolonged periods. The heated humidification of respiratory gases may be essential to maintain core temperature.

The choice of anaesthetic must take into consideration the length of the operation and the need to avoid vasoconstriction and hypotension. The toxicity of the agents and their metabolites, as well as cumulation with prolonged administration, must also be considered. Continuous regional and balanced anaesthesia are suitable techniques. Isoflurane is the volatile anaesthetic of choice.

Boredom, fatigue and inattention of the anaesthetist can be dangerous. The patient should be treated as if he were in an intensive care unit and monitored accordingly. Measurement of the CVP, haematocrit, and peripheral and core temperatures are essential.

Emergency microvascular surgery can play havoc with emergency anaesthetic rotas. Various solutions are proposed.

## REFERENCES

Amos RJ, Amess JAL, Hinds CJ & Mollin DL (1982) Incidence and pathogenesis of acute megaloblastic bone marrow change in patients receiving intensive care. *Lancet* **i**: 339–342.

Bloch EC (1986) Hyperthermia resulting from tourniquet application in children. *Annals of the Royal College of Surgeons of England* **68**: 193–194.

Caplan RA & Long MC (1984) Management and sequelae of a two day anaesthetic. *Anaesthesia and Analgesia* **63**: 353–358.

Goslinga H (1984) Blood viscosity and shock. *Anaesthesiologie und Intensivmedizin* **160**.

Holland AJC, Davies KH & Wallace DH (1977) Sympathetic blockade of isolated limbs by intravenous guanethidine. *Canadian Anaesthetic Society Journal* **24**: 597–602.

Jones BM (1983) Recent advances in circulatory monitors of the skin. *Journal of International Biomedical Information and Data* **4**: 39–48.

Khashaba AA & McGregor IA (1986) Haemodynamics of the radial forearm flap. *British Journal of Plastic Surgery* **39**: 441–450.

Macdonald DJF (1985) Anaesthesia for microvascular surgery. (A physiological approach.) *British Journal of Anaesthesia* **57**: 904–912.

Mapleson WW (1963) Quantitative prediction of anesthetic concentrations. In Papper EM & Kitz RJ (eds) *Uptake and Distribution of Anesthetic Agents*, pp 104–119. New York: McGraw Hill.

Marcus P, Robertson D & Langford R (1977) Metallized plastic sheeting for use in survival. *Aviation Space Environment Medicine* **48**: 50.

Stone DR, Downs JB, Paul WL & Perkins HM (1981) Adult body temperature and heated humidification of anesthetic gases during general anesthesia. *Anesthesia and Analgesia* **60**: 736–741.

Vandam LD (1965) The unfavourable effects of prolonged anaesthesia. *Canadian Anaesthetists' Society Journal* **12**: 107–119.

# 14

# Problems in head and neck surgery

## M. E. WARD

Major surgery in the head and neck area may be indicated for a wide range of pathologies, of which the commonest will be neoplastic lesions. Such surgery is generally of a semi-urgent nature and must be carefully planned, both individually by the surgeon and jointly between the surgeon and anaesthetist. Resection of a tumour may well be possible, but successful reconstruction to produce an acceptable cosmetic result may require a greater depth of understanding on the part of the surgeon and team work on the part of the anaesthetist, prosthetist, and other surgical colleagues such as ophthalmic surgeon, neurosurgeon, and oral surgeon (Figures 1, 2 and 3). Rarely, tumours in this area may present as emergencies when they produce symptoms as a result of involvement of the airway or intracranial contents.

Trauma involving the head and neck is clearly, at least initially, an acute emergency (Figure 4) and is regrettably an increasing part of the head and neck surgeon's workload. In the UK the introduction of seatbelt legislation has thankfully reduced this alarming rate of increase. Again, trauma of the head and neck will not infrequently overlap the field of the neurosurgeon, ophthalmic surgeon and oral surgeon, and the ideally placed head and neck surgeon will find himself working in a hospital with adequate support from the other services.

Acute infections of the head and neck, other than dental sepsis, will only rarely need surgical intervention. Also rarely, chronic low-grade infection of the facial skeleton may require radical clearance. This sort of surgery must be carefully planned and will involve co-operation not only with the other surgical specialities but also with the bacteriologist, who will advise as to appropriate antibiotic cover and who may wish to be involved more directly.

The other large part of the plastic surgeon's workload will be the purely cosmetic side. Into this category comes the 'funny looking kid' who may need surgery to improve his acceptability to society (Figures 5 and 6). Recent developments in craniofacial surgery have meant that there is a good chance of improvement for the many anomalies which may be found in approximately 1 in 4000 births. While the aetiology of the recognized syndromes such as Crouzon's and Apert's are unknown, and therefore their elimination currently impossible, these patients' only hope of acceptable survival is through major surgical reconstruction of the facial and orbital skeleton as pioneered by Paul Tessier (Tessier et al, 1967). Many of these operations are carried out for purely cosmetic reasons, but it must be understood that there are also related problems such as intracranial hypertension, visual disturbance, mental deterioration, squint and cranial nerve palsies which will need surgical treatment.

If these then are the main indications for surgery, what is the likely workload for a regional plastic surgery unit with an interest in major craniofacial and head and neck cancer surgery?

The Oxford group, which has two consultant plastic surgeons with supporting junior staff, two oral surgeons, two neurosurgeons and three ophthalmic surgeons, deals with approximately 55 craniofacial procedures a year, of which 35 are transcranial and 20 extracranial operations. In addition, about 50 major head and neck cancers are resected annually.

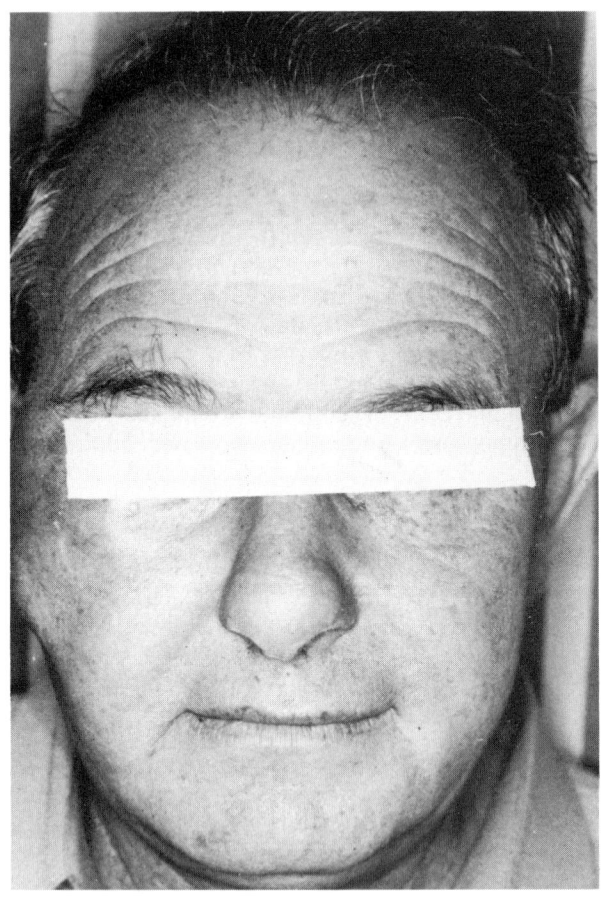

**Figure 1.** Squamous cell carcinoma of antrum.

## PREOPERATIVE ASSESSMENT

Many older patients will be suffering from intercurrent medical problems which must be completely and fully evaluated prior to surgery. As one of the factors in the aetiology of serious oral pathology is chronic alcoholism, the normality or otherwise of the liver function must be assessed. Where alcohol abuse is a factor, consideration must be given to the possibility that patients may suffer withdrawal symptoms in the postoperative period, and arrangements for suitable management must be made *in advance*. Respiratory and cardiovascular function should be carefully assessed, and any appropriate preoperative treatment commenced. Patients referred as a result of trauma must have their neurological status carefully assessed, with particular

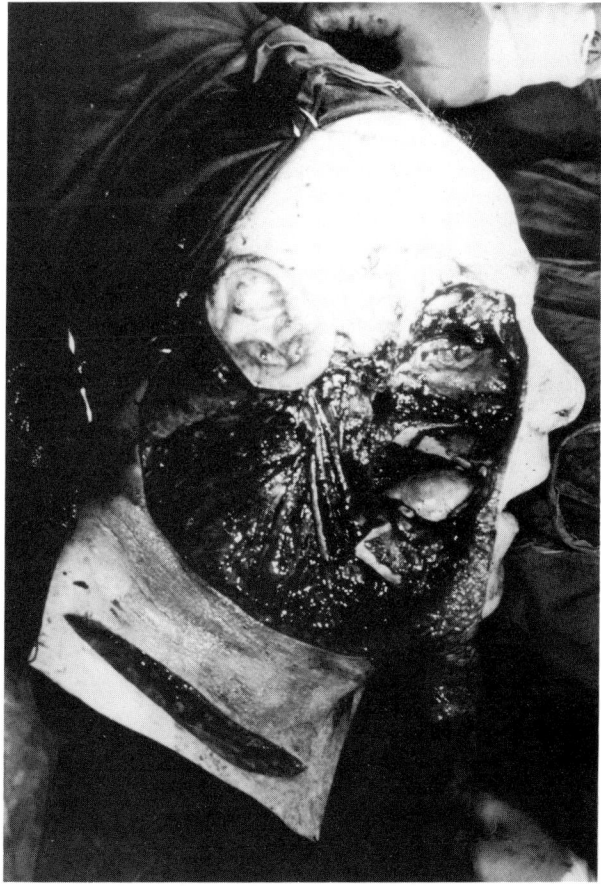

**Figure 2.** Extensive resection of maxilla, orbit and contents as a result of extra-antral spread.

reference to the level of consciousness and the pupillary behaviour, so that a preoperative baseline can be established.

## The airway

The airway must be carefully assessed preoperatively. Many patients with intraoral lesions may suffer trismus for which they have learnt to compensate in normal speech, and which therefore must be specifically looked for (Figure 7). Neck mobility must also be studied prior to induction of anaesthesia, and if there are any anticipated problems then the full armamentarium for dealing with a difficult intubation should be at hand. Recent experience with transtracheal cannulation and jet ventilation (Figure 8) allows plenty of time for careful assessment of the patient once

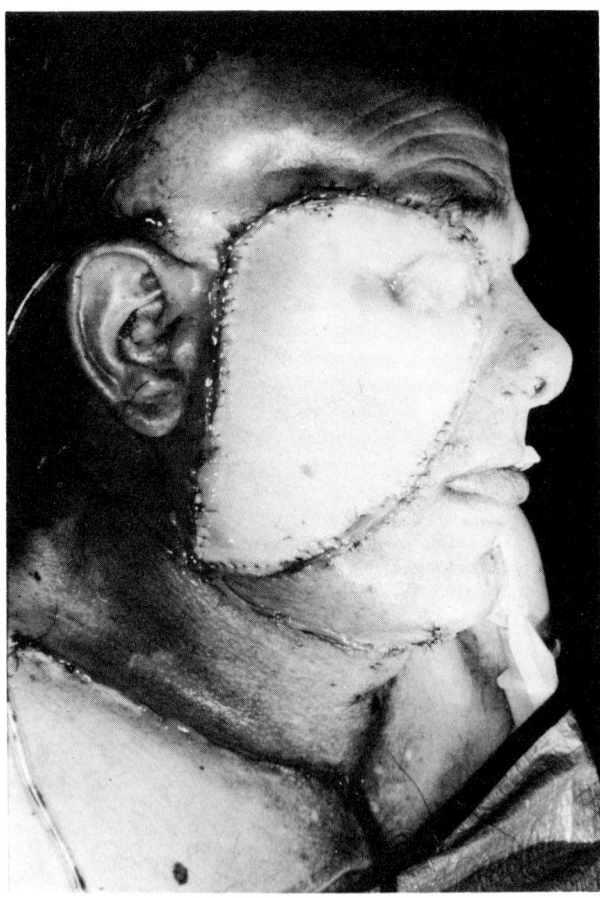

**Figure 3.** Cosmetically acceptable free flap repair.

general anaesthesia has been induced, and this has made induction of these patients much less stressful for the anaesthetist and less risky for the patients. A full description of the management of a difficult intubation is described elsewhere in this volume (Chapter 15).

### Previous anaesthesia

Many of these patients will have had anaesthesia for surgery in the recent past, for assessment and biopsy of the lesion. As these preliminary interventions may have taken place in other hospitals, careful review of the anaesthetic records must be made, and if necessary the anaesthetist involved should be consulted. This is essential in assessing airway problems or other possible intraoperative anaesthetic difficulties which, when anticipated,

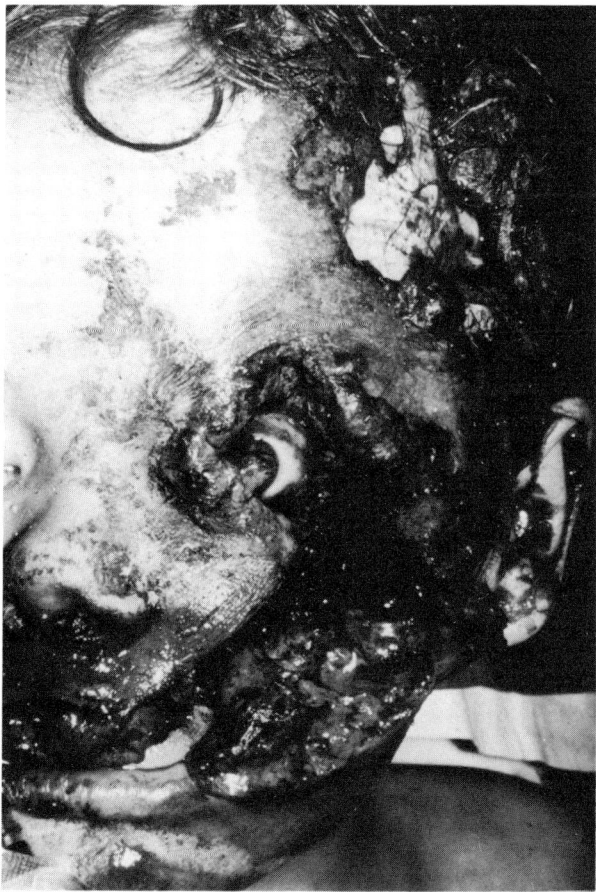

**Figure 4.** Severe facial trauma requiring major reconstructive surgery.

can be avoided. Furthermore, the hazards of repeated halothane anaesthesia can be avoided only by a full knowledge of previous anaesthetic techniques.

### Assessment

Once the above problems have been properly covered, it is necessary to discuss with the patient the planned procedure and the planned anaesthetic sequence. It is also necessary before too many promises are made to the patient to have discussed with the surgeon whether there will be any restriction of access to the patient either surgically or anaesthetically. For example, some reconstructive procedures require the use of a radial bone flap, which will limit the anaesthetist to the other arm or possibly to the lower limbs only. Having decided on a plan of anaesthetic management, it is

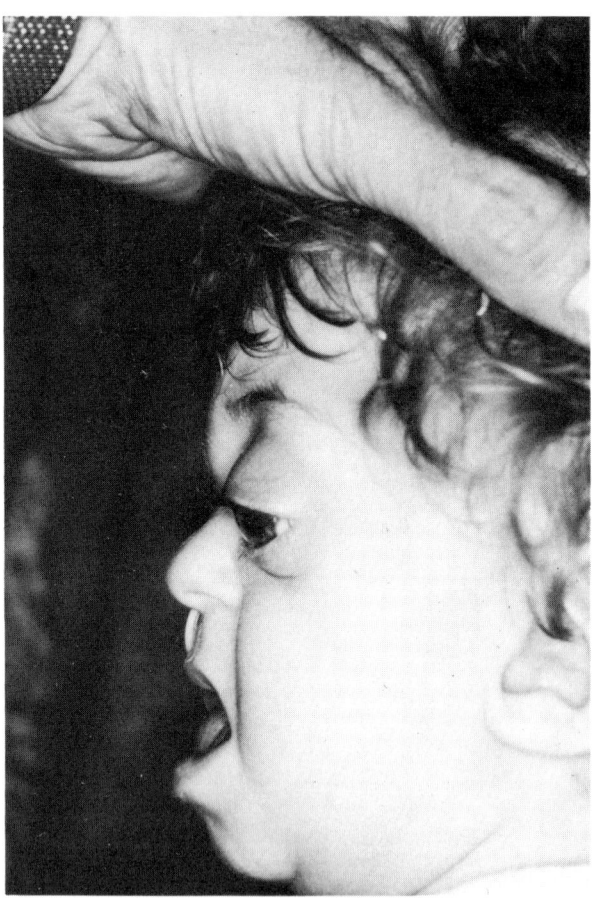

**Figure 5.** Severe Crouzon's Syndrome.

worth explaining to the patient in full what cannulae or other instrumentation will be required and what the patient should expect on recovery from anaesthesia.

Many of these patients will have their eyes covered and bandaged and the patient should be fully cognizant of this well before induction. The possibility of a nasogastric feeding tube and/or drainage tube should also be discussed, as should the possibility of a continuous indwelling urinary catheter. If bone grafts are to be taken, then the patient should be told to anticipate pain from these surgical sites far removed from the main operation site, and that, where possible, you will attempt to reduce postoperative pain by the use of local or regional anaesthetic techniques.

If a radial arterial pressure monitoring system is to be used, then the patients' radial and ulnar collateral circulations must be tested preoperatively and this should be explained to him so that he actually sees it done and

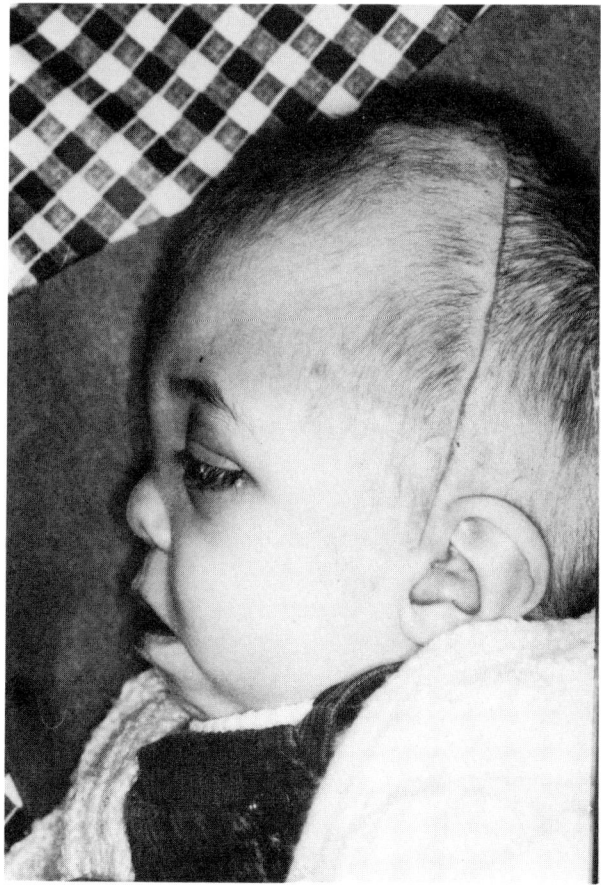

**Figure 6.** After craniofacial reconstruction.

understands the reasoning behind it.

Finally, the patient must also understand any special airway problems that are anticipated, and what procedures are planned so that where possible he does not awaken from surgery with an unexpected tracheostomy or unanticipated jaw wiring.

## INTRAOPERATIVE PROBLEMS

### Access to patients

As access by the anaesthetist to the patient is going to be severely restricted during surgery, all lines and endotracheal tubes etc. must be firmly fixed, and it may be helpful to suture tubes and venous cannula in place so that they

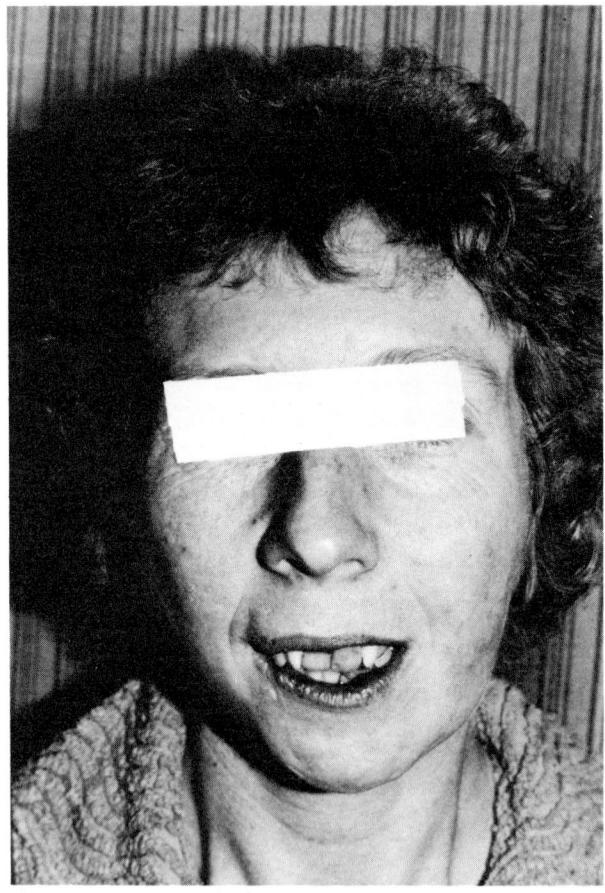

**Figure 7.** Severe trismus which was not apparent until direct questioning revealed limited jaw opening.

cannot be easily displaced. A well-placed oropharyngeal pack will often be essential. The choice of oral or nasal intubation must be made in conjunction with the surgeon. All endotracheal tube and breathing tube connections must be either fixed with strapping or be of the locking variety, or stitched in place. As many of these are prolonged procedures, some sort of humidification system should be included in the breathing circuit.

## Temperature control in long procedures

Many of these procedures last several hours, and consideration must be given to maintaining patient temperature. To minimize heat losses, a warming coil is included in the intravenous infusion lines, and a vapour condenser in the breathing circuit, and warming blankets and 'space blankets' should be used. The positioning of the patient on the table may require a large skin area to be uncovered, which will make the control of heat loss even more of a problem, and in these situations it may be neces-

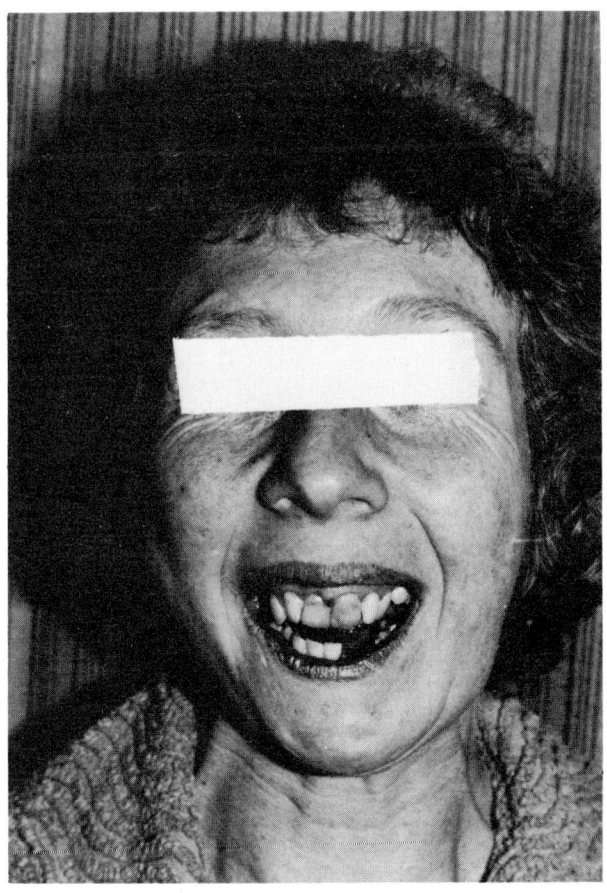

sary, particularly in small children, to increase the ambient theatre temperature. On occasions when the ventilation system to the operating theatre actually produces a cool draught across the length of the operating table, it may be necessary to erect a screen using a towel hung from two dripstands, to divert the draught from the patient and so minimize the cooling effect of the ventilation.

### Vagal reflexes

One problem that has been experienced in this area is the occurrence of profound bradycardia in response to certain surgical manoeuvres around the head and neck. While this may be anticipated in operations around the teeth and eye, there have on occasions been unexpected, and quite profound, falls in heart rate in response to such trivial procedures as washing out the mouth

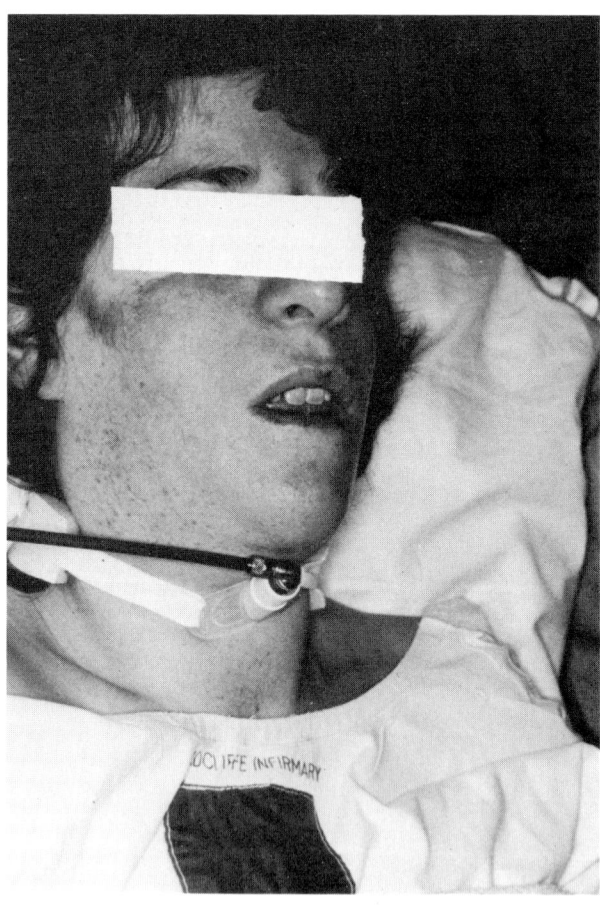

**Figure 8.** Transtracheal jet ventilation cannula in situ.

with dilute hypochlorite solution as a form of preoperative cleansing prior to surgery. Such reflex bradycardias may be minimized by insisting that the solutions used are not at room temperature but at body temperature. Furthermore, after a cancer has been excised, many surgeons like to irrigate the area liberally with water as a way of rupturing any remaining isolated cancer cells. Similar reflex bradycardias may occur unless this solution also is kept at body temperature.

Surgery around the eye, particularly orbital exenterations or orbital reconstructions, may produce bradycardia which can be prevented by adequate vagal blockade.

### Free flaps

The maintenance of patient temperature throughout a long procedure is of importance in all surgical procedures but is vital in the presence of a free flap. Of nearly equal importance is maintenance of tissue perfusion, and this will be reduced if the patient's pH or $PCO_2$ are allowed to wander far outside normal limits. A number of techniques have been devised to optimize free flap perfusion, and these are considered in detail in Chapter 13. In the present context, it should be noted that while sympathetic tone to the limbs can be controlled by the use of brachial plexus blockade or spinal or paraspinal techniques, vascular tone control in the head and neck region may require the use of a long-acting alpha-blocker such as phenoxybenzamine. This can be administered slowly over a period of 40 min at the dose of 1 mg/kg. It produces 24 h of profound alpha-blockade, which may require the administration of a large volume of colloidal fluid to maintain blood volume.

Agents such as dipyridamole (Persantin), aspirin, or Dextrans have been tried in a number of centres to prevent clotting in the free flap. Dextrans are unfortunately associated with generalized venous oozing which may be severe and result in haematoma formation beneath the flap, lifting it from its bed. Aspirin, however, has been of some value when started 12 h postoperatively in the dose of 600 mg daily, given orally or rectally.

### Monitoring

The scale of monitoring undertaken depends upon both the preoperative status and the anticipated procedure. Since many of these procedures are of several hours duration, and normal physiology may be interfered with to produce hypotension, monitoring should always include ECG, blood pressure, airway pressure and urine output, but will often also include temperature and intra-arterial pressure monitoring. End-tidal $CO_2$ monitoring is simple and can be of great value in detecting air embolism, disconnection, and adequate ventilatory function.

### Endotracheal tubes

There is an increasing choice of suitable endotracheal tubes available to the specialist anaesthetist. The Child's Anatomical Tube (Portex) has some advantages, as does the RAE (Ring Adair Elwyn, manufactured by Mallinckrodt) preformed endotracheal tube. These advantages include a degree of rigidity not present in modern red rubber tubes, a low-pressure high-volume cuff, and distancing of the tube to catheter-mount junction away from the immediate face area. The RAE tube has been our tube of choice in many situations for some time now, but has some disadvantages. Apart from being a fixed length from bend to tip, it is of limited value in children having intraoral surgery, where the surgeon wishes to use a Boyle–Davies Gag, as there is a tendency for the tube to be compressed between the lower teeth and the edge of the gag. In major craniofacial surgery a specially made, extra-long latex reinforced tube may be helpful so that all connections may be away from the immediate facial region. Where a tube is made extra long in this way, it is of course essential to stitch it in place and to mark it at the lip after checking bilateral air entry. Nasal disposable tubes may be only partially withdrawn at extubation and so used as postoperative naso-pharyngeal airways. Where this is anticipated it is helpful to mark the tube at the nares during intubation, as the tip passes the cords.

### Hypotensive anaesthesia

Many operations can be simplified or indeed made possible by the careful use of hypotensive anaesthesia, a subject that is covered in Chapter 12. It must be said here, however, that it is a technique which has been denigrated in part by its association with cosmetic surgery. There is no doubt that in operations around the head and neck, where an injudicious incision can jeopardize vital structures, surgery can be made both safer and quicker if the surgeon is able to see at all times what structures are present. However, many of the patients presented for major facial skeletal reconstructions are children, and it is often unjustified to take the added risks necessary to hypotense very young patients. Also, ganglion-blocking drugs may be relatively contraindicated in craniofacial surgery or surgery around the eyes, as they result in pupillary dilatation which persists into the postoperative period. The fixed dilated pupil, due to ganglion blockade, removes from the postoperative period an important and early warning sign of developing retro-orbital or intracranial complications.

### Air embolism

In a head-up position, any operation around the great neck veins or cranial venous sinuses may result in air embolism. It is not uncommon during head and neck surgery to see small bubbles in the internal jugular vein, something that the inexperienced anaesthetist or surgeon may find disturbing but which, unless gross, may be totally asymptomatic. By maintaining blood volume and by the use of controlled ventilation, the possibility of these small bubbles entering the chambers of the heart and producing cardiovascular symptoms is reduced. However, in the presence of an arteriovenous fistula, air may be carried into the arterial circulation.

### Urine output

Monitoring of urine output both intraoperatively and postoperatively can be a good indication of the adequacy of blood replacement and should be mandatory during major head and neck surgery. It must be remembered, however, that in the presence of hypotensive anaesthesia urine output will cease so long as the blood pressure is below the glomerular filtration pressure. Urine flow should rapidly return when the blood pressure returns to normal levels and this can be a useful extra monitoring sign. In the more major craniofacial and head and neck reconstructive procedures, post-operative urine output can be the most valuable indicator of adequacy of blood replacement.

### Nerve stimulator

Any procedure around the facial nerve may require careful dissection and preservation of the nerve intact. To this end the surgeon may wish to use a peripheral nerve stimulator and may request that the patient not be given neuromuscular blocking drugs. In this situation an anaesthetic technique which has been found to be suitable involves the combination of neuro-leptanaesthesia with short-acting relaxants such as atracurium and a volatile agent such as enflurane (Ward and Poole, 1983). The relaxant is given in minimal doses to permit endotracheal intubation and initial control of ventilation, but will have largely worn off prior to the use of the nerve stimulator. Atracurium is an ideal drug as it does not require reversal. Neuroleptanaesthesia can be achieved with droperidol 50 µg/kg and fentanyl 3 µg/kg.

### Multiple surgical input

Many major head and neck procedures require the combined effort of more than one surgeon or group of surgeons, including ophthalmic surgeons, plastic surgeons, neurosurgeons, and oral surgeons. This may mean that at any one time there may be two, three, or four different surgical specialties all trying to operate on the same patient. This inevitably leads to prolongation of the procedure and will also cause on occasions conflicting demands on the skills of the anaesthetists in altering or maintaining normal homeostasis. Careful planning by the whole team in advance of the procedure will allow for the best utilization of the anaesthetic skills available (Figure 9). Multiple points of surgical attack will also limit anaesthetic access.

### Extubation

At the end of a prolonged procedure, it may be necessary to continue positive pressure ventilation for up to 24 h to allow proper control of haemorrhage and normalization of vital signs, prior to reversal of the patient and extubation. In children particularly, it may be advisable to ventilate overnight so that stabilization can take place before the added insult of extubation. Consideration must also be given to any movement that has taken place around the airway; this may result in oedema in the immediate postoperative period, which may jeopardize the airway. It is all too easy to extubate the patient at the end of the procedure, to be satisfied that the airway is sound and then, over the next 12 h, to observe increasing dyspnoea due to swelling, which may be the normal response to surgery or a result of coughing and straining. Intubation in this situation is going to be more hazardous and may actually put at risk the success of the surgical procedure just carried out. All cases are different, each patient must be assessed on merits, and consideration must be given to transferring the patient to the intensive care unit for overnight ventilation and reassessment of the airway on the following day.

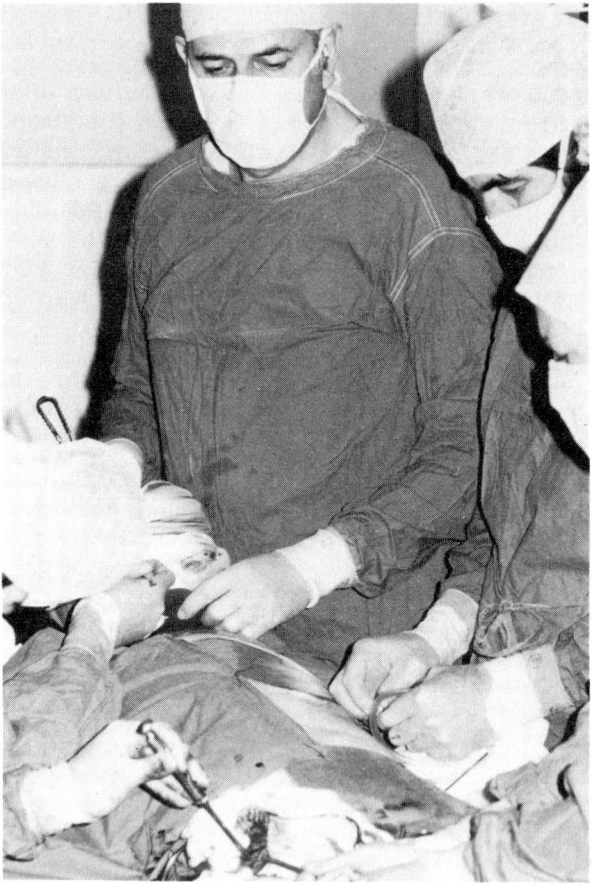

**Figure 9.** Three operations at once; mandibulectomy, preparation of rib for free flap, and harvesting of bone from iliac crest.

## RECOVERY

### Airway

As mentioned above, the airway may be hazardous in any surgery around the head and neck, both from oedema and because the anatomy may have been disturbed. It may be desirable to elect for temporary tracheostomy in the immediate postoperative period, and if so the patient should have been warned preoperatively that this would take place. In the absence of a tracheostomy, it is recommended that a nasopharyngeal airway be used, and if nasotracheal intubation has been the route of administration of anaesthetic gases, this can be left in situ, having been withdrawn from the larynx cut and trimmed and fixed in place with a safety pin. This will facilitate good tracheal and laryngeal toilet and provide a good airway in the postoperative period. Recovery nurses must be well trained and must understand that they may need to exert great diligence over airway care.

### Neurological

Neurological observations should be continued in the postoperative period and for the first 24 h. Pupils should be examined on a regular basis, and the patient's level of consciousness be assessed where possible, taking into account the interference of anaesthetic drugs. Blood loss should be carefully assessed also in the postoperative period. The recent use of Redivac and Portavac type drains has made this very much simpler. Large-bore drains should be inserted where possible, and these should be measured half-hourly for the first 3 h, and hourly thereafter if the blood loss is minimal. Any continuing haemorrhage through the drains or into the airway should be reported to both the anaesthetist and the surgeon, as it may be necessary to re-explore the wound. Pressure should be used with great care, particularly in the presence of free flap repairs, as external pressure may interfere with tissue perfusion.

Pain relief and sedation should be used sparingly in the postoperative recovery ward. The use of prochlorperazine intravenously (0.1 mg/kg) has been found to be useful, as it will gently sedate the patient and also reduce nausea. If analgesia is required, then it should be provided by the intra-venous administration of small increments of narcotic analgesics titrated against the analgesic response.

## CRANIOFACIAL SURGERY

The majority of patients presenting for major craniofacial surgery will be small children. The Oxford Craniofacial Unit has carried out major surgery on more than 23 children under 4 years of age during the last two years. This experience has been summarized in a paper by Drs Uppington and Goat (Uppington and Goat, 1987). Many of these patients with gross disturbance of the upper airway and jaws had obvious preoperative airway problems, and intubation difficulties were anticipated. Preoperative tracheostomy was essential. Recently in Oxford, we have used the Transtracheal Jet Ventilator inserted either under local anaesthetic prior to general anaesthesia or immediately after a gaseous induction, allowing plenty of opportunity to intubate the patient under general anaesthesia (Ward and Goat, 1986). The patients were all anaesthetized using techniques familiar to the neuro-anaesthetist, anaesthesia being maintained with oxygen and nitrous oxide supplemented by the volatile agent isoflurane. Isoflurane was used deliberately to assist in the production of hypotension. Analgesia was provided by the use of fentanyl in the dose of 10–20 µg/kg, and ventilation was facilitated by the use of the muscle relaxant D-tubocurarine. Thiopentone infusion was administered at the rate of 2 mg/kg/h, and was continued until skin closure.

As these patients were almost entirely small children, deliberate hypotension was not employed. One of the anxieties in operating on these children was the massive blood loss that occurred, and unfortunately no technique has been found for accurate measurement of blood loss during surgery. We rely entirely upon indirect signs of blood loss, such as blood pressure, heart rate and urine output. During surgery, dextrose 4.5% with 0.5 normal saline was infused through one peripheral line with a standard paediatric fluid regime. This was doubled for the first 2 h of anaesthesia in an effort to compensate for preoperative starvation. A second peripheral line was used for blood administration, and immediately after induction of anaesthesia all patients received a bolus of human albumin solution, which was followed by warmed microfiltered whole fresh blood, when available, at a rate sufficient to maintain cardiovascular stability.

Blood loss was always large and continuous and is, not surprisingly, related to the complexity and duration of surgery. Swab weighing was inaccurate, since moist swabs were used throughout, and saline and wet packs were applied to the wound edges on top of already blood-soaked swabs. The maintenance of cardiovascular parameters seems to have been adequate, since a postoperative estimation of blood loss by the use of haemoglobin and potassium levels showed us to be reasonably successful at blood replacement management. These markers are, however, of no use for intraoperative purposes. The use of a central and a peripheral temperature probe giving an indication of core to shell temperature gradient was also helpful in this respect. Cerebral dehydration was achieved by the use of hyperventilation and intraoperative frusemide. In other cases where intracranial pressure was normal, spinal drainage was also used. Antibiotic prophylaxis using ampicillin/flucloxacillin was given to all patients, and they also received anticonvulsants routinely commencing preoperatively and continuing for six months following surgery.

In the postoperative period, many children were electively transferred to the paediatric intensive care unit where intubation was either continued and ventilation maintained, or the patients were carefully extubated and monitored. Alternatively, they were sent back to the paediatric ward and nursed by a dedicated specially trained paediatric nurse. Codeine phosphate or paracetamol was given for pain relief to these children, and humidified oxygen administered where possible for the first 24 h.

## SUMMARY

It is clear that in order to manage successfully the special problems which may be encountered during head and neck surgery, a thorough understanding of the surgical procedure is essential. Close co-ordination between the various surgeons involved and the anaesthetic team is necessary. Attention to detail in this field, as in all others in anaesthesia, pays the expected dividends.

## REFERENCES

Tessier P, Guiot G, Rougerie J, Delbet JP & Pastorra J (1967) Osteotomies cranio-naso-orbitales hypertelorism. *Acta Chirurgiae Plasticae* **12:** 103.

Uppington J & Goat VA (1987) *Annals of the Royal College of Surgeons* **69:** 175–178.

Ward ME & Goat VA (1986) Use of transtracheal jet ventilation for patients with difficult intubation. Paper presented to Plastic Surgery and Burns Anaesthetists. *Today's Anaesthetist* **1**(4): 22.

Ward ME & Poole MD (1983) An anaesthetic technique for cross-face nerve grafting. *British Journal of Plastic Surgery* **36:** 51.

# 15

## Difficult intubation

### C. J. BARHAM

It is now over 100 years since William MacEwen first passed an oral endotracheal tube in order to operate on a patient with a tumour on the base of his
tongue, and subsequent developments have ensured that the majority of our
patients can be intubated with ease. Recently, there has been an increasing
interest in those patients who present a problem in securing their airway, but
a difficult intubation can still be one of the most challenging and exciting
procedures in anaesthetic practice.

This chapter will attempt to review some of the difficulties with intubation
presenting in plastic and maxillofacial surgery, and discuss how they may be
managed with the equipment and techniques that are now available.

### WHAT IS A DIFFICULT INTUBATION?

Cormack and Lehane (1984) have suggested the following classification of
difficult intubation:

1. Most of the glottis is visible. No difficulty.
2. Only the posterior extremity of the glottis is visible. Slight difficulty.
   Pressure on the neck may be helpful.
3. No part of the glottis can be seen, but the epiglottis is visible. Severe
   difficulty.
4. Not even the epiglottis can be seen. Special procedures may be
   required.

The incidence of difficult intubation in general anaesthetic practice has
been reported to be 2.3% (Aro et al, 1974), and in patients with burns or
presenting for plastic or maxillofacial surgery it will almost certainly be
higher than this. However, the vast majority of 'difficult' intubations in these
specialties can be anticipated.

### PROBLEMS CAUSING DIFFICULTY WITH INTUBATION

There are many factors that may contribute towards difficulty in passing an
endotracheal tube, and given a full preoperative examination, most of these
can be anticipated.

**Anticipation of difficulty**

The patient may volunteer a history of difficult intubation—and indeed, if any problem is encountered it is most important that the patient is informed postoperatively, so that any anaesthetist unfortunate enough to meet them on a subsequent occasion can be alerted.

On examination, the most important points to note are the following: the degree of mouth opening; the patency of the nasal airways; the size of the base of the tongue; the shape of the mandible and neck; limitation of movement or instability of the neck.

*Mouth opening*

Limitation of mouth opening, if severe, will clearly make direct oral intubation impossible, and so some specialized techniques will have to be employed. Prominent teeth, especially incisors, may obstruct laryngoscopy and passage of the tube; and a narrow mouth with a high arched palate may also cause difficulty.

*Patency of nasal airways*

The patient should be asked whether there is any difficulty with breathing through either nostril, and any history of nasal trauma, surgery, or pathology such as nasal polyps should be noted. On examination, the patency of each nostril can be assessed audibly, and also visibly by the degree of misting produced on a stainless steel tongue depressor. If there is reason to expect significant obstruction, especially when there is also limitation of mouth opening, the nasal passages can be examined preoperatively under local anaesthesia with a fibreoptic nasendoscope.

*Size of tongue*

A clinical sign has recently been described (Mallampati et al, 1985) to evaluate the degree of concealment of the faucial pillars and uvula by the tongue when it is maximally protruded in a seated patient. This, it is suggested, is related to the size of the base of the tongue. A classification is described as follows:

1. Faucial pillars, soft palate and uvula can be visualized (Figure 1)
2. Faucial pillars and soft palate can be visualized, but uvula is masked by the base of the tongue
3. Only the soft palate can be visualized (Figure 2)

Of 210 patients studied, 155 were in the first category, and all had adequate exposure of the larynx. Fifteen were in the third category, and in only one of these could the glottis be exposed. Thus, failure to visualize the faucial pillars or the uvula under these circumstances can indicate potential difficulty with intubation.

*Shape of the mandible*

The shape of the mandible has been studied extensively with regard to anticipating intubation problems. Cass et al (1956) identified the length, anterior depth and angle of the mandible as indicators of difficulty.

White and Kander (1975) determined various measurements of the mandible from the lateral skull X-ray to try to predict difficulty. They found that if the ratio of the effective mandibular length (incisors to condyle) to the posterior depth (third molar to angle of mandible) is less than 3.6, then direct visualization of the larynx is likely to be difficult. They also identified increased anterior mandibular depth (incisors to pogonion) as a relevant factor. However, there is no evidence that there will be any difficulty with blind nasal intubation, or other specialized techniques if these values are abnormal.

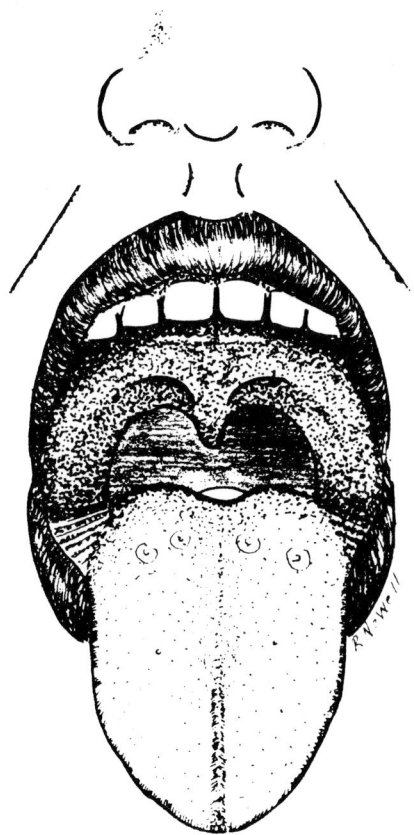

**Figure 1.** Class 1. Faucial pillars, soft palate and uvula are visible. From Mallampati et al (1985) with kind permission of the editor of the Canadian Anaesthetists' Society Journal.

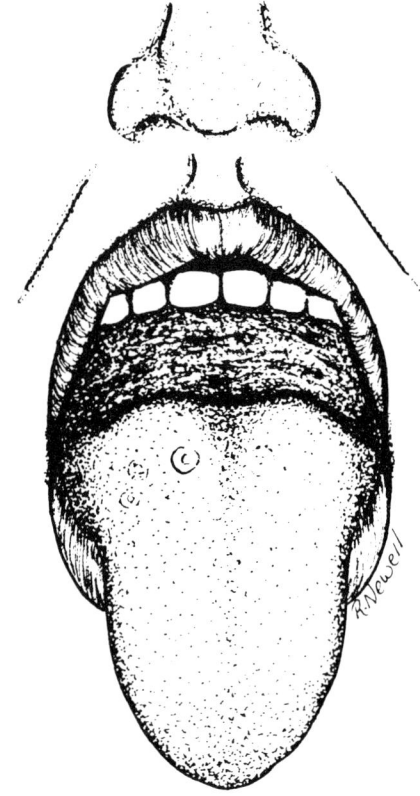

**Figure 2.** Class 3. No pharyngeal structures are visible. From Mallampati et al (1985) with kind permission of the editor of the Canadian Anaesthetists' Society Journal.

## Neck movements

The ability to flex the cervical spine and extend the atlanto-occipital joint is required to bring the glottis into alignment with the mouth and pharynx. Thus any injury or degenerative disease causing stiffness or instability of these joints should be determined. Clinically, the ability to adopt the 'sniffing the morning air' position should be assessed, and lateral X-rays of the neck should be taken in the neutral position and in flexion. Any slippage occurring at the joints should warn of potential problems, and if it is severe, intubation should be performed with the patient awake. Reduction of the atlanto-occipital distance, or to a lesser extent the c1–c2 interspinous gap may indicate reduced ability to extend the head, and indicates that difficulty may be encountered (White and Kander, 1975; Nichol and Zuck, 1983).

Cormack has derived an equation (Zuck, 1985) relating the atlanto-occipital gap to the posterior depth of the mandible:

$$Y = 27.1 - 12.2X_1 + 1.3X_2$$

Where $X_1$ = Posterior depth of mandible (cm)

$X_2$ = Atlanto-occipital gap (mm)

A negative value for $Y$ indicates difficulty with laryngoscopy and intubation.

## Other problems

The patient with an old burn injury may present with a variety of contractures around the mouth, face and neck which may make direct visualization of the larynx impossible. Similarly, previous surgery or radiotherapy for malignancy may have distorted the anatomy considerably. Surgery around the chin and the front of the neck can be most deceptive, especially when the patient has a normal degree of mouth opening. However, it must be remembered that the ability to expose the larynx in the anaesthetized patient is largely dependent upon the ability to lift the tongue and mandible forward, and any contracture of the skin or soft tissues here will inhibit this.

There are many specific conditions known to give difficulty with intubation. Some of these are listed in Table 1.

**Table 1.** Specific conditions leading to difficulty with intubation.

| |
|---|
| Achondroplasia |
| Acromegaly |
| Ankylosing spondylitis |
| Cleft palate |
| Craniofacial dystoses |
|    Apert's syndrome |
|    Crouzon's syndrome |
| Cystic hygroma |
| Engelmann's disease |
| Goitre |
| Hemifacial microsomia |
| Klippel–Feil syndrome |
| Mucopolysaccharide diseases |
|    Hurler's syndrome |
|    Hunter's syndrome |
|    Morquio's syndrome |
| Pierre Robin syndrome |
| Rheumatoid arthritis |
| Treacher Collins syndrome |

Pathology in the mouth, pharynx, larynx and trachea may give rise to problems. Abscesses especially may rupture and contaminate the respiratory tract.

Finally, a number of factors remote from the face and neck may cause difficulty. Large breasts, in full term pregnancy for example, are a common problem; and tumours on the occiput (Sale and Skyrme-Jones, 1983), unusual hairstyles (Famewo, 1983), or tissue expanders (Fergusson, 1985) may prevent extension of the atlanto-occipital joint. External fixation of facial or neck fractures may also prevent access for intubation.

## CONDUCT OF THE DIFFICULT INTUBATION

### Local anaesthesia

In the elective case with an anticipated difficulty, the approach of choice will usually be to perform the intubation under local anaesthesia with the patient awake. Given adequate co-operation from the patient, visualization of the larynx is likely to be much easier technically than in the anaesthetized patient due to the fact that the patient is maintaining the tone of the jaw and neck muscles in order to keep the airway patent. Certainly, fibreoptic laryngoscopy and intubation are far more easily performed in the awake patient, which explains why respiratory physicians apparently find the technique easier than anaesthetists!

There are, however, two major obstacles to intubation in the awake patient—operator experience and patient compliance. All specialized techniques for intubation should preferably be practised on normal patients before being used in a difficult situation, but it is difficult to ask a patient to submit to awake intubation by a novice. However, without such experience, the anaesthetist is unlikely to develop the skill and confidence to assure the patient that intubation can be performed with the minimum of discomfort, which indeed it can.

Several local and regional anaesthetic techniques are available to assist intubation. In summary, they are as follows:

1. Topical anaesthesia
2. Transtracheal injection
3. Maxillary nerve block
4. Glossopharyngeal nerve block
5. Superior laryngeal nerve block

These are described in detail by Murrin (1985). While the regional blocks listed can produce excellent anaesthesia using minimal quantities of local anaesthetic agents, the topical anaesthetic techniques, in combination with suitable sedation, are the simplest and most practical to perform. Care must be exercised, however, to avoid systemic toxicity with local anaesthetic drugs.

### General anaesthesia

If there is no alternative but to attempt a difficult intubation in a patient under general anaesthesia, it is essential that the approach to the procedure should be well planned, and that all equipment likely to be required should be to hand before induction of anaesthesia. In the anaesthetized patient, continuous attention must be paid to oxygenation and the presence of adequate anaesthesia and there may also be the added risk of aspiration of gastric contents. A suggested plan is shown in Figure 3.

The first and most vital necessity in this situation is a skilled assistant. It could also be considered mandatory to have a second anaesthetist, as the intubation procedure may be prolonged. The anaesthetist performing the intubation must be free to concentrate fully on the task in hand, and thus the presence of a second anaesthetist should ensure adequate oxygenation, anaesthesia and monitoring of the patient.

It is important to induce anaesthesia cautiously, and if there is pre-anaesthetic evidence of upper airway obstruction, an inhalation induction is mandatory. However, the majority of difficult intubations can safely be anaesthetized with an intravenous agent of choice, after suitable premedi-cation. If the patient cannot be ventilated at this stage, it is axiomatic that they should not be paralysed, as the only way out will be at best transtracheal jet ventilation, and at worst an unduly hasty tracheostomy. The anaesthetic should thus be deepened with the patient breathing spontaneously and

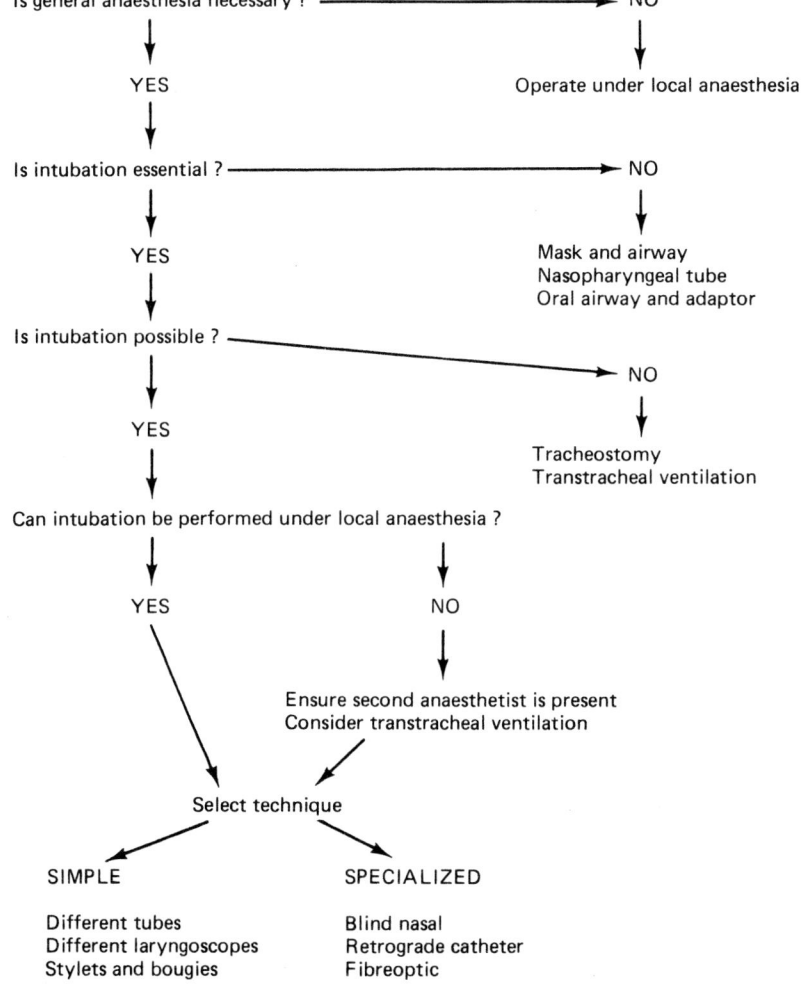

**Figure 3.** Plan for anticipated difficult intubation.

intubation performed without muscle relaxants. It is extremely rare, however, that this is necessary.

If a muscle relaxant can be given, the choice will depend on the individual circumstances. Intermittent doses of suxamethonium may be used for the less difficult cases, but where it has been established that the patient can be ventilated with mask and airway, and there is no risk of gastric regurgitation, it is perfectly safe, and probably preferable, to give a non-depolarizing relaxant such as atracurium or vecuronium.

It is essential to ensure that the patient remains oxygenated and anaesthetized while an endotracheal airway is being secured. The simplest method of achieving this is to administer oxygen and anaesthetic gases intermittently during the procedure. This allows relative hypoxia to develop progressively, and may demand interruption of the intubation procedure at a critical moment, but for intubations where only a mild degree of difficulty is anticipated, this remains the most widely adopted method.

The nasal route can be used for the uninterrupted administration of anaesthetic gases during intubation, either by the use of a single naso-pharyngeal tube, or a binasal airway. Alternatively, the patient can be ventilated using a mask with a special endoscopic port, through which a fibreoptic scope may be passed (Patil et al, 1982). All these techniques are simple but not universally satisfactory, and constant attention is necessary to maintain the airway.

An elegant method of ensuring adequate oxygenation during prolonged and difficult intubation is the use of transtracheal jet ventilation (Smith et al, 1974). This technique has also been used as an alternative to intubation in difficult cases (Layman, 1983). A purpose designed cannula* is now available (Figure 4) which can be easily secured to the neck, like a mini-tracheostomy (Ravussin and Freeman, 1985). It can be inserted either through the crico-thyroid membrane, as described by Layman, or alternatively through the upper part of the trachea, like a conventional tracheostomy. The latter choice allows a retrograde catheter technique to be used without fear of damaging the ventilating cannula. Once it has been correctly positioned, as confirmed by aspiration of air into a liquid filled syringe, it can be connected to a high pressure oxygen source for intermittent ventilation (Figure 5).

The following hazards should be borne in mind:

1.  There is no protection of the airway other than the flow of expiratory gases, and thus contamination of the airway is possible with stomach contents should the patient regurgitate, or with blood if there is bleeding in the upper airway.
2.  A pack cannot be used to protect the larynx, as this would obstruct the expiratory gasflow.
3.  High pressures may be transmitted to the respiratory tract with the danger of barotrauma, including tension pneumothorax, especially in children. Great care must therefore be exercised with the technique.

---

* Transcricothyrotomy Device. VBM, Medizintechnik, D-7247 Sulz/Nectar, Germany.

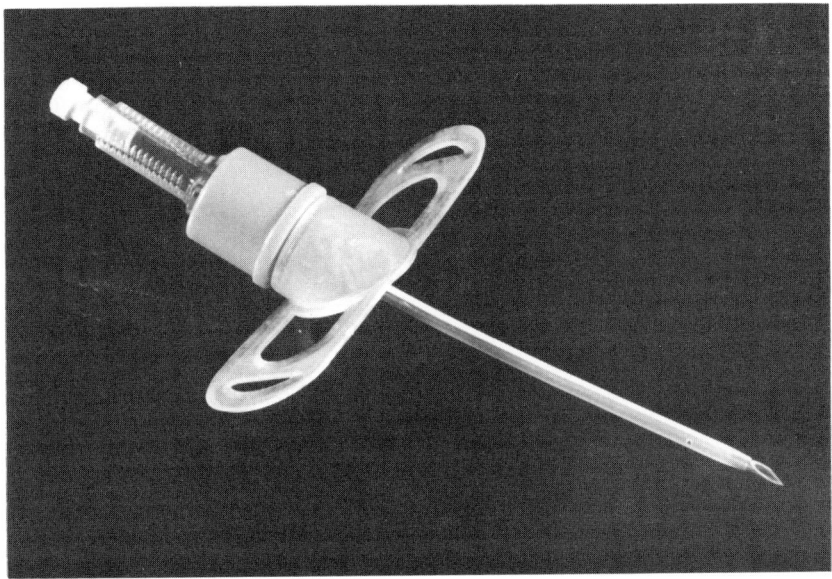

**Figure 4.** The Transcricothyrotomy Device.

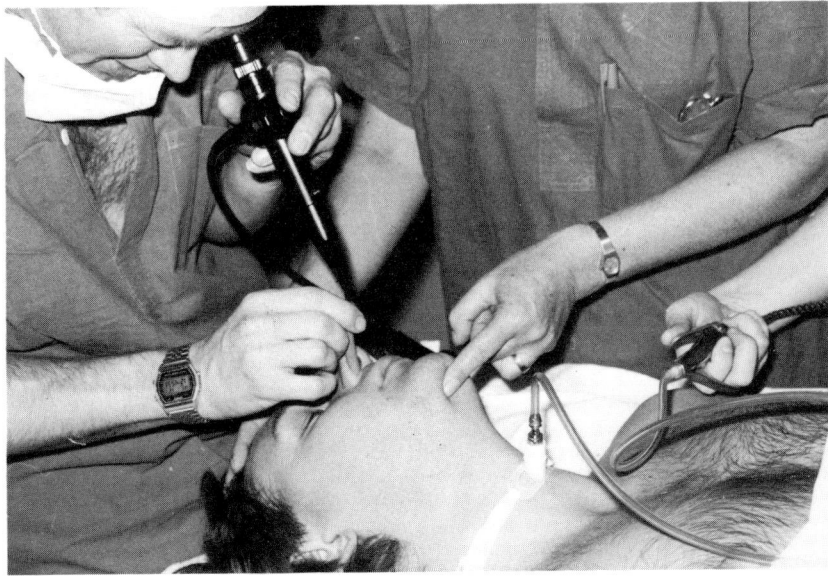

**Figure 5.** Transcricothyrotomy Device in use for fibreoptic intubation. Note assistant elevating the jaw to aid visualization of the larynx.

## METHODS AVAILABLE FOR DIFFICULT INTUBATION

Whilst it is possible to identify many of the factors that may lead to a difficult intubation, it is often difficult to predict the method with which intubation will finally be achieved. Every case is different. The basic techniques of intubation will not be described here in detail, but several points are worth noting.

### Alternative route of intubation

Sometimes the anatomy of the mouth, jaw and pharynx may make oral intubation difficult, in that whilst at least part of the larynx is visible, an oral endotracheal tube cannot be passed. Under these circumstances a tube advancing from the nose may be successful, as it may approach the glottis at a more favourable angle.

If it is mandatory that a particular route of intubation is used, as for example in surgery to the nose, this does not necessarily exclude that route to achieve intubation. It may be possible to intubate via the nose, and then change to an oral tube, as the following case history demonstrates.

*Case 1:*
A 27-year-old lady was admitted to hospital for surgery to her nose. She gave a history of apparently uneventful previous anaesthesia and there was no reason to suspect difficult intubation. After induction, laryngoscopy revealed only the tip of the epiglottis, and attempts at oral intubation were unsuccessful. Whilst resting a fatigued left arm (important in any prolonged intubation procedure) it was found that a plain Magill tube could be passed blindly into the larynx from the nose at the first attempt. This was then advanced into the trachea until the distal end appeared in the pharynx, whence it was retrieved through the mouth with Magill intubation forceps. Using a gum elastic bougie as a guide, the plain tube was then changed for a cuffed oral tube without difficulty.

### Alternative tubes

It is a matter of personal preference as to which tube to use initially in any intubation—the important point is to use one that is familiar. However, a tube with different qualities may be required with some complex techniques. For example, when using a guided technique (bougie, catheter, fibreoptic endoscope, etc.), a flexible armoured tube may be easier to advance over the guide than a plastic or rubber one.

### Alternative laryngoscopes

Again, it is wise to use a familiar instrument initially, and for most British anaesthetists this will be a Macintosh blade. In many cases an alternative blade will confer no advantage, especially if it is unfamiliar. Certain circumstances, however, may favour a straight blade, for example where mouth opening is limited.

Occasionally, if there is a large pharyngeal mass, a diagnostic otolaryngological laryngoscope, such as the Negus, may have advantages over standard anaesthetic blades. The tubular-shaped speculum will prevent the mass obstructing the view of the larynx, and when the tube has been passed, the laryngoscope can be removed by dismantling the slide.

## SPECIALIZED TECHNIQUES

There are many specialized techniques and many items of equipment have been developed for difficult intubations in a variety of situations. Not all of these are practical for use in surgery on the head and neck, and so three techniques will be considered in detail that are of particular use under these circumstances.

### Blind nasal intubation

The technique of blind nasal intubation was pioneered by Rowbotham and Magill, whilst working at the plastic surgery unit at Sidcup during and after the First World War (Rowbotham and Magill, 1921). They were using insufflation anaesthesia, and had found it desirable to pass a second tube into the trachea in order to remove the escaping vapour. This allowed them to pack off the pharynx, and also prevented the gases interfering with the surgery.

It was a serendipitous finding that this tube, which was larger than the insufflation catheter, would frequently pass from the nose directly into the larynx during aspiration. The technique achieved considerable popularity, especially in cases where laryngoscopy was not possible. However, the advent of muscle relaxants, which allowed atraumatic laryngoscopy and oral intubation to be performed at lighter levels of anaesthesia, caused the popularity of the technique to decline (Gillespie, 1941). In fact, Sir Ivan Magill, when in his eighties, is reputed to have remarked at a meeting whilst watching a demonstration of blind nasal intubation: 'I can see no indication for blind nasal intubation in modern anaesthetic practice!' (Personal communication).

The technique is, however, still widely practised, and the author finds it extremely useful, not only for the difficult cases, but also for routine use.

It has been suggested that increased trauma may result from prolonged and rough attempts at blind nasal intubation (Latto, 1985). This may well be true, but it is equally true for oral laryngoscopy and intubation under similar conditions. If performed skilfully, however, it is both quick and atraumatic, avoiding the undesirable effects of laryngoscopy (Prys-Roberts et al, 1971). The principal complication is that of epistaxis, the incidence of which can be reduced by the use of 10% cocaine spray. Even in the absence of this, the incidence of severe nasal haemorrhage is exceedingly rare, especially if a soft, well-lubricated tube is used. Trauma to the nasal passages and pharynx may occur, and polyps or adenoidal tissue may be dislodged. An increased incidence of bacteraemia has been reported after nasal intubation (Berry et al, 1973). Prolonged nasal intubation may result in paranasal sinusitis (Arens et al, 1974).

A rubber tube, of the type marketed as a Magill plain oral tube, is still in the author's opinion the best tube to ensure a successful blind intubation. If necessary, this can always be changed for another tube using a bougie as a guide once intubation has been achieved.

The classical technique of blind nasal intubation under general anaesthesia is conducted with the patient breathing spontaneously, usually with the addition of up to 10% carbon dioxide to stimulate respiration. The tube is then advanced slowly towards the glottis, using the breath sounds heard via the tube to indicate the direction. This method therefore relies almost entirely on the sense of hearing (Gillespie, 1941).

The technique which has been in use at East Grinstead for many years differs considerably from this, using visual and tactile signs to position the tube correctly (Edridge, 1980).

The patient is anaesthetized with the induction agent of choice, and then paralysis is obtained using a short-acting muscle relaxant, in exactly the same manner as for a normal oral intubation. After spraying the nares with 10% cocaine spray, the tube is passed through one nostril (the right by preference unless contraindicated). The head of the patient is placed in the 'sniffing the morning air' position with the head tilted slightly to the right. If the tube is now advanced smoothly but positively, it will in about 30% of cases enter the larynx. The signs of success are: the tip of the tube will be seen to run down the front of the neck in the midline; there will be a sensation transmitted to the hand produced by the tube running down the rings of the trachea; and small movements in the neck similar to coughing may be observed. Confirmation of successful tracheal intubation may of course require observation and auscultation of the chest, fibreoptic endoscopy (down the tube) or capnography.

If the tube is not in the trachea, one of four things will have happened, and it is quite easy to determine which by observation of the neck and the sensation of the obstruction.

1. The tube may pass to the left or to the right of the glottis, and lodge in one or other piriform fossa. If this occurs, the sensation will be of a soft compliant obstruction, and a slight bulge will also be observed on the appropriate side of the larynx. It should be emphasized that only the lightest pressure is required to do this—no more than occurs in the average oral intubation under direct vision. This can nearly always be corrected by withdrawing the tip of the tube into the nasopharynx, rotating either the patient's head or the tube, and then reinserting the tube. Usually three or four attempts at the most are all that is necessary.

2. The tube passes smoothly onwards in the midline, none of the initial signs of success are observed, and positive pressure on the bag produces a belch. The tube is in the oesophagus, and the corrective action on withdrawing the tube is to extend the head further, and possibly apply some light cricoid pressure. Persistent failure here is usually due to limitation of neck movement, and it will quickly become apparent if the tube is not even touching the posterior extremity of the larynx.

3. The tube passes in the midline, and meets a firm and definite obstruction. Here it has passed into the glottis and the tip has obstructed on the anterior ring of the cricoid cartilage. The simplest way to overcome this is to rotate the tube gently, through 360° if necessary. An alternative method is to pass a catheter down the tube as a guide. In the young patient, extension of the head will facilitate this, and by contrast, flexion of the neck will be of assistance in the elderly.

4. The tube may meet a relatively hard resistance, with slight distortion of the larynx to one side or other. Here it may have lodged on one or other false cord, or possibly on an arytenoid cartilage. Whichever it is, slight rotation of the tube towards the midline will usually allow it to pass onwards into the trachea.

It has also been suggested that the tube may on occasions become lodged in the vallecula. If this should occur, rotation of the tube together with some degree of flexion of the neck are required. This rarely occurs in practice.

With experience, a success rate of over 95% can be achieved, and many potentially difficult intubations can be performed easily and elegantly. The major drawback of the technique is that it does require practice. The description given above can only give a mere taste of the skill that can be acquired by regular use of blind nasal intubation. However, most anaesthetists, and especially those working in the field of plastic and maxillofacial surgery, regularly have cause to intubate patients via the nasal route, and thus have the opportunity to acquire the necessary expertise.

## Fibreoptic intubation

The use of fibreoptic instruments has revolutionized endoscopic practice, and the examination of the respiratory tract is no exception to this.

The technique of using a fibreoptic endoscope for difficult intubation was first described by Murphy (1967), who used a choledochoscope, and since then there have been numerous reports of the successful use of fibreoptic intubation. However, despite the recommendation of enthusiasts that the technique should be more widely adopted, only a minority of anaesthetists regularly use it. At a recent meeting of the South East Thames Regional Anaesthetic Society, less than 10% of those present had ever performed a fibreoptic intubation.

The two major factors preventing the wider use of the technique are availability of the instruments, and the allegation that proficiency is difficult to achieve.

### Availability of fibreoptic endoscopes

A variety of instruments are now available, designed for the differing requirements of examining the nasal cavities, pharynx, larynx and bronchial tree. Whilst only the most affluent anaesthetic departments may possess their own dedicated fibreoptic laryngoscope, most hospitals possess a fibreoptic bronchoscope or nasendoscope, either of which can be used for intubation purposes in most circumstances.

The bronchoscope is thicker and more cumbersome than the laryngoscope, and thus more difficult to use. It has a suction channel through which secretions can be cleared. In children, the channel can be used to pass a guide wire into the larynx, which can then be used to guide an endotracheal tube after removal of the bronchoscope (Stiles, 1974).

The nasendoscope is light and easy to manipulate, but is too short to thread a nasal tube of adequate length for most adult patients. This problem can be overcome using a standard Magill plain oral tube with a triangular fenestration cut halfway down its length on the concave surface. The nasendoscope can be threaded through this hole, and can now protrude sufficiently beyond the tip to allow successful intubation of the larynx (Figure 6). The fenestrated tube is advanced into the larynx, the nasendoscope removed, and a bougie is passed down the lumen of the tube. The original tube is then replaced with an appropriate endotracheal tube, using the bougie as a guide.

The typical laryngoscope has a length of 830 mm and a diameter of 4 mm, is relatively stiff, and is ideal for the passage of an endotracheal tube. However, its optics are inferior to the diagnostic instruments.

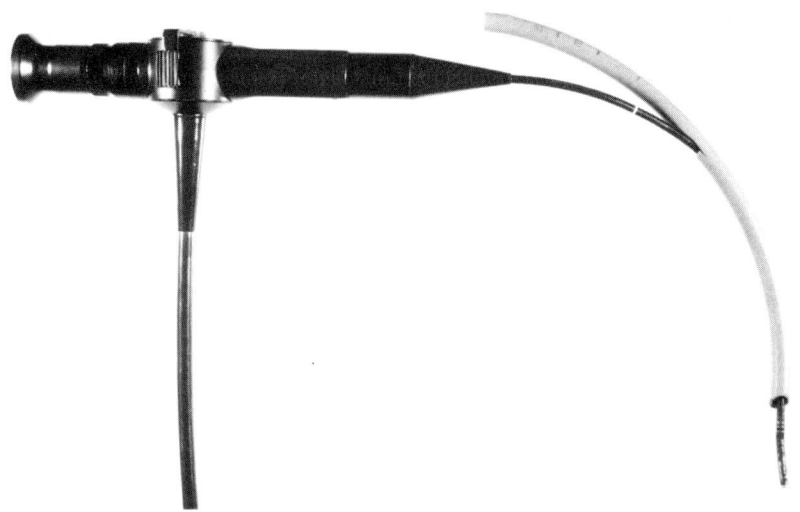

**Figure 6.** Nasendoscope passed through fenestration in plain Magill oral tube. (See text for explanation.)

## Ease of use

As with any specialized skill used in anaesthesia, it is constant practice that leads to proficiency. It can therefore be argued that it is no more difficult than conventional direct laryngoscopy. If a suitable instrument is available, there is no reason why it should not be used routinely to intubate patients, and thus skill and confidence will be acquired to deal with the more difficult problem. It is, however, asking for trouble to bring it out only when difficulty is encountered. A minimum of 30 successful routine intubations has been recommended before attempting a difficult intubation (Sia and Edens, 1981).

## Training in fibreoptic intubation

Before using the instrument for intubation it is advisable to become completely familiar with its controls, and then practise on a training model until confident of its characteristics.

Ovassapian et al (1983) have developed a training programme using awake patients under local anaesthesia. After initial experience on a training model, it progresses on to visualization of the epiglottis and vocal cords in six patients, followed by intubation of a further six patients. The use of awake patients carries two major advantages: firstly, there is no need to ventilate the patient during the procedure, and secondly, the technique is easier, as the maintenance of muscular tone allows an unobstructed view of the larynx from the postnasal space.

However, it is also possible to gain experience on patients under general anaesthesia (Davies and Holloway, 1986), and it is desirable to be able to use the technique under general anaesthesia for the unexpected difficult intubation. In this situation, there are some practical points that will greatly increase the chance of success.

*Posture.* Although some authorities recommend facing in a cephalad direction with respect to the patient (Rogers and Bumenof, 1983), the author would agree with those who advocate the conventional position for laryngoscopy, facing the patient's feet (Williams, 1984). The anatomy will then be as one is accustomed to seeing it, and also the actual intubation will be easier to perform.

*Route.* When the oral route is used, the fibrescope has to undertake a more acute angle in the pharynx, thus limiting manoeuvrability. Access can be improved, however, if an assistant elevates the tongue and jaw with a Macintosh laryngoscope. Williams and Maltaby (1982) describe a device for directing the fibrescope towards the larynx when passed through the mouth. Alternatively a modified Guedel airway (Hogan et al, 1984) or a mouth gag (Pellimon and Simunovic, 1985) may be used.

The nasal route is easier to use than the mouth, as the approach to the vocal cords is more favourable. Also, the nasal passages provide support for the proximal part of the instrument, allowing better manipulation of the tip. It is advisable to ensure that the endotracheal tube passes into the pharynx before advancing the tip of the laryngoscope into the larynx.

*Clear the airway.* The tongue is one of the major impediments to fibreoptic intubation of the anaesthetized patient by the beginner. The position of the head is as important here as it is for blind nasal intubation or conventional laryngoscopy. If the 'sniffing the morning air' position is adopted, the tongue will be elevated and the larynx brought into alignment with the naso-pharynx, giving as clear a view from the nasopharynx as in the awake patient.

### Retrograde catheterization

Retrograde laryngeal catheterization has now become established as a useful technique for dealing with an otherwise difficult intubation. It has two advantages: firstly, it can be employed in a situation when the larynx cannot be visualized by either direct or fibreoptic laryngoscopy, and secondly, that it requires no expensive equipment.

Originally described in a patient with an existing tracheostomy (Butler and Cirillo, 1960), when the endotracheal tube itself was passed retrogradely, the technique has since been developed for intubation, using a catheter passed percutaneously through the cricothyroid membrane as a guide for orthograde intubation.

It can be employed under local or general anaesthesia, but once again local anaesthesia is preferable in the compliant patient. The method used by the author is similar to that described by Latto (1985). After making a small incision above the midpoint of the cricoid cartilage, a Tuohy needle is inserted into the trachea, and its position confirmed by aspirating air. An epidural catheter is then passed through the needle in a cephalad direction, and its end retrieved through the mouth in the unconscious patient, or is spat out if the patient is awake. The Tuohy needle is removed, and a refrigerated suction catheter is threaded over the epidural catheter and into the trachea, in order to make a reasonably rigid guide for the endotracheal tube, which can now be advanced over the catheter.

It is this stage which is most likely to cause problems, as difficulty is frequently encountered in advancing the tip of the tube into the larynx. Using as rigid a catheter as possible will help to minimize this, as will the use of a soft tube, such as one of reinforced latex. If the tube will not pass easily into the trachea, it may be helpful to pass a bougie through the tube and remove the catheters. Rotation of the tube may be of assistance, as with blind nasal intubation. If a rubber or plastic tube is being used, positioning it so that the bevel points downwards (i.e. with the tube rotated 90° anticlockwise) will allow an easier passage into the larynx (Cossham, 1985).

Complications are rare, minor bleeding from the puncture site being the most frequent problem.

## WHEN TO ABANDON

When a difficult intubation occurs unexpectedly, there can be no hard and fast rule as to how long to persist. Each case must be treated on its own merits, taking into account the urgency of the operation, the trauma that has occurred, and the experience of the anaesthetist. In general, any attempt that has lasted an hour is unlikely to succeed on that occasion, and further attempts will be hampered by fatigue on the part of the operator and trauma to the patient.

If an endotracheal tube is not mandatory, or if delay in performing the operation carries considerable risk, early consideration must be given to either performing the operation under local anaesthesia, or maintaining the airway by alternative means—facemask, oral or nasal airways, transtracheal ventilation or tracheostomy.

The possibility that intubation may have to be abandoned must always be entertained, and to this end a failed intubation drill should be adopted, as in obstetric emergencies (Rosen, 1985). This should include:

1.  Maintaining the patient's position (semi-lateral if necessary)
2.  Continue ventilation via mask **and** maintain cricoid pressure, until spontaneous respiration returns
3.  Add volatile anaesthetic (preferably halothane, enflurane or isoflurane), and deepen if necessary when spontaneous respiration returns
4.  Commence operation
5.  Avoid gastric intubation, especially if active vomiting is likely

## THE PLACE OF TRACHEOSTOMY

Tracheostomy is the final resort of any intubation attempt, but must be treated with great respect. The morbidity of the procedure is not inconsiderable, and at the very least it is likely to delay the patient's discharge from hospital in all but the most major surgery. It will be very rare that a failed intubation cannot be resolved by one of the methods mentioned previously, or by deferring the operation.

If a tracheostomy is to be performed, it should be as an elective procedure for which there are definite indications. These may include major resection or injury involving the posterior tongue, pharynx or larynx; preoperative or anticipated postoperative swelling of these structures; or where postoperative chest care is likely to be a problem in the presence of a compromised airway.

## MAXILLOFACIAL INJURIES

The patient with severe maxillofacial injuries may present considerable problems to the anaesthetist, but these will usually be related to maintaining and protecting the airway prior to intubation rather than technical difficulty in performing it. Uncomplicated fractures of the mandible or maxilla rarely present a problem, and most surgical procedures can be deferred for at least 24 hours, both to monitor any concomitant head injury, and allow more favourable conditions for intubation.

Soft tissue injuries may present a more challenging problem, as the normal anatomy may be distorted, but again this will not usually produce difficulty in exposing the larynx. Local anaesthesia is difficult and indeed hazardous in the presence of upper airway bleeding, so intubation under general anaesthesia is usually required. Sometimes, however, intubation may have to be performed in unconventional fashion, as the following case-history illustrates:

*Case 2:*
A young man was admitted with severe shotgun injuries to his face following a suicide attempt. The blast had entered beneath his mandible and exited between his eyes, thus destroying the bony skeleton of his anterior mandible, middle third of his maxilla, and nose. The soft tissues of his face were left as unsupported flaps. Thus he was only able to maintain his airway in the prone position, which allowed the skin flaps to hang forward and also caused the bleeding to gravitate away from the pharynx.

Anaesthesia was induced, after preoxygenation, with halothane in oxygen. The position allowed an airway to be maintained until anaesthesia was deep enough for intubation. As Figure 7 shows, whilst the position was unusual, intubation was accomplished without difficulty. Tracheostomy was then performed prior to initial repair of the injuries.

It is important to be alert to other associated injuries that may present a hazard in these circumstances. Any blow to the head severe enough to fracture the facial skeleton may also cause an intracranial injury, and should be treated as such. Injury to the cervical spine should also be suspected, and great care exercised in manipulation of the neck, especially in positioning for intubation. Injury to the larynx may cause severe problems both in maintaining the airway and intubation. An inhalational induction is the approach of choice, and muscle relaxants should be avoided.

## POSTOPERATIVE CARE

Any patient who has had a difficult intubation, or where attempts at intubation have failed, should be observed for signs of laryngeal oedema postoperatively. It is wise to admit any such patient to an Intensive Care or High Dependency ward for 24 hours postoperatively.

### Difficult extubation

The maintenance of the difficult airway postoperatively, especially after

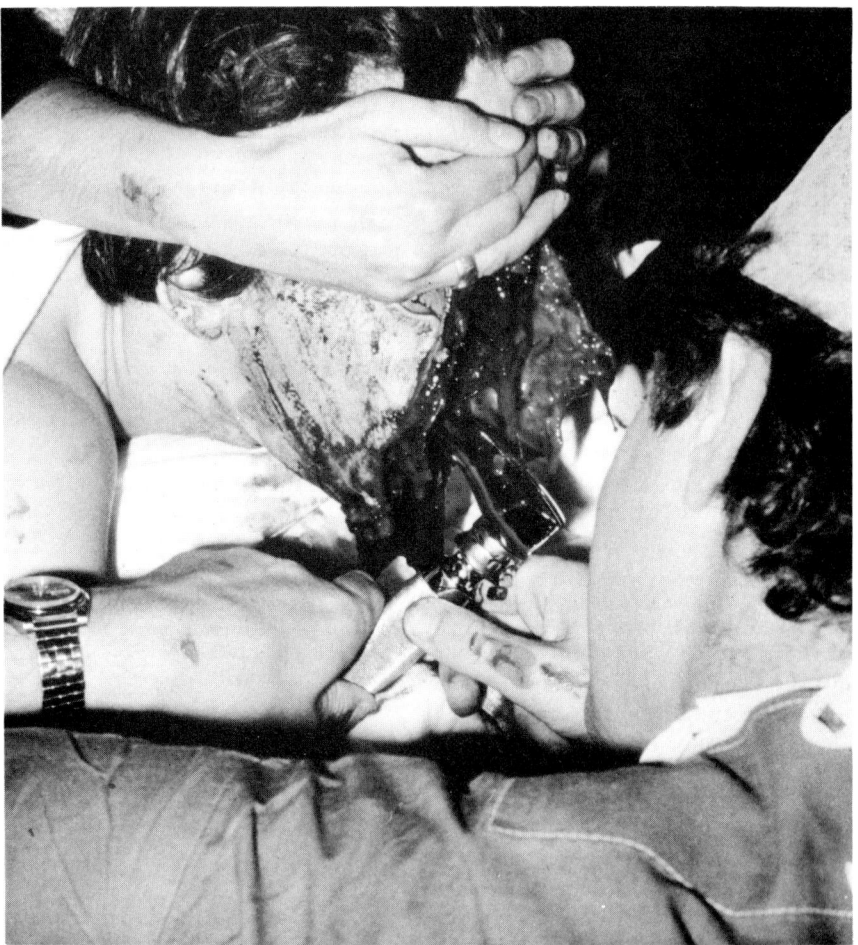

**Figure 7.** Intubation in the prone position in a case of severe facial shotgun injury.

major surgery to the head and neck, presents a number of different options, and a logical plan is required to provide the best management.

## Tracheostomy

In most cases, a decision will have been made preoperatively as to whether a tracheostomy will be required postoperatively, based among other things on the extent of the surgery. Where this has been more extensive than anticipated, it may of course be necessary to review this at the end of the operation.

## Prolonged intubation

If maintenance of the airway and control of secretions are not likely to be a persistent problem postoperatively, it may be preferable to keep the patient intubated for a while, until recovery is complete and swelling has subsided. This may be especially important where intermaxillary fixation has been applied. A nasopharyngeal airway can be useful in the period after extubation if the patient still has difficulty in breathing. This will also allow the nasopharynx to be suctioned without undue discomfort.

Great care must obviously be exercised in the extubation of a patient who has been difficult to intubate. Generally the patient should have recovered from anaesthesia—extubation while still asleep may be asking for trouble. If the patient rejects the tube this almost invariably indicates that they can maintain their own airway, and conversely, a patient who cannot will usually tolerate the presence of a tube with the minimum of sedation.

## SUMMARY

The skills required for dealing with difficult airway problems are especially relevant in the fields of plastic and maxillofacial anaesthesia. It is usually possible to identify those patients in whom problems will occur, and the factors causing such difficulty have been reviewed. The importance of a clear plan of action has been emphasized, together with the advantages of using local anaesthesia for intubation where possible.

Where general anaesthesia has to be employed, the need to provide continuous oxygenation, ventilation and anaesthesia has been underlined, and various methods discussed.

The techniques of blind nasal, fibreoptic and retrograde intubation have been examined in detail.

## REFERENCES

Arens JF, Lejeune FE & Webre DR (1974) Maxillary sinusitis, a complication of nasotracheal intubation. *Anesthesiology* **40:** 415–416.
Aro L, Takki S & Aromaa U (1974) Technique for difficult intubation. *British Journal of Anaesthesia* **43:** 1081.

Berry FA, Blankenbaker WL & Bull CG (1973) A comparison of bacteraemia occurring with nasotracheal and orotracheal intubation. *Anesthesia and Analgesia* **52**: 873–876.

Butler FS & Cirillo AA (1960) Retrograde tracheal intubation. *Anesthesia and Analgesia* **39**: 333–338.

Cass NM, James NR & Lines V (1956) Difficult direct laryngoscopy complicating intubation for anaesthesia. *British Medical Journal* **i**: 488–489.

Cormack RS & Lehane J (1984) Difficult tracheal intubation in obstetrics. *Anaesthesia* **39**: 1105–1111.

Cossham P (1985) Difficult intubation. *British Journal of Anaesthesia* **57**: 239.

Davies NJH & Holloway TE (1986) Training in fibreoptic intubation. *Anaesthesia* **41**: 1265.

Edridge AW (1980) *Sniffing the morning air*. Unpublished data presented to Southern Society of Anaesthetists.

Famewo CP (1983) Difficult intubation due to a patient's hairstyle. *Anaesthesia* **38**: 165–166.

Fergusson DJM (1985) Tissue expanders complicating intubation. *Anaesthesia* **40**: 822.

Gillespie N (1941) *Endotracheal Anaesthesia*, University of Wisconsin Press.

Hogan K, Harpur MH & Pollard BJ (1984) Use of a pharyngeal guide to intubation with the fibreoptic laryngoscope. *Anaesthesia and Intensive Care* **12**: 18–21.

Latto IP (1985) Management of difficult intubation. In Latto IP & Rosen M (eds) *Difficulties in Tracheal Intubation*, pp 99–141. London: Baillière Tindall.

Layman PR (1983) Transtracheal ventilation in oral surgery. *Annals of the Royal College of Surgeons of England* **65**: 314–318.

Mallampati SR, Gatt SP, Gugino LD et al (1985) A new sign for predicting difficult intubation? *Canadian Anaesthetists' Society Journal* **32**: 429–434.

Murphy P (1967) A fibreoptic endoscope used for nasal intubation. *Anaesthesia* **22**: 489–491.

Murrin KR (1985) Awake intubation. In Latto IP & Rosen M (eds) *Difficulties in Tracheal Intubation*, pp 90–98. London: Baillière Tindall.

Nichol HC & Zuck D (1983) Difficult laryngoscopy—the 'anterior larynx' and the atlanto-occipital gap. *British Journal of Anaesthesia* **55**: 141–144.

Ovassapian A, Yelich S, Dykes MHM & Golman ME (1983) A training programme for fibreoptic nasal intubation. Use of model and live patients. *Anaesthesia* **38**: 795–798.

Patil V, Stehling LC, Zauder HL & Koch JP (1982) Mechanical aids for fibreoptic endoscopy. *Anesthesiology* **57**: 69–70.

Pellimon A & Simunovic Z (1985) Mouth gag and tongue holder for fibreoptic laryngoscopy. *Anaesthesia* **40**: 386–387.

Prys-Roberts C, Greene LT, Meloche R & Foex P (1971) Studies of anaesthesia in relation to hypertension. 11 Haemodynamic consequences of induction and endotracheal intubation. *British Journal of Anaesthesia* **43**: 531–547.

Ravussin P & Freeman J (1985) A new transtracheal catheter for ventilation and resuscitation. *Canadian Anaesthetists' Society Journal* **32**: 60–64.

Rogers SN & Bumenof JL (1983) New and easy techniques for fibreoptic endoscopy aided tracheal intubation. *Anesthesiology* **59**: 569–574.

Rosen M (1985) Difficult and failed intubation in obstetrics. In Latto IP & Rosen M (eds) *Difficulties in Tracheal Intubation*, pp 152–155. London: Baillière Tindall.

Rowbotham ES & Magill IW (1921) Anaesthetics in the plastic surgery of the face and jaws. *Proceedings of the Royal Society of Medicine* **14**: 17.

Sale JP & Skyrme-Jones S (1983) An unusual cause for difficult intubation. *Anaesthesia* **38**: 1228.

Sia RL & Edens ET (1981) How to avoid problems when using the fibreoptic bronchoscope for difficult intubations. *Anaesthesia* **36**: 74–75.

Smith RB, Myers EN & Sherman H (1974) Transtracheal ventilation in paediatric patients. *British Journal of Anaesthesia* **45**: 313–314.

Stiles CM (1974) A flexible fibreoptic bronchoscope for endotracheal intubation in infants. *Anesthesia and Analgesia* **53**: 1017–1019.

White A & Kander PL (1975) Anatomical features in difficult direct laryngoscopy. *British Journal of Anaesthesia* **47**: 468–474.

Williams RT (1984) Comments from an experienced user of the airway intubator. *Anesthesiology* **61**: 108–109.

Williams RT & Maltaby JY (1984) Airway intubator. *Anesthesia and Analgesia* **61**: 309.

Zuck D (1985) Difficult tracheal intubation. *Anaesthesia* **40**: 1016–1017.

# Index

Note: Page numbers of article titles are in **bold** type.